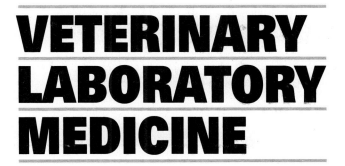

VETERINARY
LABORATORY
MEDICINE

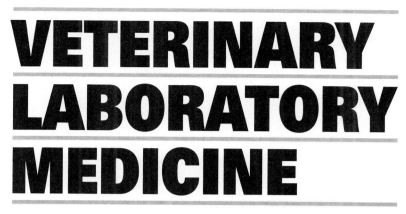

VETERINARY LABORATORY MEDICINE

Interpretation & Diagnosis

SECOND EDITION

DENNY J. MEYER, DVM
DIPLOMATE, ACVP, DIPLOMATE, ACVIM
Senior Clinical Pathologist
CVD/Idexx Veterinary Services
West Sacramento, California
and Courtesy Associate Professor
Department of Small Animal Clinical Sciences
College of Veterinary Medicine
University of Florida
Gainesville, Florida

JOHN W. HARVEY, DVM, PhD
DIPLOMATE, ACVP
Professor and Chair
Department of Physiological Sciences
College of Veterinary Medicine
University of Florida
Gainesville, Florida

W.B. SAUNDERS COMPANY
A Division of Harcourt Brace & Company
Philadelphia ▪ London ▪ Toronto ▪ Montreal ▪ Sydney ▪ Tokyo

W.B. SAUNDERS COMPANY
A Division of Harcourt Brace & Company

The Curtis Center
Independence Square West
Philadelphia, Pennsylvania 19106

Library of Congress Cataloging-in-Publication Data

Meyer, Dennis J.
    Veterinary laboratory medicine : interpretation and diagnosis /
Denny J. Meyer, John W. Harvey.—2nd ed.
        p.   cm.
    Includes index.
    ISBN 0-7216-6222-6
    1. Veterinary clinical pathology.   I. Harvey, John W.   II. Title.
SF772.6.M49   1998
636.089′6075—dc21   98-7725

VETERINARY LABORATORY MEDICINE   ISBN 0–7216–6222–6

Printed in the United States of America

Last digit is the print number: 9   8   7   6   5   4   3   2   1

Denny dedicates this work to Jae, his wife, for her altruistic tolerance, support, and devotion to family; you are special and wonderful . . . and to Chris and Jen, his favorite son and daughter, for providing me with the definition of life and making it all worthwhile.

John dedicates not only this effort, but his whole professional career to his wife Liz, daughter Ashley and son Thad. I greatly appreciate the many family sacrifices you have made for me to be able to devote the long hours necessary to be successful in academia.

PREFACE

Tempora mutantur, nos mutamur in illis. *Times change and we change with them.*

—Anon, Roman

There are numerous changes in the second edition; one of which was not in the outline. Embert Coles died on August 13, 1993 in Topeka, Kansas, just prior to his 70th birthday. During our final communication the day before his death, in reply to the question of book cover color preference for the second edition, he had the nurse in the Intensive Care Unit fax the reply "green." He leaves behind a long legacy of contributions to the discipline of clinical pathology. I am pleased to have had the opportunity to collaborate with him on the first edition.

John Harvey is internationally recognized for his expertise in clinical pathology, notably hematology. We worked together for 13 years at the College of Veterinary Medicine, University of Florida and this collaboration is, in many ways, 'poetic justice'. John's contributions reflect his decades of clinical and investigative experiences in hematopathology and immunohematology. The information is pathophysiologically contemporary, yet it retains a clinical pragmatism, a difficult task that few, other than he, could achieve. I am excited and honored to collaborate with him on the second edition.

In addition to the new chapters contributed by John, most of the other chapters have been either completely rewritten or updated. The changes reflect the suggestions from practitioners, clinical pathologists, and students, notably the Classes of '95 & '96, the College of Veterinary Medicine, Colorado State University. During my two enjoyable years with these students, they took equal pleasure in making suggestions for improvements, and in finding mistakes in their professor's first edition! My thanks to each one of them, and to the Classes of '80 through '92, the College of Veterinary Medicine, University of Florida, for being concerned and caring professionals who, in their own way, influenced both editions through their questions, comments, and opinions expressed during the courses I taught.

> *I desire no other epitaph, no hurry about it may I say, than I taught medical students in the wards, as I regard this as by far the most useful and important work I have been called upon to do.*
>
> —Sir William Osler, M.D.

A list of recommended reading that supports the content of the chapters has been provided in response to other suggestions. The magnitude and diversity of the 67 case studies in the first edition have not been repeated. The cases in this edition were chosen to illustrate the interpretative approach to the assessment and synthesis of the clinical pathology findings in the formation of a diagnosis.

We have tried to retain the user-friendly format to facilitate the 'quick look' need of the busy practitioner, yet provide sufficient physiology and pathophysiology to accommodate the both inquisitive clinician and student. The objective is to provide a guide that links the clinical pathology findings to the underlying pathophysiological consequences of disease and propose differential diagnostic considerations that ultimately lead to a diagnosis. It is also intended to serve as a 'bridge' to the other veterinary medical textbooks in W.B. Saunders Company portfolio. Your critical suggestions are again invited.

When a man's knowledge is not in order, the more of it he has the greater will be his confusion.

—Herbert Spenser, *The Study of Sociology*

Denny Meyer

ACKNOWLEDGMENTS

If I have seen further, it is by standing on the shoulders of giants before me.
—Sir Isaac Newton

The first edition was dedicated to veterinary clinicians, researchers, and students, the foundation of our profession and its future. Again we thank this constituency for providing the case-related material, published information, and stimulating questions that contributed to the architecture of this edition. Denny reiterates his sincere appreciation to those specifically mentioned in the first edition for their mentorship. A special thank you goes to David Twedt, David Williams, Bob Washabau, Greg Ogilvie, Steve Withrow, Morrow Thompson, and John Mara for opportunities that contributed to my professional growth and their outward expressions of friendship and support in various aspects of my career and life. I wish to extend a special recognition to Tim Terrell, Ken Kagan, and Steve Hines for their emotional hugs and to Mary Jo Burkhard for her valuable contributions to this book and her valued friendship.

What's more valuable than gold? Diamonds. Than diamonds? Friendship.
—Ben Franklin

John wishes to acknowledge those most responsible for this development as a clinical pathologist. Few people have the opportunity to receive training from the giants of their profession, but I was blessed in being trained by Jerry Kaneko, the father of veterinary clinical biochemistry and Oscar Schalm, the father of veterinary hematology. I also want to thank the many other veterinary clinical pathologists I have interacted with over the years. I have especially enjoyed the give-and-take sessions with Victor Perman and Alan Rebar.

Finally, this book would not have become a reality without the assistance of the professionals at W.B. Saunders Company, notably Cass Stamato and Ray Kersey. Ray, thank you for believing in our effort, accommodating our timeline, and your personal support.

Bits and pieces. God moves people in and out of each other's lives. And each leaves his mark on the other. You find you are made up of bits and pieces of all who ever touched your life, and you are more because of it, and you would be less if they had not touched you. Accept the bits and pieces in humility and wonder, and never question, and never regret. Bits and pieces.
—Mary Jo Burkhard

CONTENTS

NOTICE

Companion animal practice is an ever-changing field. Standard safety precautions must be followed, but as new research and clinical experience grow, changes in treatment and drug therapy become necessary or appropriate. The authors and editors of this work have carefully checked the generic and trade drug names and verified drug dosages to assure that dosage information is precise and in accord with standards accepted at the time of publication. Readers are advised, however, to check the product information currently provided by the manufacturer of each drug to be administered to be certain that changes have not been made in the recommended dose or in the contraindications for administration. This is of particular importance in regard to new or infrequently used drugs. Recommended dosages for animals are sometimes based on adjustments in the dosage that would be suitable for humans. Some of the drugs mentioned here have been given experimentally by the authors. Others have been used in dosages greater than those recommended by the manufacturer. In these kinds of cases, the authors have reported on their own considerable experience. It is the responsibility of those administering a drug, relying on their professional skill and experience, to determine the dosages, the best treatment for the patient, and whether the benefits of giving a drug justify the attendant risk. The editors cannot be responsible for misuse or misapplication of the material in this work.

THE PUBLISHER

COLOR PLATES

Color Plate I

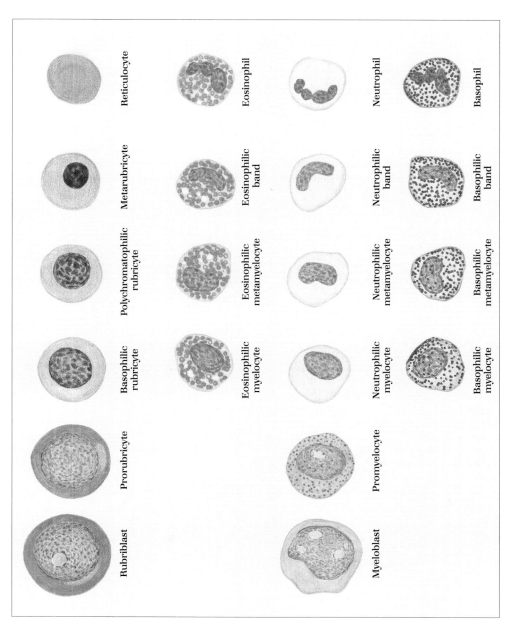

Maturation of canine erythroid and granulocytic cells as they appear in Wright-Giemsa-stained bone marrow aspirate smears. Drawing by Dr. Perry Bain.

Color Plate II

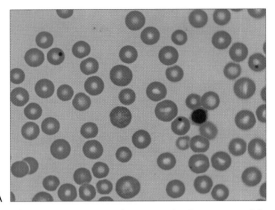

A

Plate 2A. Regenerative anemia in a cat with increased polychromasia and anisocytosis. A metarubricyte and 3 RBCs containing Howell-Jolly bodies are present. Wright-Giemsa stain.

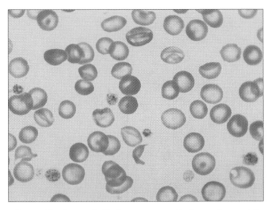

B

Plate 2B. Iron deficiency anemia in a dog with hypochromic RBCs. Moderate poikilocytosis is also present. Wright-Giemsa stain.

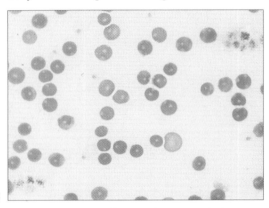

C

Plate 2C. Heinz body hemolytic anemia in a cat, resulting from acetaminophen toxicity. Pale spots present within RBCs are poorly stained Heinz bodies. Some lysed RBCs with red-staining Heinz bodies are also present. Wright-Giemsa stain.

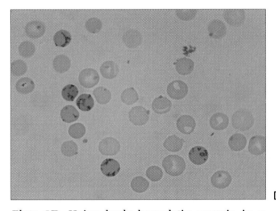

D

Plate 2D. Heinz body hemolytic anemia in a dog, resulting from onion toxicity. Reticulocytes containing dark-blue-staining material and RBCs containing small light-blue-staining Heinz bodies are present. Reticulocyte stain.

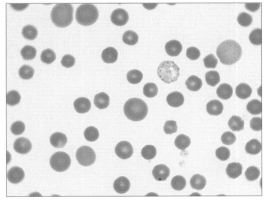

E

Plate 2E. Regenerative anemia with increased anisocytosis in a cow with anaplasmosis. A single *Anaplasma marginale* organism is present in a RBC at the bottom and a RBC with basophilic stippling is present in the top portion of the photograph. Wright-Giemsa stain.

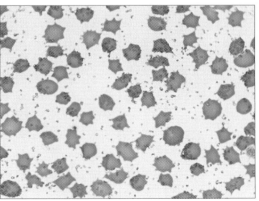

F

Plate 2F. Eperythrozoonosis in a pig. Large numbers of *Eperythrozoon suis* organisms are present on and between RBCs. Most RBCs are echinocytes, an expected finding in porcine blood films. Wright-Giemsa stain.

Color Plate III

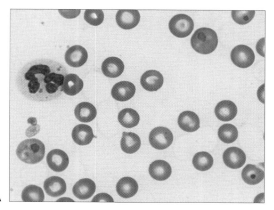

Plate 3A. Blood from a dog with distemper. Red-staining distemper inclusions are present in a neutrophil and several RBCs. Diff-Quik stain.

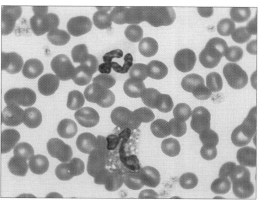

Plate 3B. A neutrophil and an eosinophil in blood from a dog. Wright-Giemsa stain.

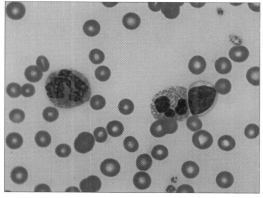

Plate 3C. A basophil, eosinophil and lymphocyte in blood from a cat. Wright-Giemsa stain.

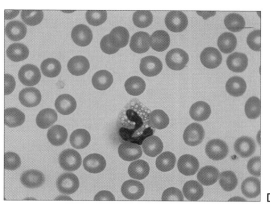

Plate 3D. An eosinophil with vacuolated cytoplasm in blood from a greyhound dog. Wright-Giemsa stain.

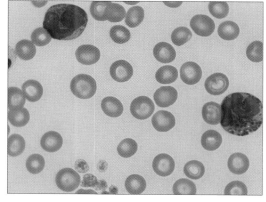

Plate 3E. Two basophils in blood from a dog with a noncutaneous mast cell tumor. Wright-Giemsa stain.

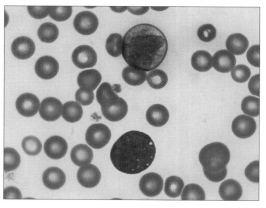

Plate 3F. An intensely basophilic reactive lymphocyte (bottom) and a monocyte (top) in blood from a dog.

Color Plate IV

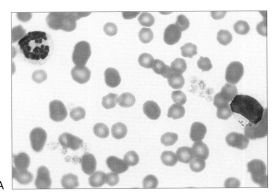

Plate 4A. A neutrophil and a granular lympho-cyte in blood from a horse. Wright-Giemsa stain.

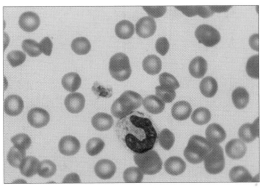

Plate 4B. A toxic band neutrophil in blood from a dog with a bacterial infection. The cytoplasm exhibits increased basophilia and a Doehle body. Wright-Giemsa stain.

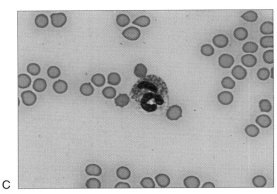

Plate 4C. A neutrophil in blood from a cat with mucopolysaccharidosis type VI, an inherited lysosomal storage disease. Wright stain.

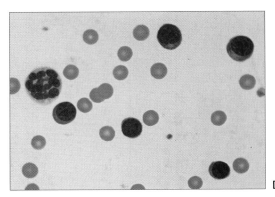

Plate 4D. Blood from an anemic cat with a myelodysplastic syndrome with excessive pro-liferation of nucleated RBCs (MDS-Er). A hyper-segmented neutrophil and several nucleated RBCs are present, but polychromasia is absent. Wright-Giemsa stain.

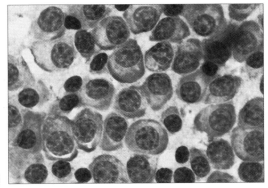

Plate 4E. Plasma cells in a bone marrow aspi-rate from a dog with multiple myeloma. Wright-Giemsa stain.

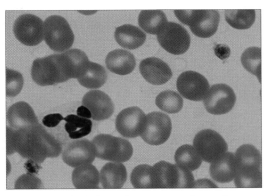

Plate 4F. *Ehrlichia platys* organisms in two platelets in blood from a dog. Wright-Giemsa stain.

Part I

GENERAL DISCUSSIONS

1

Laboratory Medicine Testing: Specimen Interferences and Clinical Enzymology

A physician who depends on the laboratory to make his diagnosis is probably inexperienced; one who says that he does not need a laboratory is uninformed. In either instance the patient is in danger.

— J.A. Halsted

Laboratory medicine often complements the clinical examination of the veterinary patient. Normal and abnormal laboratory findings provide objective information in the process of differential diagnosis, monitoring treatment, and formulation of a prognosis. Abnormal laboratory measurements and examinations are defined clinically as those values that lie outside the limits of the reference range. The reference range is obtained by sampling a representative population, statistically eliminating outliers, with the resultant limits defining "normal" values equivalent to health. What constitutes "normal" is more complex than initially apparent as every clinician knows who has experienced the frustration of trying to decide if a value just slightly outside of the reference range is indicative of disease or physiologic variation. Some of this indecision can be alleviated by using a reference range that is specific for age, species (in some cases breed), physical disposition (stress), geographic locale, husbandry practices, reproductive status, and laboratory methodology. Properly collected specimens permit one to have confidence in the data generated and to focus on their interpretation. The interjection of artifact can produce erroneous test values that guide one down the wrong road of differential diagnostic possibilities, especially if ignorant of its presence.

An artifact is suspected when the laboratory data are incongruent with the clinical assessment or there is an inappropriate relationship between tests. For example, lipemia frequently causes an increased serum bilirubin value determined by commonly used methods. A serum concentration greater than

3.0 mg/dL should be associated with clinical findings of icterus. A serum concentration greater than 1.0 mg/dL should be associated with a concomitant bilirubinuria in the dog. If bilirubinuria is not present, the validity of the serum bilirubin value must be questioned. Similarly, a sample with moderate to marked hemolysis should be accompanied by hemoglobinuria if it is an *in vivo* phenomenon. The absence of hemoglobinuria suggests an *in vitro* lysis of the erythrocytes perhaps due to rough handling or water-contaminated syringe or tube. An implicit value in these examples is the added interpretive information obtained from simultaneous measurements in blood and urine. Some laboratories provide numerical indices of lipemia, hemolysis, and icterus which sensitize one to their presence and can suggest if the magnitude is sufficient to alter laboratory measurements.

PHYSIOLOGIC CONSIDERATIONS

Age

Selected laboratory results that are normal for immature animals are outside the reference range for mature animals (Table 1–1). Maturity is attained by 6 to 8 months for dogs, a couple of months longer for giant breeds, and by 4 to 6 months for cats. The increased concentration of growth hormone is, at least in part, responsible for the increased serum phosphorous and the decreased serum urea nitrogen concentrations of growing animals. Between 3 and 14 years of age most hematologic and biochemical values are relatively constant, although trends of change are noted for some analytes (Table 1–1).

Stress and Epinephrine Responses

Stress can cause changes in the leukogram and serum biochemical analytes that mimic findings associated with inflammation and disease. The "stress response" is associated with the release of endogenous glucocorticoids or the administration of exogenous corticosteroids. It is more consistent in the dog; variable in other species. Excitement or exercise-induced epinephrine release causes a demargination of neutrophils resulting in a physiologic leukocytosis. The response is accentuated in cats because of a greater marginated neutrophil "pool." Another prominent feature in cats is a marked lymphocytosis, probably a consequence of a temporary alteration of lymphocyte recirculation, which can mimic lymphocytic leukemia. A transient hyperglycemia with or without a transient glucosuria can occur because of epinephrine-stimulated hepatic glycogenolysis and corticosteroid-induced insulin resistance. Because of the propensity of the canine to develop an increased serum alkaline phosphatase (ALP) activity secondary to the presence of increased corticosteroid concentrations, prolonged stress may be one cause.

Hydration and Diet

The hydration state will affect expressed concentration or activity of an analyte due to the reduced water content of the plasma. This is not usually of

Table 1–1. The Effect of Various Factors on the Measurement of Constituents in Serum and Plasma

Patient/Collection Variables	BUN	Creatinine	ALT	AST	ALP	GGT	Total Bilirubin	Bile Acids	Glucose	Cholesterol	Triglycerides	Calcium	Phosphorus	Total Protein	Globulins	Albumin	Sodium	Chloride	Potassium	Magnesium	Amylase	Lipase	CPK	SDH	Iron	PCV	Hemoglobin	MCV	MCHC
Lipemia	V	⇑	⇑	⇑	⇑	V	⇑	⇑	⇑	V		⇑	⇑	⇑[7]		⇓	⇓[1]	⇓[1]	⇓[1]		⇓						⇑		⇑
Hemolysis		⇓	⇑	⇑	⇓		⇑	⇓[2]	⇑			⇑	⇑	⇑[7]		⇑		V	⇑[3,4]	⇑	⇑	⇑	⇑		⇑	⇓	⇑	⇓	⇑
Icterus		⇓			⇑	↓			V	V	⇓		⇑	⇑[7]				⇑		⇓	V	V							
Hyperglycemia																			⇓[3]										
Hyperproteinemia														⇑[7]			⇓[1]	⇓[1,3]		⇓									
Ketonemia		⇑		⇑						⇑																			
Severe azotemia							⇑		⇑					⇑[7]		↓			⇓[3]										
Immature animals	↓	↓			↑	↑[9]							↑	↓	↓				↑									↑	↑
Aging changes (3–12 yr)	↓	↓				↓								↑	↑										↓	↓			
Anticoagulants																													
EDTA	⇑[8]	⇓			⇓							⇓	V				⇓[6]		⇑[5]		⇓	⇓	⇓	⇓	⇓				
Oxalate	⇑[8]	⇓			⇓							⇓	V							⇓[6]	⇓	⇓	⇓	⇓	⇓				
Citrate	⇓[6]				⇓							⇓	V							⇓[6]	⇓	⇓	⇓	⇓	⇓[6]				
Fluoride	⇓				⇓				⇓[6]	⇑		↓					⇓[6]		⇑[5]	⇓[6]	⇓				↓				
Heparin	⇑[8]							⇓									⇓[6]		⇑[5]										
Sample dehydration														⇑			↑									⇑			
UV light							⇓																⇓						

↑, value increased due to physiologic change; ↓, value decreased due to physiologic change; ⇑, value increased due to interference with methodology or collection changes; ⇓, value decreased due to interference with methodology or collection changes; V, variable change depending on methodology; 1, flame photometric methods only, ISE not affected; 2, RIA not affected; 3, dry reagent methods; 4, Akita dogs; 5, sodium salt; 6, potassium salt; 7, refractometer; 8, ammonium; 9, if nursing.

clinical importance due to the wide reference range. However, dilutional changes will occur for serially monitored measurements during the rehydration. A practical application of this concept is by the assessment of the hydration state using sequential determinations of the packed cell volume (PCV) and plasma protein. Hemoconcentration secondary to dehydration results in an improper citrate-to-blood ratio, which will prolong the activated partial thromboplastin time (APTT). Diet can alter several biochemical measurements. A high-protein diet can increase the serum urea nitrogen concentration. The prolonged use of a low-protein diet can cause decreased serum albumin and urea nitrogen concentrations, increased bile acid concentration, and increased serum ALP and alanine aminotransferase (ALT) activities.

SPECIMEN INTERFERENCES

Lipemia

Lipemia causes a number of changes in hematology and chemistry measurements by light scattering in spectrophotometric methods (Table 1–1). Refractometer readings of the plasma protein concentration will be increased and cause a discrepancy between it and the total serum protein value measured biochemically. The serum electrolyte values measured by flame photometry are decreased, while those measured by ion-specific electrodes (ISE) are not affected. The lipid can be partially cleared by ultracentrifugation techniques or precipitating agents (polyethylene glycol, liposol, lipoclear), although clearing agents may themselves induce artifacts. The removal of the lipid may in itself adversely affect the validity of the test value. For example, lipoproteins bind bile acids which would be discarded along with the lipid following ultracentrifugation. This may be one factor that contributes to the occasional measurement of a postprandial value less than the fasted. Lipemia predisposes to hemolysis *in vitro*, which may further confound the effect on the test value. This is especially bothersome for analytes that are measured following a meal. Again using bile acids measured with spectrophotometric methodology as an example, lipemia artifactually increases the value (as much as four-fold) due to the light scattering effect of turbidity while hemolysis has a decremental effect. This may be another factor that contributes to the measurement of a postprandial bile acid concentration that is less than the fasting value. The best approach is to visually examine the sample for lipemia (or hemolysis) prior to its submission. A 12-hour (overnight) fast will usually provide a clear serum sample. The subsequent persistence of lipemia may be in itself indicative of a disease (hypothyroidism, diabetes mellitus, hyperadrenocorticism, pancreatitis, primary lipid disorder).

Hemolysis

Hemolysis can directly interfere with the spectrophotometric absorbance reading and alter the pH of enzymatic reactions. Constituents that are higher in erythrocytes than in serum will be increased, *e.g.*, aspartate aminotransferase (AST) and lactate dehydrogenase (LD) activities. Laboratory changes associated with hemolysis are presented in Table 1–1. Thrombin time, plasminogen concentration, and antithrombin III measurements are increased. Rocket immunoelectrophoresis for the measurement of von Willebrand's factor are decreased and fibrinogen values are increased. Thyroxine (T_4) and adrenocorticotropic hormone (ACTH) determinations are not usually affected by hemolysis but insulin values are decreased. A mean cell hemoglobin concentration (MCHC) that is greater than the reference range, a physiologic improbability, is a numerical indication of hemolysis.

Hyperbilirubinemia, Bile Acids, and Hyperglobulinemia

Bilirubin increases the concentration of albumin assayed by the 2-*p*-hydroxyphenylazobenzoic acid (HABA) procedure, cholesterol using the ferric chloride reagents, glucose using *o*-toluidine method, and the total protein measured by the biuret method. Severe hyperbilirubinemia can artifactually decrease the serum creatinine (Jaffe reaction). Bile acids can adversely affect the measurements for serum secretin, glucagon, insulin, and gastrin determined by radioimmunoassay (RIA).

Marked hyperglobulinemia can falsely increase the inorganic phosphate value and falsely decrease the serum electrolyte measurements obtained by flame photometry. Hyperglobulinemia does not affect the ISE measurement of these values (Table 1–1).

Anticoagulants

Anticoagulants can alter the measurements of a variety of analytes (Table 1–1). Values are increased if the anticoagulant contains the analyte being measured or activates enzymes and decreases the value if it binds the analyte. Ethylenediaminetetraacetic acid (EDTA) alters the morphology of neutrophils with prolonged storage resulting in a "toxic" appearance. An improper EDTA to blood ratio (underfilling the tube) causes shrinkage of erythrocytes, which results in decreased packed cell volume (PCV) and mean cell volume (MCV) values and an increased MCHC value. Heparin results in poorly stained leukocytes; it is acceptable for most chemistries, blood gas, and ammonia determinations. Notable exceptions include ammonium heparin for the measurement of plasma ammonia concentrations, sodium and potassium heparin for the measurement of those respective electrolytes, and heparinized plasma for bile acid determinations (both false increases and decreases have been reported; it is, therefore, an unreliable measurement).

PHARMACOLOGIC AND THERAPEUTIC AGENTS

A wide variety of drugs alter urine dipstick, specific gravity, and sulfosalicylic acid measurements (Table 1–2). Endogenous metabolites, *e.g.*, nitrites and ascorbic acid in the dog, can adversely affect urine reagent strip measurements (Table 1–2). Drug-induced alterations are numerous. Mechanisms include enzyme induction, direct interference with the test methodology, and indirect systemic influences caused by changes in blood pressure or acid-

Table 1–2. The Effect of Drugs and Other Factors on the Measurement of Constituents in Urine

Urinalysis Alterations	Specific gravity	Urine pH	Proteinuria	Glucosuria (Dipstick)	Ketonuria	Bilirubinuria	Urobilinogen	Hemo/Myoglobinuria	Nitrituria	Pyuria
Acetazolamide		↑	⇑1				⇑			
Aminoglycosides			⇑2	↑						⇑1
Ascorbic acid		↓		⇓		⇓	↓	⇓	⇓	
Cephalosporins			⇑2							⇑1
Chlorpromazine			⇑2			⇓				
Colchicine	↓									
Corticosteroids	↓									
Dipyrone				⇓						
Diuretics	↓									
Methionine		↓			↑					
Penicillins			⇑2							
Phenazopyridine			⇑1		⇑	⇑	⇑		⇑	
Phenolphthalein					⇑					
Phenothiazines						⇑	⇑			
Procaine							⇑			
Radiographic contrast media	⇑		⇑2							
Salicylates			⇑2		⇓	⇓				
Sodium bicarbonate		↑	⇑1				↑			
Sulfobromophthalein (BSP)						⇑	⇑			
Sulfonamides			⇑2				⇑			
Urinary acidifiers		↓					↓			
Acetoacetate (ketonuria)				⇓						
Alkaline urine	⇓1		⇑1⇓2							⇓3
Bilirubinuria							⇑			
Highly concentrated urine								⇓		
Nitrituria						⇓	⇓	⇓		
Proteinuria	⇑1									
Refrigerated urine				⇓						
Time		⇑								
UV light						⇓	⇓			

↑, value increased due to physiologic change; ↓, value decreased due to physiologic change; ⇑, value increased due to interference with methodology; ⇓, value decreased due to interference with methodology; 1, dipstick; 2, sulfosalicyclic acid method; 3, sediment.

base status. Commonly used medications and their potential effects are listed in Table 1–3.

Corticosteroids

Topical, oral, and parenteral preparations cause changes in the hemogram, biochemistry profile, urinalysis, endocrine, and immunologic tests (Table 1–3). Although the changes are usually predictable, the magnitude of change is not. An increase in the serum activities of hepatic enzyme tests in dogs is most consistent. Less commonly, megestrol acetate in cats and corticosteroids in cats and horses can cause small increases in serum hepatic enzyme tests. The former can cause hyperglycemia and glucosuria in cats. The renal tubular concentrating mechanism can be impaired resulting in an inappropriate urine specific gravity for the hydration state, *i.e.*, inability to respond to water depravation. Some of the corticosteroids (such as prednisone) are measured as cortisol by certain assays while dexamethasone is not. Even topically administered corticosteroids suppress the hypothalamic-pituitary-adrenal axis, adversely resulting in serum cortical values consistent with hypoadrenocorticism. The thyroid function in dogs is suppressed secondary to corticosteroid administration. The Coombs' test and antinuclear antibody test (ANA) can be negative in a patient with an immune-mediated disease if measured 2 to 3 days after the start of immunosuppressive therapy.

Nonsteroidal Anti-inflammatory Drugs (NSAIDs)
(Table 1–3)

Aspirin causes platelet dysfunction resulting in an increased bleeding time; an unexpected hematoma following venipuncture may be a clinical observation. Aspirin and acetaminophen artificially decrease serum glucose values measured by the oxidase system. Intravenous dipyrone can negatively interfere with measurement of creatine kinase, lactate dehydrogenase, triglyceride, cholesterol, and creatinine concentrations.

Antibiotics (Table 1–3)

Cephalosporins and penicillins can artifactually increase the serum creatinine concentration (Jaffe reaction), while chloramphenicol decreases the actual serum urea nitrogen concentration. Sulfonamides appear to increase some serum enzyme activities through enzyme induction in the tissue. Trimethoprim/sulfamethoxazole has been shown to decrease thyroid function in dogs. Many antibiotics will cause false positive protein measurements on the urine reagent strip and by the sulfosalicylic acid procedure (Table 1–2).

Anticonvulsants

Anticonvulsant medications, particularly phenobarbital, can cause increases in serum hepatic enzyme activities probably by their induction in the tissue

Table 1–3. The Effect of Drugs and Hormones on the Measurement of Constituents in Serum and Plasma

Biochemical Alterations	BUN	Creatinine	ALT	AST	ALP	GGT	Total Bilirubin	Bile Acids	Glucose	Cholesterol	Triglycerides	Calcium	Phosphorus	Total Protein	Albumin	Sodium	Chloride	Potassium	Magnesium	Amylase	Lipase	CK	Thyroxine	ACTH	Cortisol	Gastrin
Corticosteroids	↑		↑	↑		↑			↑	↑	↑	↓		↑		↑		↓		↓	↑	↑	↓	↓	V	
Mineralcorticoids																↑		↓								
Anabolic steroids	↑		↑		↑		↑				V	↑	V	↑		↓		↑								
NSAIDs		↑																								
Acetaminophen	↑	⇓	↑															↑								
Aspirin	↑	⇑	↑																							
Dipyrone									⇓	⇓	⇓											⇓				
Ibuprofen	↑		↑						⇓																	
Phenylbutazone	↑		↑				↑									↑							↓			
Antibiotics																										
Aminoglycosides	↑	↑	↑																↓							
Cephalosporins		⇑	↑				↑																			
Chloramphenicol	V																									
Penicillins		⇑																								
Sulfonamides			↑		↑		↑		↑	↑										↑	↑					
Tetracycline					↑					⇑			V				⇑			↑	↑					
Anticonvulsants																										
Phenobarbital			↑	↑	↑		↓					↓	↓										↓			
Phenytoin			↑			↑																	↓		↑	
Potassium bromide			↑																							
Primidone																										
Hormones																										
Androgens									↑			↑											↓			
Estrogen									↓		↑	↑	↑		↑	↑	↑	↓		↑			↑	↑	↑	↑
Insulin									⇑																	
Progesterone									↑	↓		↑							↑							
Thyroxine																							↑			
Amphotericin B	↑	↑							↑									↓	↓							
Ascorbic Acid	⇑	⇑		V			⇓		⇓		↓															

Biochemical Alterations	BUN	Creatinine	ALT	AST	ALP	GGT	Total Bilirubin	Bile Acids	Glucose	Cholesterol	Triglycerides	Calcium	Phosphorus	Total Protein	Albumin	Sodium	Chloride	Potassium	Magnesium	Amylase	Lipase	CK	Thyroxine	ACTH	Cortisol	Gastrin
Asparaginase	↑		↑						↑	↓	↓									↑	↑		↓			
Azathioprine		⇑	↑	⇓	↑															↑	↑					
Barbiturates		⇑	↑		↑																					
β-Adrenergics	↑	⇑							↑																	
Captopril	↑	⇑																↑								
Cholestyramine				↑				↓		↓	↑						↑									
Cimetidine			↑																							↑
Cisplatin		↑																	↓							
Colchicine										↓																
Flucytosine	↑	⇑																								
Furosemide	↑	⇑							↑		↓		↑			↓	↓	↓	↓	↑						
Glucose		⇑							⇑				↑			↓		↓								
Heparin									↑	↑	↓							↑					↓			
Methimazole				↑	↑				⇑	↑											↑		↓			
Metronidazole				⇓					↑											↑	↑		↓			
Phenothiazines					↑				↑	↑			⇓													
Propranolol									↓									↑					↑			
Radiographic contrast media	↑	↑					⇑						↑			↑							↑			
Salicylates	↑	↑	↑						V									↓					↓			
Sodium bicarbonate																	↓	↓								
Sulfobromophthalein (BSP)		⇑			⇓		⇓																			
Theophylline			↑						↑																	
Thiacetarsamide			↑																							

↑, value increased due to physiologic change; ↓, value decreased due to physiologic change; ⇑, value increased due to interference with methodology or collection changes; ⇓, value decreased due to interference with methodology or collection changes; V, variable change depending on methodology.

and may decrease serum thyroxine concentrations. Patients on potassium bromide may have increased serum chloride concentrations; bromide is measured as chloride by flame photometry and ISE methods. Bromide also interferes with the cholesterol measurement (Table 1–3).

Blood Transfusions

The use of citrate blood transfusion products has been associated with decreased serum ionized calcium concentrations in dogs, especially with greater than 40% blood replacement.

Radiographic Contrast Media (Table 1–2)

Following a myelogram, the specific gravity and Pandy score may be falsely increased and the quantitative protein concentration and white blood cell count can be increased subsequent to an irritant effect. The radiographic contrast media can also affect urine measurements, increasing the specific gravity and protein concentration. Radiographic dyes can form pleomorphic crystals in acid urine up to 3 days following their administration.

Hormones (Table 1–3)

Numerous *in vivo* effects are mediated by hormones that can affect laboratory test results. For example, the administration of insulin not only decreases the plasma glucose concentration but also decreases the plasma potassium and phosphorous concentrations.

Vitamins

Ascorbic acid has been shown to decrease serum glucose (oxidase method), increase serum creatinine concentration (Table 1–3), and cause false negative glucose and nitrate reactions on the urine reagent strip (Table 1–2).

COLLECTION AND STORAGE

Prior to collection, the appropriate sample container is labeled with the names of the owner and patient and the signalment. Color-coded, rubber stoppered, evacuated tubes are well standardized: lilac-colored containing EDTA for hemogram measurements, red-colored without an anticoagulant to harvest serum, green-colored containing heparin to harvest plasma, and robin's egg blue-colored containing citrate to harvest plasma for the measurement of coagulation tests. The serum or plasma should be removed within 20 to 30 minutes and kept refrigerated or frozen. Prolonged contact of erythrocytes with serum will decrease the serum glucose concentration at a rate of about 10% per hour. Most biochemical parameters are stable in serum or plasma stored at 4° C for at least 24 hours. EDTA-anticoagulated blood can be stored at 4° C; the MCV will increase and the MCHC decrease after approximately 12 hours. Decreased stability of certain analytes occurs with exposure to UV light (Table 1–1). Urine bilirubin is oxidized to biliverdin with exposure to fluorescent light; green-colored urine and a negative test for bilirubin on the reagent strip test is a consequence. Likewise, fluorescent lighting can cause an oxidation of the colorless urobilinogen to urobilin resulting in a negative reagent strip test and a greenish color may develop.

Some hormones are adversely affected by prolonged or inappropriate storage. ACTH, insulin, and gastrin degrade quickly at room temperature and should be immediately placed on ice following collection. Some, such as ACTH, adhere to glass surfaces, and the plasma must be collected and stored using plastic containers or, if collected in an EDTA-filled glass tube, separated and stored in a plastic container within 15 minutes of collection. The laboratory should be contacted for their recommendations regarding the nuances associated with the submission of the less frequently measured hormones.

Sample evaporation during transportation can cause an increase in the PCV, plasma protein concentration, and white blood cell count. The biochemical changes are usually limited to increases in the serum sodium and potassium concentrations. In an arid environment, increases in these measurements that could be interpreted as clinically important can occur within 2 hours. Bacterial contamination of a sample or collection tube can cause a decreased serum glucose concentration if sent by standard mail.

Vitreous and Aqueous Humor Specimens

Postmortem blood undergoes rapid chemical change and is easily contaminated, precluding its use for the reliable measurement of analytes. Selected serum constituents can be measured in the vitreous or aqueous humor after death for diagnostic purposes. In canine vitreous humor, the increase of the potassium concentration of vitreous humor is dependent on time and temperature and can be used to assess the time of death. The chloride concentration is stable for up to 24 hours at both 4° C and 20° C. The sodium concentration fluctuates during this time and temperature range, but raised values suggest hypernatremia antemortem. The urea nitrogen and creatinine concentrations are stable for up to 24 hours at both 4° C and 20° C, the former being the most reliable of the two. The glucose concentration decreases by approximately 50% within 3 hours at both temperatures and by approximately 75% of the antemortem concentration by 24 hours. Therefore, a normal or raised value in the vitreous humor would be suggestive of antemortem hyperglycemia. In bovine vitreous humor, the magnesium, sodium, and chloride concentrations are stable at ambient temperature for up to 24 hours postmortem. The urea nitrogen and creatinine concentrations in bovine vitreous humor are reliable indicators of azotemia for up to 24 hours after death at ambient temperature. Similarly, in equine aqueous humor, the urea nitrogen and creatinine concentrations can be used as markers of azotemia for up to 24 hours postmortem at ambient temperature. γ-glutamyltransferase (GGT) activity is stable for up to 4 hours at ambient temperature in rabbit aqueous humor. The measurement of the other serum enzyme and biochemical constituents are not valid markers of antemortem disease.

In summary, the interpretation of laboratory medicine test results begins with proper sample management and reliable reference ranges.

DIAGNOSTIC ENZYMOLOGY

We know that half of what we teach will be proved false in ten years; the hard part is that we do not know which half.

—Wise Medical Pedagogue

Enzymes are protein catalysts that accelerate biochemical reactions within cells. They undergo a physical change during a reaction and revert to their original state when the reaction is complete. A variety of pathophysiologic processes, notably injury to the cell, result in an increase in their measurable activity in plasma. Diagnostic enzymology is the area of laboratory medicine that is involved in the study and application of plasma enzyme activity as a diagnostic aid, as a monitor of disease activity, and in the evaluation of the response to treatment. The catalytic property is sensitive and specific for each enzyme and is used for their own measurement. The rate of the reaction it catalyzes is proportional to the quantity of the enzyme present. The rate of appearance of a product, disappearance of a substrate, or change in concentration of a coenzyme is usually used for the quantification. The result is expressed in enzyme units. One international unit (IU) is defined as the amount of enzyme that catalyzes the conversion of 1 micromole (micro-equivalent) of substrate or coenzyme per minute under the defined conditions of the test (temperature with optimal pH and substrate concentration). The katal (kat) is also used to denote catalytic activity; 1 katal represents 1 mole catalyzed per second. One unit equals 16.67 nanokatals.

Since temperature and hydrogen ion concentration influence the reaction, they must be optimized and held constant for consistency. If one or more of these variables are changed, the value for the plasma enzyme activity will change. This may happen, for example, if a sample is analyzed both "in-house" as well as sent to a commercial laboratory and the methodologies use different reaction conditions. Two different values for the same analyte, both correct, will be generated! The disparity can occur if two different methodologies are used; for example, "wet" and "dry" reagent systems. The clinical impact is obvious. Other factors can cause more subtle changes in the measurements. The use of quality control specimens (lyophilized) charted daily on a Levey-Jennings quality control graph and replicate measurements to evaluate assay precision are essential for detecting inconsistency associated with analytical bias, random analytical variability, and mistakes.

The interpretive meaning associated with the diagnostic use of enzymes is impregnated by experimental studies, clinical studies, and clinical experience. Certain applications for diagnostic enzymology developed for use in humans were directly incorporated into veterinary medicine without adequate interrogation. We now know that some of these diagnostic uses are inappropriate due to species differences. Examples of differences between humans and domestic animals include corticosteroid-associated increases in plasma alkaline phosphatase activity in the dog, bilirubin metabolism in the dog, horse, and bovine, and the paucity of hepatic ALT activity in the horse and bovine. The classic experimental work for the study of enzyme kinetics initiated in the 1950s provides an important base for their clinical utility. The clinical studies supplement this information by expanding, clarifying and, sometimes, complicating the interpretive possibilities as a consequence of the biologic complexities associated with disease. Continued investigative attention needs to be given to this intriguing area of medicine in order to unravel the remaining mysteries for diagnostic enzymology and enhance its clinical value.

Factors Affecting the Activity of Enzyme in Plasma

Enzymes are the constituents of the cells that form organs. Some enzymes tend to be prominent in only one organ while others are present in multiple organs. Those present in multiple organs have different molecular forms referred to as isoenzymes (isozymes). In the liver, the same enzyme can have multiple forms that differ for each of the three acinar zones. They are physically distinct forms with the same catalytic activity. They can be separated electrophoretically based on their differing charge in the pH-adjusted assay media to indicate the specific tissue of origin or subcellular component. In general, their measurement is no longer diagnostically popular in veterinary medicine with the exception of investigative work.

The location of the enzyme within the cell affects its release. They may be located in the cytoplasm, "attached" to organelles, be present in both of these locations, or "attached" to an area of the cell membrane (see Fig. 7–1 and Table 1–4). Those present in the cytoplasm are soluble and released with relative ease. They tend to be relatively "sensitive" markers of altered cellular integrity, i.e., a "marker" of cell injury. An example is ALT in the cytosol of the hepatocyte. The plasma ALT activity readily increases subsequent to hepatocellular damage in the dog and cat. An example of the second enzyme location is glutamate dehydrogenase (GD, GLDH), which is found only in mitochondria of the hepatocyte. Sufficient cellular damage to cause injury to

Table 1–4. Distribution in the Cell of Some Clinically Used Enzymes[a]

Cellular Location	Enzyme
Cytoplasm	ALT
	AST_1 (cystolic isoenzyme)
	SD
	CK (isoenzymes 1–3)
	LD (isoenzymes 1–5)
Mitochondria	AST_2 (mitochondrial isoenzyme)
Endoplasmic reticulum	GGT
Membrane	ALP
	GGT
Zymogen (intracytoplasmic) granules	Amylase
	Lipase
	Immunoreactive trypsin

[a]Modified from Boyd, JW: The mechanism relating to increases in plasma enzymes and isoenzymes in disease in animals. Vet Clin Pathol 1982;12:9–24.

these little "factories" of the cell is required for its release. An example of the third situation is AST. For the hepatocyte, the majority of its activity is located in the cytoplasm for most species, with the remainder associated with mitochondria. Two additional concepts will be broached in the context of this enzyme. First, despite relatively similar molecular weights (~110,000) for both cytosolic ALT and AST, an increase in the plasma ALT activity is the first to occur with mild hepatocellular injury. This suggests that factors other than size are involved in release subsequent to the alteration of cell membrane integrity. Second, studies have demonstrated that the mitochondrial isoenzyme of AST is released at the time of necrobiosis, providing a "marker" of cell death. The correlation of the intracellular source of the enzyme in the plasma with organelle injury remains investigative, with clinical relevance, if any, to be determined. An example of the fourth cellular enzyme location is ALP, which is associated with the canilicular membrane of the hepatocyte. Membrane enzymes are firmly attached, may have relatively low tissue activity, and can be shed with fragments of the cell membrane following injury. However, it is not this process that results in the diagnostic utility. A poorly understood, complex process of increased synthesis and release subsequent to the appropriate stimulus is usually responsible for their increased plasma activity and contribution to diagnostic enzymology.

The intracellular activity for cytosolic enzymes is usually thousands of times greater than in the plasma. The "normal" serum enzyme activity probably reflects a balance between some leakage through the dynamically metabolic membrane and its degradation or excretion. It is unlikely that physiologic or "self-programmed" cell death (apoptosis) has a significant contribution. It appears that most enzymes pass into the interstitial fluid and then into the lymphatic circulation prior to their appearance in the blood. Their kinetics may be even more complex in disease. Using pancreatitis as an example, studies have suggested amylase makes its way from the inflamed organ into the peritoneal fluid followed by its absorption into the diaphragmatic lymphatic circulation on its way to the peripheral blood.

Most plasma enzymes are degradated by the macrophage system or parenchymal cells and others are excreted in the urine. There is species variation for the elimination of enzymes that can impact on their diagnostic and investigative uses (see Table 7–1). For example, amylase is excreted in the urine of humans where it can be used as a "marker" of pancreatitis but appears to be metabolized by the canine kidney precluding a similar diagnostic application. Subtle changes in the physiochemical characteristics of the enzyme can prolong its rate of removal. A macroenzyme is an enzyme that occasionally forms in plasma as a high-molecular-mass by binding with an immunoglobulin or other nonimmunoglobulin components in plasma. They have been described for most diagnostic enzymes in humans and macroamylasemia in dogs with renal insufficiency. The change in molecular configuration can dramatically prolong its presence in the plasma and lead to misdiagnoses. There are two more examples that relate to alkaline phosphatase, an enzyme with multiple isoenzymes. The intestinal isoenzyme of ALP is degradated by the hepatocyte in the dog but by the Kupffer cell in the rat; each using a different receptor-mediated uptake system. The appearance in the plasma of an ALP isoenzyme unique to the dog is associated with hyperadrenocorticism or the administration of corticosteroids. Its molecular weight, amino acid content, and peptide maps are nearly identical to the canine intestinal ALP isoenzyme but differs dramatically in its carbohydrate content. The hyperglycosylation of this unique enzyme is probably the reason that its plasma half-life is approximately 66 hours in contrast to approximately 6 minutes for the intestinal isoenzyme. A similar mechanism may be responsible for a mysterious, spontaneous, transient increase in the plasma ALP activity in humans. While the impact on diagnostic enzymology of the last example for the dog is well known, the importance of this phenomenon for other enzymes in veterinary medicine is unknown but should be kept in mind when the abnormal enzyme value does not "fit" the patient.

The magnitude of increase in the plasma activity of most enzymes following injury is dependent on several factors—its innate tissue activity (Table 1–5), the amount of tissue damaged, the type of injury, the rate of its removal from the plasma (Fig. 1–1), and its cellular location. The rate of removal of the enzyme from the circulation seems to have molecule-specific and species-specific properties. For a few enzymes such as ALP and GGT, the increase in plasma activity is dependent on an increased rate of production by the tissue (cell) in which it is located. For example, the plasma ALP is increased during growth because of the increased osteoclastic activity associated with the growth plates of the bone.

Those plasma enzymes with the greatest clinical utility will be discussed in detail with each organ system. We will see that their increase is often secondary to multiple causes. By understanding the kinetics of each one, you will be able to triage clinically the possibilities into probabilities and, by combining the information obtained from other tests, the history, and physical examination, usually into a diagnosis.

SENSITIVITY, SPECIFICITY, AND PREDICTIVE VALUE— DIAGNOSTIC CONSIDERATIONS

A clinical test should be safe and practical, and should accurately indicate the presence or absence of a specific disease or pathology for which its use is defined. Sensitivity, specificity, and predictive value constitute the measures of test accuracy. Diagnostic sensitivity is the likelihood that a patient with the disease has a positive test result indicative of the presence of that disease in a population known to have the disease. Diagnostic specificity is the likelihood that a patient without the disease being tested for has a test value that remains within the reference range when that disease is not present in a population without the disease. The predictive value (PV) of a test is determined by its measurement in a population that have and do not have the disease. As an indication of accuracy; a positive test result is obtained when the disease is present (positive PV), and a negative test result is measured when the disease is not present (negative PV). The PV is dependent on the sensitivity and specificity of a test and the prevalence of the disease being tested for in a given population. The formulas for the determination of these measures are listed in Table 1–6.

The sensitivity and specificity are inherent properties of the test that the clinician cannot affect. The likelihood (prevalence) of the disease being tested for in a given population can be manipulated by use of the history, physical examination, and adjunctive diagnostic aids. This narrows the possibilities into probabilities, referred to as a list of differential diagnoses or "rule-outs"

Table 1–5. Enzyme Activities in Tissues[a,b]

Enzyme	Dog	Cat	Horse	Bovine	Pig	Rat
Alanine aminotransferase						
Liver	32	29.8	0.9	0.3	0.9	2.4
Heart	8.7	1.4	1.7	1.7	3.1	1.7
Muscle	1.8	1.0	4.4	2.0	1.3	2.8
Kidney	2.9	3.7	0.4	0.3	0.5	1.6
Intestine	0.4	0.5	0.03	0.3	—	4.5
Pancreas	1.5	0.9	0.7	—	—	—
Sorbitol dehydrogenase						
Liver	11.7	0.60	5.2	9.7	9.5	31
Heart	1.0	0.20	0.2	0.1	0.00	0
Muscle	0.4	0.05	0.0	0.1	0.03	0
Kidney	6.5	0.10	1.0	3.0	3.70	11
Intestine	0.7	0.04	0.1	0.4	0.20	0
Pancreas	0.4	0.06	0.2	—	0.00	—
Glutamate dehydrogenase						
Liver	6.8	125	10.4	19.0	1.3	36
Heart	2.3	10.0	0.1	2.1	0.1	3
Muscle	0.6	2.0	0.1	0.7	0.01	2.4
Kidney	5.1	40	0.7	8.5	0.3	7.9
Intestine	2.0	3.0	—	1.2	—	3.3
Pancreas	0.5	—	0.3	—	—	—
Aspartate aminotransferase						
Liver	53	59	33	70	57	88
Heart	67	69	32	48	115	269
Muscle	46	22	54	70	44	69
Kidney	24	17	7	30	47	57
Intestine	12	7	6	6	—	25
Pancreas	22	10	—	—	—	—
Lactate dehydrogenase						
Liver	130	127	82	57	25	212
Heart	320	89	354	97	60	360
Muscle	169	259	155	336	591	453
Kidney	256	40	122	69	30	167
Intestine	58	47	18	20	29	185
Pancreas	52	16	52	—	12	—
Creatine kinase						
Liver	50	1	7	—	—	10
Heart	1150	518	1710	—	—	644
Muscle	2500	692	4300	—	—	3516
Kidney	50	1	97	—	—	31
Intestine	200	20	254	—	—	223
Pancreas	—	15	—	—	—	—
Alkaline phosphatase						
Liver	0.3	0.30	0.74	0.09	0.3	1.17
Heart	0.8	0.05	0.07	0.01	0.1	—
Muscle	0.1	0.05	0.10	0.02	0.1	0.5
Kidney	6.4	3.79	10.20	0.80	13.0	300
Intestine	220	7.98	2.24	—	10.1	—
Pancreas	1.3	0.19	2.15	0.07	—	0.6
γ-Glutamyltransferase						
Liver	0.90	—	2.40	4.97	2.69	0.13
Heart	—	—	0.12	0.31	0.02	0
Muscle	0.00	—	0.28	0.01	0.02	0
Kidney	86.10	—	38.66	60.50	16.45	189
Intestine	1.50	—	0.59	0.59	1.47	—
Pancreas	41.70	—	6.80	22.18	8.58	—

[a] Modified from Boyd, JW: The mechanism relating to increases in plasma enzymes and isoenzymes in disease in animals. Vet Clin Pathol 1982;12:9–24.

[b] Measurements given in IU/g throughout.

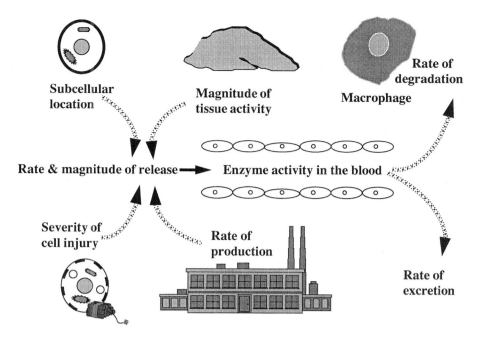

FIGURE 1–1. The *in vivo* plasma enzyme activity is dependent on a variety of factors. The type and severity of tissue injury impacts its magnitude of change as does an alteration in its rate of production and release into the plasma in concert with its elimination.

Table 1–6. Formulas for the Calculation of Diagnostic Sensitivity, Diagnostic Specificity, Positive Predictive Value, and Negative Predictive Value[a]

$$\text{Diagnostic sensitivity} = \frac{TP}{TP + FN}$$

$$\text{Diagnostic specificity} = \frac{TN}{TN + FP}$$

$$\text{Positive predictive value} = \frac{TP}{TP + FP}$$

$$\text{Negative predictive value} = \frac{TN}{TN + FN}$$

[a] TP, true positive (the number of patients with the disease being tested for that have a test result outside the reference range indicative of that disease); TN, true negative (the number of patients without the disease being tested for that have a test result within the reference range); FP, false positive (the number of patients without the disease being tested for that have a test result outside the reference range indicative of that disease); FN, false negative (the number of patients with the disease being tested for that have a test result within the reference range).

that effectively enhance the PV of a test without changing its sensitivity or specificity.

Perhaps the impact of disease prevalence on the predictive value of a test can be better appreciated with a "what-if" example. Let's say that previous clinical trials have determined that both a test's sensitivity and specificity for the diagnosis of a specific disease is 90%, relatively quite good. If the prevalence of that disease is 1/1000 (0.1%), the predicative value of a positive test is a miserable 1% (0.01). If the prevalence is 25/100 (25%), the positive predictive value improves to a diagnostically reasonable 75% (0.75). If the patient population is further triaged to provide a prevalence of 50/100 (50%), the positive predictive value is 90% (0.90)—an excellent diagnostic probability is achieved. A directly applicable clinical paradigm for this effect on testing can be applied to canine hyperadrenocorticism. Its occurrence in the general patient population is approximately 0.1%. Prior to the use of tests of adrenal function, patient culling after a careful examination can increase its prevalence to 25%. Following the evaluation of additional differential diagnostic information to eliminate other disease possibilities, its prevalence in the patient population can be increased up to 50%. Consequently, the positive (and negative) predictive value for the selected adrenal function test is greatly accentuated in supporting or denying the presence of the disease.

Additional Reading

Burkhard M, Meyer D: Causes and effects of interference with clinical laboratory measurements and examinations. In Kirk R, Bonagura J (eds): Current Veterinary Therapy XII. Philadelphia, WB Saunders Co, 1995, pp 14–20.

Cantor GH, Palmer GH, Fenwick BW: Analysis of post mortem aqueous humor chemistry in the horse, with particular reference to urea nitrogen and creatinine. Equine Vet J 1989;21:288–291.

Ceryak S, Bouscarel B, Fromm H: Comparative binding of bile acids to serum lipoproteins and albumin. J Lipid Res 1993;34:1661–1674.

Chauvet A, Feldman E, Kass P: Effects of phenobarbital administration on results of serum biochemical analyses and adrenocortical function tests in epileptic dogs. J Am Vet Med Assoc 1995;207:1305–1307.

Corazza M, Tognetti R, Guidi G, et al: Urinary a-amylase and serum macroamylase activities in dogs with proteinuria. J Am Vet Med Assoc 1994;205:438–440.

Dial S: Hematology, chemistry profile, and urinalysis for pediatric patients. Comp Contin Educ Small Anim Pract 1992;14:305–308.

Fettman M, Allen T: Developmental aspects of fluid and electrolyte metabolism and renal function in neonates. Comp Cont Educ Small Anim Pract 1991;14:392–403.

Gerstman B, Cappucci D: Evaluating the reliability of diagnostic test results. J Am Vet Med Assoc 1986;188:248–251.

Grasbeck R: Reference values, why and how. Scand J Clin Lab Invest 1990;201:45–53.

Hall I, Campbell K, Chambers M, et al: Effect of trimethoprim/sulfamethoxazole on thyroid function in dogs with pyoderma. J Am Vet Med Assoc 1993;202:1959–1962.

Halsted JA, Halsted CH: The Laboratory in Clinical Medicine, Interpretation and Application. Philadelphia, WB Saunders Co, 1981.

Hoffmann W, Dorner J: Disappearance rates of intravenously injected canine alkaline phosphatase isoenzymes. Am J Vet Res 1977;38:1553–1556.

Kamimoto Y, Horiuchi S, Tanase S, et al: Plasma clearance of intravenously injected AST isozymes: Evidence for preferential uptake by sinusoidal liver cells. Hepatology 1985;5:367–375.

Kuhlenschmidt M, Hoffmann W, Rippy M: Glucocorticoid hepatopathy: Effect on receptor-medicated endocytosis of asialoglycoproteins. Biochem Med Metab Biol 1991;46:152–168.

Lake-Bakaar G, Tovoli S, Straus E, et al: The effects of bile salts on the radioimmunoassay of hormonal peptides. J Lab Clin Med 1982;99:740–745.

Lee D, Lamb S, Reimers T: Effects of hyperlipemia on radioimmunoassays for progesterone, testosterone, thyroxine, and cortisol in serum and plasma samples from dogs. Am J Vet Res 1991;52:1489–1491.

Lekhakula S, Boonpisit S, Amornkitticharoen B: Total bile acids in hyperlipidaemic serum determined by bioluminescent and spectrophotometric methods. J Biolumin Chemilumin 1991;6:259–262.

Lincoln SD, Lane VM: Postmortem chemical ananlysis of vitreous humor as a diagnostic aid in cattle. Mod Vet Pract 1985;9:883–886.

Lott J, Mitchell L, Moeschberger M, et al: Estimation of reference ranges: How many subjects are needed? Clin Chem 1992;38:648–650.

Lowseth L, Gillett N, Gerlach R, et al: The effects of aging on hematology and serum chemistry values in the beagle dog. Vet Clin Pathol 1990;19:13–19.

Pappas N Jr: Theoretical aspects of enzymes in diagnosis. Why do serum enzymes change in hepatic, myocardial, and other diseases? Clin Lab Med 1989;9:595–626.

Pappas N Jr, Qureshi A: Liver AST activity as a power function of body weight. Biochem Med Metab Biol 1988;39:121–125.

Reimers T, Lamb S, Bartlett S, et al: Effects of hemolysis and storage on quantification of hormones in blood samples from dogs, cattle, and horses. Am J Vet Res 1991;52:1075–1080.

Remaley A, Wilding P: Macroenzymes: Biochemical characterization, clinical significance, and laboratory detection. Clin Chem 1989;35:2261–2270.

Saris N: Approved recommendation (1978): Quantities and units in clinical chemistry. J Clin Chem Clin Biochem 1979;17:807–821.

Schoning P, Strafuss AC: Postmortem biochemical changes in canine vitreous humor. J Forensic Sci 1980;25:53–59.

Solter P, Hoffmann W, Hoffman J: Evaluation of an automated serum bile acids assay and the effect of bilirubin, hemoglobin, and lipid on the apparent bile acid yield. Vet Clin Pathol 1992;21:114–118.

Statland B, Winkel P: Preparing patients and specimens for laboratory testing. In Henry J (ed): Clinical Diagnosis and Management by Laboratory Methods, 18th edition. Philadelphia, WB Saunders Co, 1991, pp 68–71.

Sugimoto Y, Hayakawa T, Kondo T, et al: Peritoneal absorption of pancreatic enzymes in bile-induced acute pancreatitis in dogs. J Gastroenterol Hepatol 1990;5:493–498.

Thoresen S, Havre G, Morberg H, et al: Effects of storage time on chemistry results from canine whole blood, heparinized whole blood, serum and heparinized plasma. Vet Clin Pathol 1992;21:88–94.

Tietz N: Clinical Guide To Laboratory Tests, 2nd edition. Philadelphia, WB Saunders Co, 1990.

Wolf P: The significance of transient hyperphosphatasemia of infancy and childhood to the clinician and clinical pathologist. Arch Pathol Lab Med 1995;119:774–775.

Hematopoiesis and Evaluation of Bone Marrow

OVERVIEW

Sites of Blood Cell Production

Hematopoiesis begins outside the body in the yolk sac of the embryo. At the time of early fetal development, the liver and spleen are major hematopoietic organs. The bone marrow and peripheral lymphoid organs become the major sites of blood cell production in mammals during the second half of fetal development. Throughout adult life, all blood cell types are continuously produced from primitive stem cells within extravascular spaces of bone marrow in mammals. Leukocytes are also produced within the extravascular spaces of bone marrow in birds, but erythrocytes and thrombocytes are produced within the vascular spaces.

Stem Cells and Progenitor Cells

By definition, stem cells are capable of proliferation, continuous self-renewal, and differentiation. The term progenitor cell will be used for cells that form colonies in bone marrow culture like stem cells, but do not have long-term self-renewal capacities. Stem cells and progenitor cells are mononuclear cells that cannot be distinguished morphologically from lymphocytes. A totipotent hematopoietic stem cell produces a pluripotent lymphoid stem cell, as well as a pluripotent myeloid stem cell. The pluripotent myeloid stem cell gives rise to a series of progressively more differentiated progenitor cells, with limited or no self-renewal capabilities, that support the production of all nonlymphoid blood cells. When measured in an *in vitro* cell culture assay, these progenitor cells are referred to as colony-forming units (CFUs). Progenitor cells that give rise to multiple subcolonies are called burst-forming units (BFUs). A simplified working model of hematopoietic development is given (Fig. 2–1). Oligopotential progenitor cells may be bi-, tri-, tetra-, penta-,

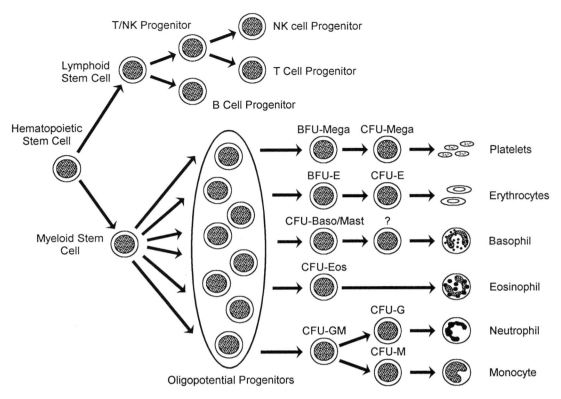

FIGURE 2–1. Simplified working model of hematopoiesis. NK, natural killer; BFU, burst-forming unit; CFU, colony-forming unit; Mega, megakaryocyte; E, erythroid; Baso, basophil; Eos, eosinophil; G, granulocyte; M, macrophage.

or hexapotential. Colony-forming unit–granulocyte, erythrocyte, macrophage, megakaryocyte (CFU-GEMM) is a tetrapotential progenitor cell that has been studied extensively *in vitro*. Although portrayed as discrete cell compartments, the transition from one cell type to another is gradual; consequently, considerable heterogeneity exists within stem cell and progenitor cell compartments.

Progenitor cells for certain tissue cells also occur in the marrow. These include progenitor cells for marrow reticular cells, osteoblasts, and osteoclasts, and for mast cells, dendritic cells, and Langerhans cells in other tissues. Some of these progenitor cells appear to be related to hematopoietic progenitor cells, while others do not.

Hematopoietic Microenvironment

Blood cell production occurs in bone marrow of adult animals because of the unique microenvironment present there. The hematopoietic microenvironment is a complex meshwork composed of various stromal cells, accessory cells, glycoprotein growth factors, and extracellular matrix components that profoundly affect stem cell and progenitor cell survival, proliferation, and differentiation. Stromal cells (endothelial cells, fibroblast-like reticular cells, and macrophages) and accessory cells (subsets of lymphocytes and natural killer cells) produce a variety of positive and negative growth factors. Stromal cells also produce components of the extracellular matrix.

The extracellular matrix (ECM) consists of broad categories of macromolecules: collagen, proteoglycans, and glycoproteins. In addition to providing structural support (collagen) the ECM is important in the binding of hematopoietic cells and soluble growth factors to stromal cells so that optimal proliferation and differentiation can occur. Adhesion molecules (primarily integrins) on progenitor cells bind to ECM glycoproteins such as hemonectin, fibronectin, thrombospondin, and vascular cell adhesion molecule-1. The spectrum of expression of adhesion molecules varies with the type and maturity of hematopoietic cells. Proteoglycans with their glycosaminoglycan moieties such as chondroitin sulfate and heparan sulfate bind growth factors and strengthen the bond between progenitor cells and stromal cells. Growth factors such as stem cell factor (c-*kit* ligand) may also be involved in the adhesion of hematopoietic cells by binding to both the extracellular matrix and to specific receptors on hematopoietic cells.

Hematopoietic Growth Factors

Proliferation of stem cells and progenitor cells cannot occur spontaneously, but requires the presence of specific hematopoietic growth factors (HGFs) that may be produced locally in the bone marrow or produced by peripheral tissues and transported to the marrow via the blood (humoral transport). Some HGFs have been called poietins (erythropoietin and thrombopoietin). Other growth factors have been classified as colony-stimulating factors (CSFs) based on *in vitro* culture studies. Finally, some have been described as interleukins (ILs). Hematopoietic cells coexpress receptors for more than one HGF on their surface, with the number of each receptor type present depending on the stage of the cell differentiation. Binding of an HGF to its receptor can stimulate proliferation and/or modulation of HGF receptors on the surface of the cell that is acted upon. Some HGFs have permissive hematopoietic effects by inhibiting apoptosis (programmed cell death). The binding of an HGF generally results in down-modulation of its own receptor and up-modulation (transactivation) of receptors for distal HGFs, which primarily act on more differentiated cell types.

HGFs vary in the type(s) of progenitor cells that they can stimulate to proliferate. Factors are often synergistic in their effects on hematopoietic cells. A factor may not directly stimulate the proliferation of a given cell type, but may potentiate its stimulation by inducing the expression of membrane receptors for a direct stimulating factor. Some glycoproteins such as IL-1 and tumor necrosis factor (TNF) can stimulate hematopoiesis indirectly by stimulating marrow stromal cells, endothelial cells, fibroblasts, and T-lymphocytes to produce HGFs. Different combinations of HGFs regulate the growth of different types of progenitor cells.

Early-acting HGFs are involved with triggering dormant (G_0) primitive progenitors to begin cycling. Stem cell factor (SCF) is important in combination with one or more other cytokines (*e.g.*, IL-6, IL-11, IL-12, G-CSF). Intermediate-acting HGFs have broad specificity. IL-3 (multi-CSF), granulocyte/macrophage-CSF (GM-CSF), and IL-4 support proliferation of pluripotent progenitor cells after they exit G_O. These factors also interact with late-acting factors to stimulate proliferation of a wide variety of committed progenitor cells. Late-acting HGFs have restricted specificity. Granulocyte-CSF (G-CSF), macrophage-CSF (M-CSF), erythropoietin, thrombopoietin, and IL-5 are more restrictive in their actions. They have their most potent effects on committed progenitor cells and later stages of development when cell lines can be recognized morphologically.

ERYTHROPOIESIS

Progenitor Cells and the Bone Marrow Microenvironment

Oligopotent progenitor cells (including CFU-GEMM cells) are stimulated to proliferate and differentiate into BFU-E by IL-3 and GM-CSF in the presence of erythropoietin (EPO). BFU-E proliferation and differentiation into CFU-E results from the presence of these same factors and may be further potentiated by additional growth factors. EPO is the primary growth factor involved in the proliferation and differentiation of CFU-E into rubriblasts, the first morphologically recognizable erythroid cells. CFU-E cells are more responsive to EPO than are BFU-E cells because CFU-E cells exhibit greater numbers of surface receptors for EPO.

Marrow macrophages appear to be an important component of the hematopoietic microenvironment involved with erythropoiesis. Both early and late stages of erythroid development occur with intimate membrane apposition to central macrophages in so-called erythroblastic islands. These central macrophages may regulate erythrocyte development by producing both positive factors such as burst-promoting activity and EPO and negative factors such as IL-1, TNF, and interferons. Macrophages may be important in the local or basal regulation of erythropoiesis, but humoral regulation is also important, with EPO production primarily occurring in the kidney and various inhibitory cytokines being produced at sites of inflammation throughout the body.

Nutrients Needed for Erythropoiesis

In addition to amino acids and essential fatty acids, several metals and vitamins are required for normal erythropoiesis. Iron is needed for the synthesis of heme, an essential component of hemoglobin and certain enzymes. Copper, in the form of ceruloplasmin, is important in the release of iron from tissue to plasma for transport to developing erythroid cells. Vitamin B_6 is needed as a cofactor in the first enzymatic step in heme synthesis.

Tetrahydrofolic acid, the active form of folic acid, is needed for the transfer of one carbon molecules in DNA and RNA synthesis. The physiologic mechanism of B_{12} involvement in erythrocyte production is not well understood, but it is interrelated with folate metabolism. Cobalt is essential for the synthesis of B_{12} by ruminants.

Maturation of Erythroid Cells

Rubriblasts are continuously generated from progenitor cells in the extra-vascular space of the bone marrow. The division of a rubriblast initiates a series of approximately four divisions over a period of 3 to 4 days to produce about 16 metarubricytes that are no longer capable of division (Fig. 2–2). These divisions are called maturational divisions because there is a progressive maturation of the nucleus and cytoplasm concomitant with the divisions.

Early precursors have intensely blue cytoplasm, when stained with Romanowsky-type blood stains, owing to the presence of many basophilic ribosomes and polyribosomes that are actively synthesizing globin chains and smaller amounts of other proteins. As these cells divide and mature, overall cell size decreases, nuclear chromatin condensation increases, cytoplasmic basophilia decreases, and hemoglobin progressively accumulates, imparting a red coloration to the cytoplasm (Color Plate 1). Cells with both red and blue coloration are described as having polychromatophilic cytoplasm. An immature erythrocyte, termed a reticulocyte, is formed following extrusion of the metarubricyte nucleus. Extruded nuclei are bound and phagocytosed by a novel receptor on the surface of bone marrow macrophages.

Early reticulocytes have polylobulated surfaces. Their cytoplasm contains ribosomes, polyribosomes, and mitochondria necessary for the completion of hemoglobin (Hb) synthesis. Reticulocytes derive their name from a net-

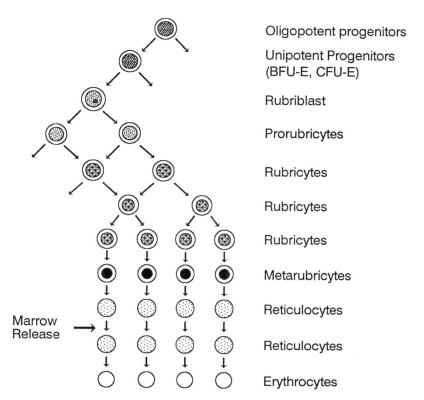

Oligopotent progenitors

Unipotent Progenitors (BFU-E, CFU-E)

Rubriblast

Prorubricytes

Rubricytes

Rubricytes

Rubricytes

Metarubricytes

Reticulocytes

Marrow Release

Reticulocytes

Erythrocytes

FIGURE 2–2. A diagram of erythropoiesis showing the release of reticulocytes into blood as it normally occurs in dogs.

work or reticulum that appears when stained with basic dyes such as new methylene blue and brilliant cresyl green. That network is not preexisting but is an artifact formed by the precipitation of ribosomal ribonucleic acids and proteins. As reticulocytes mature, the amount of ribosomal material decreases until only a few basophilic specks can be visualized with reticulocyte staining procedures. These mature reticulocytes have been referred to as punctate reticulocytes.

Reticulocyte maturation into mature erythrocytes is a gradual process that requires a variable number of days depending on the species involved. Consequently, the morphologic and physiologic properties of reticulocytes vary with the stage of maturation. The cell surface undergoes extensive remodeling with the selective loss of certain membrane protein and lipid components and ultimately the formulation of the biconcave shape of mature erythrocytes. Mitochondria and ribosomes are also lost by energy-dependent mechanisms.

Reticulocyte maturation begins in the bone marrow and is completed in the peripheral blood and spleen in dogs, cats, and pigs. As reticulocytes mature, they lose the surface receptors needed to adhere to fibronectin and thrombospondin components of the extracellular matrix, thereby facilitating their release from the bone marrow.

Reticulocytes become progressively more deformable as they mature, a characteristic that also facilitates their release from the marrow. To exit the extravascular space of the marrow, reticulocytes press against the abluminal surfaces of endothelial cells, which make up the sinus wall. Cytoplasm thins and small pores develop in endothelial cells which allow reticulocytes to be pushed through by a small pressure gradient across the sinus wall. Pores apparently close after cell passage.

Relatively immature aggregate-type reticulocytes are released from canine bone marrow; consequently, most of these cells appear polychromatophilic when viewed following routine blood film staining procedures. Reticulocytes are usually not released from feline bone marrow until they mature to punctate-type reticulocytes (Fig. 2–3); consequently, few or no aggregate re-

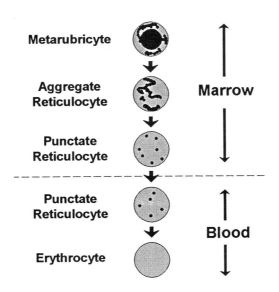

FIGURE 2–3. Drawing of cat erythroid cells (stained with the reticulocyte stain) demonstrating reticulocyte release into blood as it occurs in most normal cats.

ticulocytes (less than 0.4%), but up to 10% punctate reticulocytes, are found in blood from normal adult cats. The high percentage of punctate reticulocytes results from a long maturation time with delayed degradation of organelles. Reticulocytes are generally absent in peripheral blood of healthy adult cattle and goats, but a smaller number of punctate types (0.5%) may occur in adult sheep. Equine reticulocytes are absent from blood normally and are not released in response to anemia.

Control of Erythropoiesis

EPO production is stimulated by tissue hypoxia within the kidney (Fig. 2–4). The oxygen sensor has not been defined, but there is evidence that a heme protein may be involved. Tissue oxygen tension is determined by the oxygen consumption of the tissue and the oxygen-delivering capacity of the blood. Oxygen-delivering capacity depends on cardiovascular integrity, oxygen content in arterial blood, and Hb oxygen affinity. Low oxygen content in the blood can result from low partial pressure of oxygen (Po_2) in blood, as occurs with high altitudes or with congenital heart defects in which some of the blood flow bypasses the pulmonary circulation. Low oxygen content in blood can also occur with normal Po_2, as occurs with anemia and methemoglobinemia. An increased oxygen affinity of Hb within erythrocytes results in a decreased tendency to release oxygen to the tissues.

High titers of EPO may accelerate rubriblast entry into the first mitotic division, shortening the marrow transit time and resulting in the early release

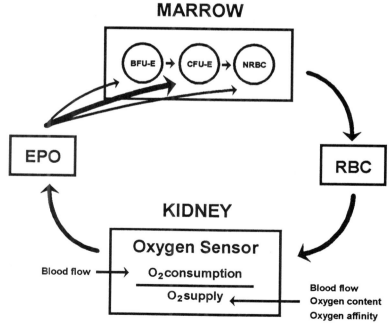

FIGURE 2–4. Central role of erythropoietin (EPO) in the control of erythropoiesis. BFU-E, burst-forming unit–erythroid; CFU-E, colony-forming unit–erythroid; NRBC, nucleated red blood cell.

of stress reticulocytes. Although EPO has been assumed to act as a mitogen because of its capacity to amplify erythrocyte production, other studies have suggested it acts primarily as a survival factor preventing apoptosis and permitting cells to proceed with programmed proliferation and maturation. In the presence of EPO, other hormones, including androgens, thyroid hormones, and growth hormone, can enhance the growth of erythroid precursor cells.

LEUKOPOIESIS

Neutrophil Production

Neutrophilic cells within the bone marrow can be included in two pools (Fig. 2–5). The proliferation and maturation pool (mitotic pool) includes myeloblasts, promyelocytes, and myelocytes. Approximately four or five divisions occur over several days. During this time primary azurophilic (reddish purple) cytoplasmic granules are produced in late myeloblasts or early promyelocytes and specific (secondary) granules are synthesized within myelocytes. Once nuclear indention and condensation become apparent, precursor cells are no longer capable of division. The maturation and storage pool (postmitotic pool) includes metamyelocytes, bands, and segmented neutrophils. Cells within this pool normally undergo maturation and storage for several more days prior to the migration of mature neutrophils through the vascular endothelium and into the circulation. The marrow transit time from mye-

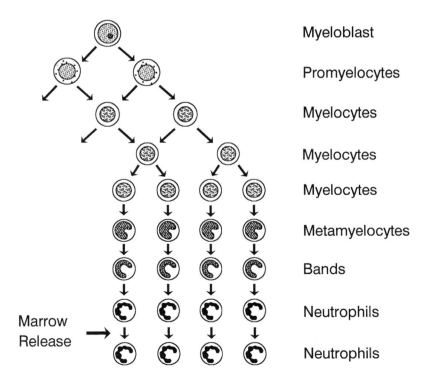

| | Myeloblast |
| Promyelocytes |
| Myelocytes |
| Myelocytes |
| Myelocytes |
| Metamyelocytes |
| Bands |
| Neutrophils |
| Neutrophils |

Marrow Release

FIGURE 2–5. A diagram of granulopoiesis.

loblast to release of mature neutrophils into blood varies by species, but is generally between 6 and 9 days. This time can be shortened considerably when inflammation is present.

The normal release of mature neutrophils from the marrow involves the maturational loss of receptors for extracellular matrix proteins such as hemonectin. The number of mature neutrophils stored in marrow is several times the number present in the circulation.

A variety of cytokines with overlapping specificities are important in neutrophil production. Oligopotent cells (e.g., CFU-GEMM) are stimulated to proliferate (and possibly differentiate) by IL-3. One progeny produced is a bipotential progenitor cell type (CFU-GM) that is the precursor of both neutrophils and monocytes (Fig. 2–1). CFU-GM cells are stimulated to proliferate and differentiate by GM-CSF. At low concentrations, GM-CSF stimulation favors the formation of mononuclear phagocytes and, at high concentrations, the formation of neutrophils. Unipotential CFU-G cells are stimulated to proliferate and differentiate into myeloblasts by G-CSF. This cytokine appears to play a role in the basal regulation of granulopoiesis, as well as function as a primary regulator of the neutrophil response to inflammatory stimuli. G-CSF increases the number of cell divisions and reduces the time for maturing neutrophil precursors to develop into terminally differentiated cells and be released into blood.

Activated helper T-lymphocytes produce various cytokines including IL-3 and GM-CSF. Mononuclear phagocytes, fibroblasts, and endothelial cells can produce GM-CSF and G-CSF when appropriately stimulated. Not only can mononuclear phagocytes synthesize HGFs when they contact bacterial products, but they can stimulate other cells to produce them. The monokines IL-1 and TNF stimulate the production of HGFs by other cell types (Fig. 2–6). These monokines are important in the inflammatory response to foreign organisms and neoplastic cells, but may not be involved in resting granulopoiesis.

Inhibition of neutrophil production is not well understood, but mature neutrophils within the marrow inhibit neutrophilic colony formation. The release of lactoferrin (an iron-chelating protein present in secondary granules of neutrophils) is one possible mediator, but results are controversial. When appropriately stimulated, neutrophils also secrete interferon-α which inhibits neutrophil production. Increased neutrophil numbers in blood are associated with increased clearance of circulating G-CSF following binding to surface receptors, thereby producing a negative feedback on granulopoiesis. Mature neutrophils also indirectly inhibit granulopoiesis by removal (phagocytosis) of invading microorganisms that would otherwise result in the production of HGFs by tissue cells.

Eosinophil and Basophil Production

Eosinophil production in marrow parallels that of neutrophils. The marrow transit time is 1 week or less, with a significant storage pool of mature eosinophils. As for neutrophils, growth factors such as IL-3 and GM-CSF are needed for proliferation of early progenitors. Activated T-lymphocytes produce IL-5, which promotes the terminal maturation of eosinophils.

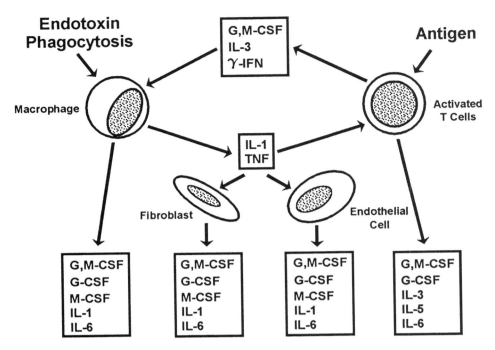

FIGURE 2–6. T-cell and macrophage activations produce cytokines that directly and/or indirectly stimulate hematopoiesis. CSF, colony-stimulation factor; IL, interleukin; γ-IFN, γ-interferon; TNF, tumor necrosis factor.

Basophils and eosinophils appear to share a common marrow progenitor cell that gives rise to precursors specific for each lineage. Eosinophil and basophil precursors become recognizable at the eosinophilic myelocyte stage when their characteristic secondary granules appear. SCF, IL-3, IL-4, IL-5, and probably other cytokines stimulate basophil production. It is unclear whether basophils and mast cells share a common progenitor cell. In contrast to basophils, which mature in the bone marrow, maturation of mast cell progenitors into mast cells occurs in the tissues. Some local proliferation of mast cells can occur in tissues if appropriately stimulated.

Monocyte Production

Monocytes are produced through the combined effects of IL-3, GM-CSF, and M-CSF on proliferation and differentiation of bone marrow precursors. M-CSF acts on later progenitor cells than the other two CSFs and induces predominantly macrophage cultures *in vitro*. Less time is required to produce monocytes than granulocytes and there is little marrow reserve of monocytes. Monocytes are not end-stage (finished) cells, but enter the tissues to become macrophages.

Lymphocyte and Natural Killer Cell Production

The totipotent hematopoietic stem cell of the bone marrow gives rise to a pluripotent lymphoid stem cell (Fig. 2–1) in addition to the myeloid stem cell.

The lymphoid stem cell gives rise to B-cell progenitor and T/NK progenitor cells, and the T/NK progenitor gives rise to T-cell progenitor and natural killer (NK) progenitor cells. The development of B-cell and T-cell progenitors in bone marrow is antigen-independent. B-cell progenitors produce B-cells in the marrow in most mammals, in ileocecal Peyer's patches in ruminants, and the bursa of Fabricius in birds. As with other blood cells, the microenvironment of the marrow and lymphoid organs is important for lymphopoiesis. The production of antigen-sensitive, surface-immunoglobulin-positive B-cells is marked by successive rearrangements of the immunoglobulin gene loci and selective expression of surface proteins. Although a number of cytokines including SCF are involved in B-cell production in marrow, IL-7 appears to be an especially important positive growth factor. B-cells migrate to the cortex in lymph nodes and within follicles in jejunal Peyer's patches and spleen in mammals.

T-cell progenitors leave the marrow and migrate to the thymus. Homing of these cells to the thymus depends on their interaction with various adhesion molecules on thymic endothelial cells and the production of specific chemotactic factors by thymic stromal cells. T-cell progenitors develop into T-cells under the influence of the thymic microenvironment and growth factors (including SCF and IL-7) produced in the thymus. After maturation in the thymus, T-cells accumulate within paracortical areas of lymph nodes, periarteriolar lymphoid sheaths of the spleen, and the interfollicular areas of jejunal Peyer's patches in mammals.

NK cells are primarily produced and undergo maturation in the bone marrow, but NK progenitor cells are also present in the thymus. Growth factors controlling their production have not been well characterized, but SCF, IL-7, and IL-2 can stimulate NK cell development from progenitor cells *in vitro*. NK cells are located primarily in blood and the spleen, with low numbers in lymph nodes in normal mammals. The mucosal lymphocytes (interepithelial lymphocytes of the small intestine) may represent a subset of NK cells.

THROMBOPOIESIS

Blood platelets in mammals are produced from multinucleated giant cells in bone marrow called megakaryocytes. The earliest definable progenitor cell committed to form megakaryocytes is termed BFU-megakaryocyte (BFU-Mega). When appropriately stimulated, this progenitor cell divides and differentiates into CFU-Mega progenitor cells, which divide and differentiate into megakaryoblasts (Fig. 2–7). Mitosis stops at this stage and endomitosis (nuclear reduplication without cell division) begins. Usually three to five reduplications occur resulting in 8 to 32 sets of chromosomes in mature megakaryocytes. Individual nuclei can be observed following the first two reduplications (promegakaryocytes), but a large polylobulated nucleus is seen when mature megakaryocytes are formed. The cytoplasm in promegakaryocytes is intensely basophilic. There is a progressive decrease in basophilia and increase in granularity as megakaryocytes mature. Cell volume increases with each reduplication; consequently, megakaryocytes are much larger than all other marrow cells except osteoclasts. In contrast to mature megakaryocytes, osteoclasts have discrete multiple nuclei.

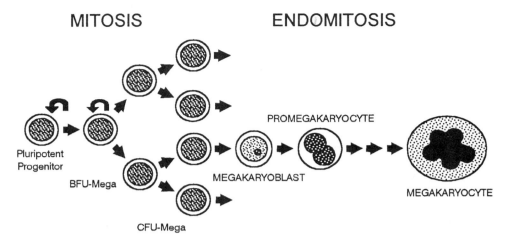

FIGURE 2–7. Stages of megakaryocyte development. BFU-Mega, burst-forming unit–megakaryocyte; CFU-Mega, colony-forming unit–megakaryocyte.

Megakaryocytes either lie just outside a vascular sinus or compose part of the wall of a sinus. Cylinders of cytoplasm from megakaryocytes form and extend into sinuses (Fig. 2–8). These beaded-appearing proplatelets eventually fragment into individual platelets within the sinuses and general circulation. It is estimated that 1000 to 5000 platelets are produced from each megakaryocyte, depending on megakaryocyte size. Megakaryocytes are not present in nonmammalian species. Like erythrocytes and leukocytes, nucleated thrombocytes are produced by mitosis of precursor cells.

A number of cytokines can stimulate or enhance the proliferation and expansion of megakaryocyte progenitor cells. Factors that may be involved include IL-3, GM-CSF, IL-6, and IL-11. Thrombopoietin (TPO), c-Mpl ligand, increases platelet production by stimulating megakaryocyte differentiation from marrow progenitor cells and by stimulating increased endomitosis, resulting in increased ploidy and megakaryocyte size. TPO may also transiently enhance the aggregatory response of platelets to agonists. The mechanisms involved in the regulation of blood TPO levels remain to be defined. It is suggested that the c-Mpl receptor on blood platelets may provide a negative feedback on platelet production by binding circulating TPO, thus preventing its action on bone marrow progenitor cells and megakaryocytes.

BONE MARROW BIOPSY AND EVALUATION

Reasons for Bone Marrow Examination

Bone marrow evaluation is indicated when peripheral blood abnormalities are detected. The most common indications are persistent neutropenia, unexplained thrombocytopenia, poorly regenerative anemia, or a combination thereof. Examples of proliferative abnormalities where bone marrow examination may be indicated include persistent thrombocytosis or leukocytosis, abnormal blood cell morphology, or the unexplained presence of

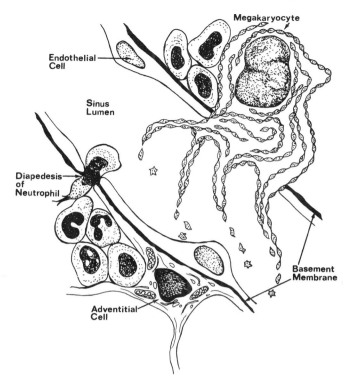

FIGURE 2-8. Extension of proplatelets into the sinus lumen and the subsequent formation of individual platelets.

immature cells in blood (*e.g.*, nucleated erythroid cells in the absence of polychromasia or a neutrophilic left shift in the absence of inflammation).

Bone marrow is sometimes examined to stage a neoplastic condition (lymphomas and mast cell tumors); estimate the adequacy of body iron stores; evaluate lytic bone lesions; and search for occult disease in animals with fever of unknown origin, unexplained weight loss, and unexplained malaise. Bone marrow examination can also be useful in determining the cause of a hyperproteinemia when it occurs secondarily to multiple myeloma, lymphoma, leishmaniasis, and systemic fungal diseases. It may also reveal the cause of a hypercalcemia when associated with lymphoid neoplasms, multiple myeloma, or metastatic neoplasms to bone.

Bone marrow aspirate biopsies are done more frequently than core biopsies in veterinary medicine. Aspirate biopsies are easier, faster, and less expensive to perform than are core biopsies. Bone marrow core biopsies require special needles that cut a solid core of material that is then placed in fixative, decalcified, embedded, sectioned, stained, and examined microscopically by a pathologist. Core biopsy sections provide a more accurate way of evaluating marrow cellularity and examining for metastatic neoplasia than do aspirate smears, but cell morphology is more difficult to assess. This section will address the collection, preparation, and evaluation of aspirate smears only.

Bone Marrow Aspirate Technique

There are few contraindications for a bone marrow aspiration biopsy. Restraint, sedation, and anesthesia (when used) generally provide more risks to the patient than the biopsy procedure itself. Postbiopsy hemorrhage is a potential complication in patients with hemostatic diatheses, but it rarely occurs. Hemorrhage may occur after the biopsy of animals with monoclonal hyperglobulinemias, but it is easily controlled by placing a suture in the skin incision and applying pressure over the biopsy site. Postbiopsy infection is also a potential but highly unlikely complication if proper techniques are used.

The usefulness of bone marrow aspirate cytology as a diagnostic aid depends on the proper collection of the bone marrow sample and preparation of high-quality marrow smears. In most cases only local anesthesia is needed for needle biopsies. Tranquilization is sometimes used in patients that resist positioning by manual restraint. Biopsy sites are prepared by clipping the hair and scrubbing the skin with antiseptic soap preparations. A local anesthetic is injected under the skin and down to the periosteum overlying the site to be biopsied, and a small skin incision is made with a scalpel blade to facilitate passing the needle through the skin. Sterile needles and gloves are always used. If general anesthesia is required for other procedures, bone marrow aspiration may be scheduled at the same time to minimize the stress on the animal.

The biopsy needle used to aspirate marrow must have a removable stylet that remains in place until the marrow cavity is entered to prevent obstruction of the needle lumen with cortical bone. A 16- or 18-gauge Rosenthal needle that is between 1 and 1.5 inches long is satisfactory. The wing of the ilium is often used as a site to biopsy marrow in dogs and large cats, unless specific lesions are to be biopsied based on radiographic findings (Fig. 2–9). For small cats and toy breeds of dogs, where the ilium is especially thin, one may aspirate from the head of the proximal femur by way of the trochanteric fossa. Aspiration of marrow from the anterior side of the proximal end of the humerus is another popular site, especially in obese patients. In horses

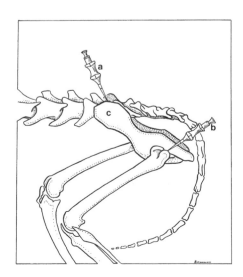

FIGURE 2–9. Bone marrow biopsy sites include (a) positioning the needle in the widened dorsal aspects of the iliac crest; (b) positioning the needle in the trochanteric fossa of the proximal femur; or (c) positioning the needle in the central depression in the wing of the ileum. (From Harvey JW: Canine bone marrow: Normal hematopoiesis, biopsy techniques, and cell identification and evaluation. Comp Contin Educ Pract Vet 1984;6:909, with permission.)

and large dogs, the third, fourth, or fifth sternebra can be biopsied. Sternebra biopsies have the risk of inadvertent penetration of the thorax and damage to structures in the thoracic cavity. A short biopsy needle (preferably with an adjustable guard) should be used, and care should be taken to remain in the center of these bones to minimize the risk of pneumothorax, uncontrolled hemorrhage, or cardiac laceration.

To enter the marrow space, moderate pressure is applied to the needle (with the stylet locked in place) as the needle is rotated in an alternating clockwise-counterclockwise motion. Once the needle is firmly embedded into the bone, it is usually within the marrow cavity. The stylet is then removed and a 10-mL or 20-mL syringe is attached to the needle. Vigorous negative pressure should be applied by rapidly pulling the plunger back as far as possible. As soon as a few drops of blood appear in the syringe, the negative pressure is released and the complete assembly is rapidly removed for smear preparation. If marrow does not appear in the syringe, the stylet is replaced and the needle is repositioned for another aspiration attempt.

It is important for accurate bone marrow evaluation that smears contain marrow particles (stroma and associated cells). Marrow particles appear as small white grains. One useful method to assist in the separation of particles from contaminating blood involves the forcible expulsion of several drops of the marrow aspirate onto one end of a glass slide that is then held vertically (Fig. 2–10). Particles tend to stick to the slide while blood runs off. A second glass slide is placed across the area of particle adherence perpendicular to the first slide and, after marrow spreads between the slides, they are pulled apart in the horizontal plane. Resultant smears are rapidly air dried. Since marrow clots rapidly, one may collect marrow into a syringe that contains several drops of 4% ethylenediaminetetraacetic acid (EDTA) as an anticoagulant. Marrow is mixed with the anticoagulant and expelled into a weighing dish or Petri dish. Particles are then collected by capillary tube or pipette, and squash preparations are made.

Smears are stained with a Romanowsky-type blood stain such as Wright, Giemsa, or a combination thereof. Satisfactory results can usually be obtained with the Diff-Quik stain, a rapid modified Wright stain. If adequate smears are available, one smear should be stained using the Prussian blue

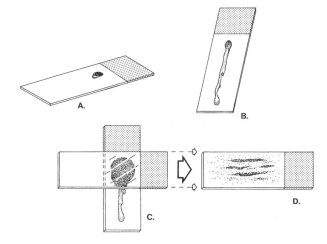

FIGURE 2–10. Preparation of a bone marrow smear involves (*A*) expelling several drops of bone marrow aspirate material onto the end of a glass slide. *B*, Contaminating blood drains down the slide as it is held vertically. *C*, Adherent marrow particles are squashed between a perpendicularly placed slide, and (*D*) the slides are pulled apart in a horizontal plane in the direction of the arrows. (From Harvey JW: Canine bone marrow: Normal hematopoiesis, biopsy techniques, and cell identification and evaluation. Comp Contin Educ Pract Vet 1984;6:909, with permission.)

procedure for iron. Additional special stains may be needed to help differentiate the type of leukemia when present.

Bone Marrow Aspirate Cytology

Bone marrow should be examined and findings recorded in a systematic manner. Smears should be scanned with lower-power objectives to gain an appreciation of overall cellularity and determine the adequacy of megakaryocyte numbers. Normal marrow appears heterogenous. As a general rule, erythroid precursors are smaller, have more nearly spherical nuclei with more condensed nuclear chromatin, and have darker cytoplasm than do granulocyte precursors at similar maturation stages (Color Plate 1). Rubriblasts have deeper basophilic cytoplasm than do myeloblasts, promyelocytes, or myelocytes. Consequently, smaller and darker cells, observed by scanning marrow smears at low power, are usually erythroid precursors (unless lymphocytes are increased in numbers) and the larger, paler cells are usually granulocyte precursors.

Complete differential cell counts are not usually done on marrow smears, but rather a number of judgments are made and recorded as presented below.

1.   The cellularity of the marrow is estimated by examining the proportion of cells *versus* fat present in particles. Marrow particles appear as bluestaining areas when viewed grossly. When examined microscopically, they contain vessels, reticular cells, macrophages, plasma cells, and blood cell precursors (Fig. 2–11). Most particles in normal animals are composed of

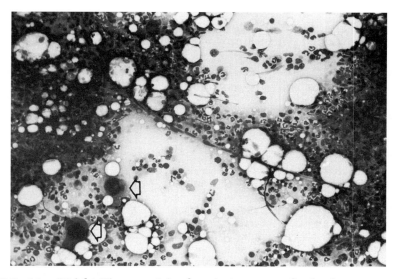

FIGURE 2–11.   Wright-Giemsa–stained aspirate smear of a dog bone marrow particle with a centrally located capillary. Two megakaryocytes are present (*arrows*). Large vacuoles represent adipocytes from which lipid was removed during fixation. (From Harvey JW: Canine bone marrow: Normal hematopoiesis, biopsy techniques, and cell identification and evaluation. Comp Contin Educ Pract Vet 1984;6:909, with permission.)

one third to two thirds cells. If few or no particles are present on smears, it is not possible to accurately estimate marrow cellularity.

2. The frequency and morphology of megakaryocytes should be evaluated. Most large particles should have associated megakaryocytes, and normally a majority of megakaryocytes are of the granular, mature type. Abnormal megakaryocyte morphology (*e.g.*, dwarf megakaryocytes) should be noted when present.

3. The distribution of granulocytic cells should be evaluated to determine whether the series is complete (*i.e.*, a normal number of mature granulocytes are present) and orderly. If there are increased proportions of cells in the proliferating pool (myeloblasts, progranulocytes, or myelocytes) compared to the later stages of development, this finding should be noted. Morphologic abnormalities, such as vacuolated cytoplasm, or increased representation of eosinophilic or basophilic series should be noted when present.

4. The maturation and morphology of the erythroid series should be evaluated to determine if it is complete (frequent polychromatophilic erythrocytes should be present) and orderly. Possible abnormal morphologic findings that should be noted include megaloblastic cells, frequent binucleate cells, and pleomorphic nuclei.

5. A myeloid to erythroid (M:E) ratio is calculated by examining 500 cells and determining the ratio of granulocytic cells (including mature granulocytes) to nucleated erythroid cells. The M:E ratio is generally between 0.75 and 2.5 in normal dogs, between 1 and 3 in normal cats, and between 0.5 and 1.5 in normal horses. One needs to have a knowledge of the overall marrow cellularity, as well as the complete blood count (CBC), to interpret the M:E ratio. Examples of dog bone marrow aspirate smears with high (Fig. 2–12) and low (Fig. 2–13) M:E ratios are shown.

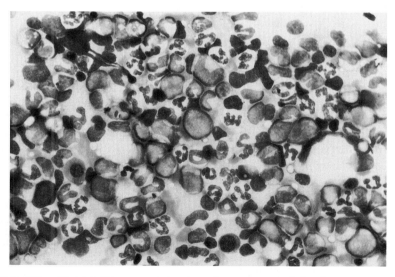

FIGURE 2–12. Wright-Giemsa–stained aspirate smear of dog bone marrow with a high myeloid to erythroid ratio. CBC results are needed to determine whether granulocytic hyperplasia or erythroid hypoplasia is present. (From Harvey JW: Canine bone marrow: Normal hematopoiesis, biopsy techniques, and cell identification and evaluation. Comp Contin Educ Pract Vet 1984;6:909, with permission.)

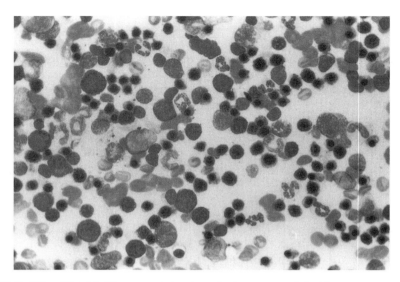

FIGURE 2–13. Wright-Giemsa–stained aspirate smear of dog bone marrow with a low myeloid to erythroid ratio. CBC results are needed to determine whether erythroid hyperplasia or granulocytic hypoplasia is present. (From Harvey JW: Canine bone marrow: Normal hematopoiesis, biopsy techniques, and cell identification and evaluation. Comp Contin Educ Pract Vet 1984;6:909, with permission.)

6. Specific comments should be made about lymphocytes, plasma cells, osteoblasts, and osteoclasts when they appear in increased numbers and/or exhibit abnormal morphology. Normal marrow may contain up to 15% small lymphocytes and 2% plasma cells. Ferrets may have considerably higher numbers of marrow lymphocytes than other species. Monocytes, macrophages, and mitotic cells normally do not exceed 1 to 2% of total nucleated cells present. Osteoclasts and osteoblasts are rarely seen except in young, growing animals. Any abnormal cells such as mast cells, neoplastic cells, or macrophages containing phagocytized cells or infective agents should be described.

7. The amount of stainable iron present is routinely evaluated using the Prussian blue reaction. Stainable iron is easily found in normal marrow aspirates from most domestic mammals, so long as particles are present. It is decreased or absent in iron-deficient animals and increased in association with hemolytic anemias and the anemia of chronic disease. Bone marrow iron increases in horses with age; consequently, normal old horses can have marked amounts of stainable iron present in the marrow. Normal cat bone marrow does not exhibit stainable iron, so its absence cannot be used to confirm a diagnosis of iron deficiency.

8. Because reticulocytes are rarely released into blood in response to anemia in horses, reticulocyte counts can be done in bone marrow aspirates from horses to assist in the differential diagnosis of anemia. Greater than 5% reticulocytes suggests a regenerative response to anemia.

9. The final step in evaluating a bone marrow aspirate is to provide an interpretation of the cytologic findings in light of the history, clinical findings, CBC, and results from other diagnostic tests and procedures. For example, a high M:E ratio could indicate the presence of either increased granulocytic cells or decreased erythroid cells. Examination of CBC results from blood

collected at the same time usually allows the correct interpretation to be made.

References

Andreasen CB, Gerros TC, Lassen ED: Evaluation of bone marrow cytology and stainable iron content in healthy adult llamas. Vet Clin Pathol 1994;23:38.

Babior BM, Golde DW: Production, distribution, and fate of neutrophils. In Beutler E, Lichtman MA, Coller BS, Kipps TJ (eds): Williams Hematology, 5th ed. New York, McGraw-Hill, 1995, p 773.

Ball TC, Hirayama F, Ogawa M: Lymphohematopoietic progenitors of normal mice. Blood 1995;85:3086.

Burstein SA, Breton-Gorius J: Megakaryopoiesis and platelet formation. In Beutler E, Lichtman MA, Coller BS, Kipps TJ (eds): Williams Hematology, 5th ed. New York, McGraw-Hill, 1995, p 1149.

Campbell AD: The role of hemonectin in the cell adhesion mechanisms of bone marrow. Hematol Pathol 1992;6:51.

Debili N, Wendling F, Katz A, et al: The Mpl-ligand or thrombopoietin or megakaryocyte growth and differentiative factor has both direct proliferative and differentiative activities on human megakaryocyte progenitors. Blood 1995;86:2516.

Dunn JS, Dunn JK, Dobson JM: Canine lymphoid leukaemia and lymphoma with bone marrow involvement: A review of 24 cases. J Small Anim Pract 1993;34:72.

Ellis MH, Avraham H, Groopman JE: The regulation of megakaryocytopoiesis. Blood Rev 1995;9:1.

Erslev AJ, Beutler E: Production and destruction of erythrocytes. In Beutler E, Lichtman MA, Coller BS, Kipps TJ (eds): Williams Hematology, 5th ed. New York, McGraw-Hill, 1995, p 425.

Födinger M, Fritsch G, Winkler K, et al: Origin of human mast cells: Development from transplanted hematopoietic stem cells after allogeneic bone marrow transplantation. Blood 1994;84:2954.

Galli SJ, Dvorak AM: Production, biochemistry, and function of basophils and mast cells. In Beutler E, Lichtman MA, Coller BS, Kipps TJ (eds): Williams Hematology, 5th ed. New York, McGraw-Hill, 1995, p 805.

Gordon MY: Physiology and function of the haemopoietic microenvironment. Br J Haematol 1994;86:241.

Hamood M, Corazza F, Bujan-Boza W, et al: Natural killer (NK) cells inhibit human umbilical cord blood erythropoiesis. Exp Hematol 1995;23:1187.

Harvey JW: Canine bone marrow: Normal hematopoiesis, biopsy techniques, and cell identification and evaluation. Comp Contin Educ Pract Vet 1984;6:909.

Huss R, Hong D-S, Beckham C, et al: Ultrastructural localization of stem cell factor in canine marrow-derived stromal cells. Exp Hematol 1995;23:33.

Hyun BH, Stevenson AJ, Hanau CA: Fundamentals of bone marrow examination. Hematol Oncol Clin North Am 1994;8:651.

Jain NC: Essentials of Veterinary Hematology. Philadelphia, Lea & Febiger, 1993.

Kinashi T, Springer TA: Adhesion molecules in hematopoietic cells. Blood Cells 1994;20:25.

Lebien TW: Lymphocyte otogeny and homing receptors. In Beutler E, Lichtman MA, Coller BS, Kipps TJ (eds): Williams Hematology, 5th ed. New York, McGraw-Hill, 1995, p 921.

Long MW: Blood cell cytoadhesion molecules. Exp Hematol 1992;20:288.

Metcalf D: Hematopoietic regulators: Redundancy or subtlety. Blood 1993;82:3515.

Nagahisa H, Nagata Y, Ohnuki T, et al: Bone marrow stromal cells produce thrombopoietin and stimulate megakaryocyte growth and maturation but suppress proplatelet formation. Blood 1996;87:1309.

Pantel K, Nakeff A: The role of lymphoid cells in hematopoietic regulation. Exp Hematol 1993;21:738.

Porter DL, Goldberg MA: Regulation of erythropoietin production. Exp Hematol 1993;21:399.

Quesenberry PJ: Hemopoietic stem cells, progenitor cells, and cytokines. In Beutler E, Lichtman MA, Coller BS, Kipps TJ (eds): Williams Hematology, 5th ed. New York, McGraw-Hill, 1995, p 211.

Qui LB, Dickson H, Hajibagheri N, et al: Extruded erythroblast nuclei are bound and phagocytosed by a novel macrophage receptor. Blood 1995;85:1630.

Rennick D, Hunte B, Holland G, et al: Cofactors are essential for stem cell factor-dependent growth and maturation of mast cell progenitors: Comparative effects of interleukin-3 (IL-3), IL-4, IL-10, and fibroblasts. Blood 1995;85:57.

Russell KE, Sellon DC, Grindem CB: Bone marrow in horses: Indications, sample handling, and complications. Comp Contin Educ Pract Vet 1994;16:1359.

Shull RM, Suggs SV, Langley KE, et al: Canine stem cell factor (c-*kit* ligand) supports the survival of hematopoietic progenitors in long-term canine marrow culture. Exp Hematol 1992;20:1118.

Spits H, Lanier LL, Phillips JH: Development of human T and natural killer cells. Blood 1995;85:2654.

Testa U, Pelosi E, Gabbianelli M, et al: Cascade transactivation of growth factor receptors in early human hematopoiesis. Blood 1993;81:1442.

Waller EK, Olweus J, Lund-Johansen F, et al: The "common stem cell" hypothesis reevaluated: Human fetal bone marrow contains separate populations of hematopoietic and stromal progenitors. Blood 1995;85:2422.

Wardlaw AJ, Kay AB: Eosinophils: Production, biochemistry and function. In Beutler E, Lichtman MA, Coller BS, Kipps TJ (eds): Williams Hematology, 5th ed. New York, McGraw-Hill, 1995, p 798.

Yoder MC, Williams DA: Matrix molecule interactions with hematopoietic stem cells. Exp Hematol 1995;23:961.

3

Evaluation of Erythrocytic Disorders

NORMAL ERYTHROCYTES

Total Blood Volume and Erythrocyte Volumes

In relation to body weight, total blood volume accounts for about 10 to 11% in hot-blooded horses; 8 to 9% in dogs; 6 to 7% in cats, ruminants, laboratory rodents, and cold-blooded (draft) horses; and 5 to 6% in pigs. The total blood volume of young growing animals often exceeds 10% of body weight. The total volume of erythrocytes present depends on the total blood volume and the fraction of blood volume that is occupied by erythrocytes or red blood cells (RBCs).

Erythrocyte Morphology

RBCs from most mammals are anucleated biconcave discs called discocytes. The biconcave shape results in the central pallor of RBCs observed in stained blood films. Of common domestic animals, biconcavity and central pallor are most pronounced in dogs. RBCs from animals in the Camellidae family (camels, llamas, vicunas, alpacas) are anucleated, thin, elliptical cells termed elliptocytes (ovalocytes). They are not biconcave. RBCs from birds, reptiles, and amphibians are also elliptical in shape. They are larger than mammalian RBCs and contain nuclei.

Erythrocyte Functions

Mammalian RBCs are anucleated cells that normally circulate for several months in blood despite limited synthetic capacities and repeated exposures to mechanical and metabolic insults. RBCs have three functions: transport of O_2 to tissue, transport of CO_2 to the lungs, and buffering of hydrogen ions. In nonanemic animals, the presence of hemoglobin (Hb) within RBCs increases the oxygen-carrying capacity of blood more than 50 times that of plasma without RBCs. The oxygen content of blood depends on the blood

Hb content, the partial pressure of oxygen (Po_2) in blood, and the affinity of Hb for oxygen.

Each Hb tetramer is capable of binding four molecules of oxygen when fully oxygenated. The initial binding of a molecule of O_2 to a monomer of tetrameric, deoxygenated Hb facilitates further binding of O_2 to the Hb molecule. The changing oxygen affinity of Hb with oxygenation results in a sigmoid oxygen dissociation curve (Fig. 3–1) when the percent saturation of Hb with oxygen is plotted against the Po_2. The steepness of the middle portion of the curve is of great physiologic significance, since it covers the range of oxygen tensions present in tissues. Consequently, a relatively small decrease in oxygen tension results in substantial oxygen release from Hb. The overall affinity of Hb for oxygen is decreased by increasing H^+, CO_2, temperature, and, in most mammals, 2,3-diphosphoglycerate (2,3-DPG). There is a direct correlation between body weight and oxygen affinity of Hb in whole blood (lower body weight, lower oxygen affinity) when various species of mammals are compared.

The O_2 affinity of fetal blood (except in the cat) is greater than that of maternal blood. Differences in fetal *versus* maternal oxygen affinity may potentiate oxygen transport from the mother to the fetus. However, the fetus is subjected to low arterial oxygen tensions and the increased oxygen affinity of fetal blood is likely needed to more fully saturate Hb with oxygen.

The ability of carrying CO_2 dissolved in plasma is small, but the carbonic anhydrase reaction in RBCs increases the carbon dioxide–carrying capacity of blood 17-fold by rapidly converting CO_2 to H_2CO_3. This carbonic acid formed spontaneously ionizes to H^+ and HCO_3^-. The HCO_3^- diffuses out of

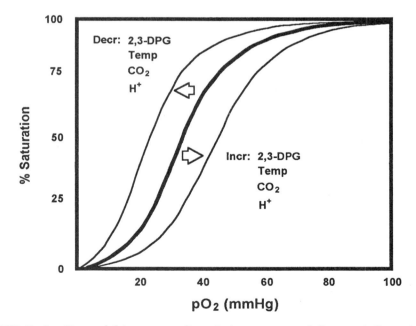

FIGURE 3–1. Hemoglobin-oxygen dissociation curve and factors influencing the position of the curve. (From Harvey JW: The erythrocyte: Physiology, metabolism and biochemical disorders. In Kaneko JJ, Bruss ML, Harvey JW [eds]: Clinical Biochemistry of Domestic Animals, 5th ed. San Diego, CA, Academic Press, 1997 [in press], with permission.)

the cell down a concentration gradient and Cl^- moves in (chloride shift) to maintain electrical neutrality. These processes are reversed at the lungs. Some CO_2 is also transported bound to Hb as carbamino groups. Deoxyhemoglobin binds about twice the CO_2 that oxyhemoglobin does.

Hb is the major protein buffer in blood. Deoxyhemoglobin is a weaker acid than oxyhemoglobin. Consequently, when oxyhemoglobin releases its O_2 in the tissues the formation of deoxyhemoglobin results in increased binding of H^+. Hb buffers the effects of carbonic acid and allows for the isohydric transport of CO_2. Hb also buffers organic acids produced during metabolism.

Erythrocyte Biochemistry

The RBC membrane contains a phospholipid bilayer with molecules of unesterified cholesterol intercalated between fatty acid chains. Phospholipids can move in various ways and contribute to membrane fluidity. Glycolipids are located on the outer layer of the membrane, with carbohydrate groups extending outward. Some blood group antigens are glycolipids, with the specificity residing in the carbohydrate moieties. (See Chapter 6 for discussion of clinically significant blood groups.)

Membrane proteins consist of integral membrane proteins that penetrate the lipid portion, often spanning the bilayer, and skeletal proteins that form or attach to the internal surface of the lipid bilayer. Glycoproteins associated with the membrane are integral membrane proteins with the carbohydrate residues extending from the outside surface of the cell membrane. They carry RBC antigens and function as receptors or transport proteins (e.g., band 3 is an anion transporter). The membrane skeleton is composed of various proteins located in a lattice-like arrangement on the inner surface of the RBC membrane. This meshwork is attached to the membrane by binding to transmembrane proteins. The membrane skeleton is a major determining factor of membrane shape, deformability, and durability. It is in a condensed configuration in intact cells and can be stretched considerably without rupturing.

RBCs lack nuclei in mammals. Therefore, they cannot synthesize DNA or RNA. They also lack ribosomes, mitochondria, and endoplasmic reticulum and, consequently, have no Krebs cycle or electron transport system and are unable to synthesize proteins or lipids (de novo). Mature RBCs depend on anaerobic glycolysis for energy (Fig. 3–2). ATP is needed for maintenance of RBC ionic composition, for maintenance of RBC shape and deformability, and for limited synthetic activities such as glutathione synthesis. RBC 2,3-DPG is produced from a side pathway of the Embden-Meyerhof pathway. No net ATP is generated when molecules traverse this pathway. 2,3-DPG is the most abundant organic phosphate in RBCs of most species, but is low in RBCs of cats and mature ruminants.

NADPH generated in the pentose phosphate pathway (PPP) provides electrons for protection against oxidants. Oxidative reactions can damage Hb, enzymes (SH groups especially), and membrane lipids. Methemoglobin forms when Hb iron is oxidized from the $+2$ to the $+3$ state. Heinz bodies are inclusions that form within RBCs following the oxidative denaturation of the globin portion of Hb. Membrane damage can result in intravascular hemolysis or erythrophagocytosis and shortened RBC life spans.

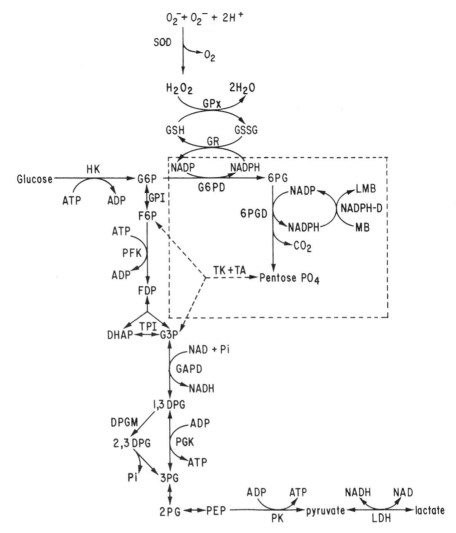

FIGURE 3–2. Metabolic pathways of the mature RBC. HK, hexokinase; GPI, glucose phosphate isomerase; PFK, phosphofructokinase; TPI, triosephosphate isomerase; GAPD, glyceraldehyde-3-phosphate dehydrogenase; PGK, phosphoglycerate kinase: MPGM, monophosphoglycerate mutase; DPGM, diphosphoglycerate mutase; PK, pyruvate kinase; G6PD, glucose-6-phosphate dehydrogenase; 6PGD, 6-phosphogluconate dehydrogenase; LDH, lactate dehydrogenase; GR, glutathione reductase; GPx, glutathione peroxidase; TK, transketolase; TA, transaldolase; GSSG, oxidized glutathione; G6P, glucose 6-phosphate; F6P, fructose 6-phosphate; FDP, fructose 1,6-diphosphate; DHAP, dihydroxyacetone phosphate; GAP, glyceraldehyde 3-phosphate; 1,3DPG, 1,3-diphosphoglycerate; 2,3DPG, 2,3-diphosphoglycerate; 3PG, 3-phosphoglycerate; 2PG, 2-phosphoglycerate; PEP, phosphoenolpyruvate; ADP, adenosine diphosphate; ATP, adenosine triphosphate; NAD, nicotinamide adenine dinucleotide; NADH, reduced nicotinamide adenine dinucleotide; NADP, nicotinamide adenine dinucleotide phosphate; NADPH, reduced nicotinamide adenine dinucleotide phosphate; GSH, reduced glutathione; P_i, inorganic phosphate; SOD, superoxide dismutase. (From Harvey JW: The erythrocyte: Physiology, metabolism and biochemical disorders. In Kaneko JJ, Bruss ML, Harvey JW [eds]: Clinical Biochemistry of Domestic Animals, 5th ed. San Diego, CA, Academic Press, 1997 [in press], with permission.)

Reduced glutathione (GSH) is a tripeptide containing one SH group. It is the substrate for the glutathione peroxidase reaction, providing electrons for the reduction of hydrogen peroxide. Glutathione peroxidase contains selenium, accounting for selenium's antioxidant properties. GSH can also react directly with various free radicals. Oxidized glutathione can be reduced back to GSH molecules by the glutathione reductase enzyme using NADPH as the source of electrons (Fig. 3–2). Catalase is an enzyme that can catalyze the conversion of hydrogen peroxide to water and oxygen without using energy. Vitamin E is lipid soluble and acts as a free radical scavenger in the membrane.

About 3% of Hb is oxidized to methemoglobin each day. Methemoglobin is unable to bind oxygen. To prevent hypoxia that would result from the accumulation of high levels of methemoglobin, it is reduced back to functional Hb in a reaction that requires NADH and the methemoglobin reductase (cytochrome-b_5 reductase) enzyme.

Iron Metabolism

More iron is needed for RBC production than for all other cells in the body combined. Developing erythroid cells generally extract 70 to 95% of the iron circulating in plasma, and 55 to 65% of the iron in the body occurs in Hb within erythroid cells (3.4 mg iron per gram of hemoglobin).

Inorganic iron is solubilized from food by hydrochloric acid (HCl) in the stomach. Acidified iron binds with mucin in the stomach, which keeps it soluble and available for absorption in the more alkaline environment of the small intestine. Mechanisms of absorption by epithelial cells of the intestine remain to be fully elucidated. Recent studies suggest that integrin molecules on the surface of the mucosal epithelial cells bind iron and facilitate its transfer through the cell membrane for binding to mobilferrin, a shuttle protein within mucosal cells. Iron can be absorbed as heme by a different mechanism. The mechanism of iron transfer from the mucosal cell to transferrin in plasma is unknown.

Iron absorption depends upon age, iron status, and health of the animal, as well as the amount and chemical form of iron ingested. Ferric (Fe^{+3}) iron is less well absorbed than ferrous (Fe^{+2}) iron. It appears that ferric iron is reduced to ferrous iron for transport into the mucosal cell. Excess iron taken up by the mucosal cell stimulates apoferritin synthesis. Following oxidation, ferric iron binds with apoferritin to form ferritin. Each ferritin molecule is composed of a protein shell of 24 apoferritin subunits surrounding a central core of up to 4500 iron atoms as ferric oxyhydroxide. Ferritin is a storage protein that prevents free iron from catalyzing oxidative reaction, which would injure the cell. Ferritin within mucosal cells is lost when these cells are shed into the intestinal lumen. Normally only a small percentage of dietary iron enters the circulation. Iron absorption is increased when total body iron is low or anemia is present and decreased when total body iron is high.

As indicated earlier, more than half of the total body iron is present in Hb. About a third is stored as ferritin and hemosiderin (primarily within macrophages), 3 to 7% is present in myoglobin (with the higher values occurring in dogs and horses), 1% is present in hemoprotein and flavoprotein enzymes, and only 0.1% is bound to transferrin in plasma.

Free cytoplasmic ferritin molecules are visible by electron microscopy, but not by light microscopy. Hemosiderin is composed of aggregates of protein and iron within lysosomes. It is insoluble in water and thought to result from the degradation of ferritin. Hemosiderin is visible by light microscopy when stained with an iron stain (Prussian blue stain). Iron stored as hemosiderin is released more slowly to transferrin in plasma than is iron stored as ferritin.

Transferrin is a β-globulin with two binding sites for Fe^{+3}. Normally, 25 to 50% of the plasma transferrin binding sites are saturated with iron. Although ferritin is released in small amounts from macrophages and can be taken up by cells (especially the liver), most iron is transported to developing erythroid cells by transferrin. Transferrin binds to transferrin receptors (TfR) on the surface of cells. After binding, the transferrin–TfR complex is internalized by endocytosis. Iron is dissociated from transferrin and the resultant apotransferrin molecule, bound to the TfR, is recycled to the cell membrane where it is dissociated from the TfR and is available for binding new iron. After release from transferrin, iron is complexed to low-molecular-weight compounds for transport to mitochondria, the site of iron incorporation into protoporphyrin to form heme. TfR and apoferritin synthesis are controlled by the amount of intracellular iron present. High iron stimulates apoferritin synthesis and inhibits TfR expression to minimize the potential of iron toxicity to the cell. Low iron results in decreased ferritin synthesis and increased TfR expression on the cell surface to maximize iron uptake and use for heme synthesis.

ERYTHROCYTE DESTRUCTION

Normal Removal of Aged Erythrocytes

Most RBCs circulate in blood for a finite time period (survival time or life span) that ranges from 2 to 5 months in domestic animals, depending on the species. RBC life spans are related to body weight (and consequently metabolic rate), with the smallest animals (highest metabolic rate) having the shortest RBC life spans. Aged RBCs are phagocytized by the mononuclear phagocyte system (MPS). A variety of changes occur in RBCs as they get older, but the nature of the factor(s) that initiates age-related changes and the mechanism(s) of removal of senescent RBCs from the circulation require further clarification. Current evidence suggests that cumulative oxidative injury to membrane components may be responsible for normal RBC aging and removal.

Although multiple mechanisms may be involved in the recognition and removal of aged RBCs, it has been suggested that removal of senescent RBCs is largely immune mediated, following the appearance of a senescent cell antigen. This senescent cell antigen is derived from alterations in the band 3 anion transporter. A natural antibody in plasma binds to senescent cell antigens on the surface of aged cells and, together with bound complement, promotes the phagocytosis of aged RBCs by macrophages which exhibit Fc

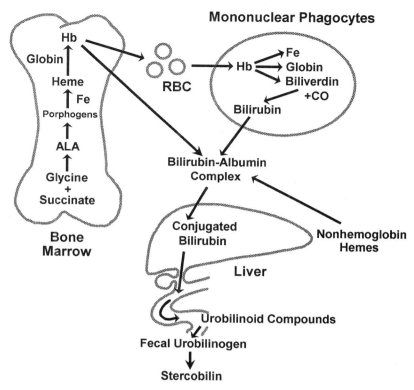

FIGURE 3–3. Overview of RBC production, RBC phagocytosis by mononuclear phagocytes, hemoglobin degradation, and bilirubin metabolism.

and C3b surface receptors. The possibility that senescent RBCs can also be removed via binding to monocyte scavenger receptors requires further study.

Following phagocytosis by macrophages of the spleen and other organs of the MPS, RBCs are lysed and Hb is degraded to heme and globin (Fig. 3–3). Globin is catabolized to constituent amino acids and the microsomal heme oxygenase reaction within macrophages degrades heme to iron, carbon monoxide, and biliverdin. Iron is conserved and stored as ferritin and hemosiderin in the macrophages. It can be released to the circulation and transported back to developing erythroid cells bound to transferrin. Biliverdin is reduced to bilirubin via biliverdin reductase. Bilirubin is then released from the macrophage and bound to albumin for transport to the liver for conjugation and excretion. Approximately 85% of the bilirubin produced in the body comes from Hb, with the remaining coming from heme in other heme-containing proteins.

Pathologic Destruction of Erythrocytes

Increased membrane injury associated with pathologic disorders can result in increased phagocytosis of RBCs. Anemia develops if the rate of destruction exceeds the ability of the bone marrow to respond by producing new RBCs. Lysis of RBCs within macrophages is sometimes referred to as extravascular hemolysis. Hyperbilirubinemia may be present within a few hours following substantial RBC destruction.

Almost no lysis of RBCs occurs within the circulation in normal individuals, but intravascular hemolysis can be present when severe membrane damage occurs in disease states (Fig. 3–4). Following lysis, Hb in plasma (hemoglobinemia) reversibly dissociates into dimers that bind nearly irreversibly to haptoglobin (Hp), an α_2-glycoprotein. The Hb–Hp complex is too large to be filtered through the kidney and is removed from the circulation following binding to receptors on hepatocytes. As in macrophages, the Hb is degraded and iron is conserved. Once plasma Hp is saturated (about 50 to 150 mg/dL Hb-binding capacity in dogs, cats, and horses), remaining free Hb dimers are small enough to readily be filtered by the kidney. Some Hb is reabsorbed by the proximal tubules, but once that capacity is exceeded, Hb appears in the urine (hemoglobinuria). Plasma appears red when as little as 50 mg/dL Hb is present; consequently, hemoglobinemia may be observed in the absence of hemoglobinuria. Hb absorbed by the proximal tubules is rapidly catabolized and iron is stored as ferritin and hemosiderin. Iron not reutilized is lost when tubular epithelial cells slough into the urine, producing hemosideriuria.

Free Hb in plasma can spontaneously oxidize to form methemoglobin, which tends to dissociate into hemin (ferriheme) and globin. Free hemin binds to a plasma β-globulin called hemopexin for transport to the liver. This

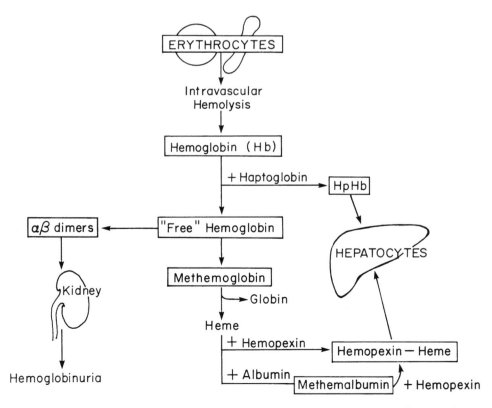

FIGURE 3–4. Pathophysiology of intravascular hemolysis. Methemalbumin forms in primates, but not in common domestic animals.

protects cell membranes from toxic effects of free hemin and it also conserves iron. Albumin from primates can also bind hemin to form methemalbumin, but albumin from common domestic animals does not bind hemin.

The measurement of low plasma Hp in dogs, cats, and horses suggests that recent or ongoing intravascular hemolysis is present. Plasma Hp in cattle and sheep is usually very low or unmeasurable in normal individuals; consequently, this assay cannot be used to examine for evidence of intravascular hemolysis in these species. Haptoglobin is an acute-phase reactant protein and the measurement of increased concentrations in plasma provides evidence of inflammation in all domestic animals examined, although increased values can also result from glucocorticoid administration in some species. Not only does Hp prevent some Hb loss (and therefore iron loss) when intravascular hemolysis occurs, but it binds to free Hb in infected tissues and makes the iron unavailable to bacteria for growth.

EVALUATION OF ERYTHROCYTES

RBCs in blood are quantified by cell counting (RBCs/μL), by determining blood Hb content (g/dL), and by determining the hematocrit (HCT) or packed cell volume (PCV) as a percentage. Because essentially all Hb is present within RBCs, the RBC count, HCT, and Hb content parallel each other when change occurs. Of these measurements, the HCT is the easiest to measure and most reproducible in clinical practice. The other measurements need only be done when RBC indices are to be calculated. The HCT is easily measured by centrifugation of blood in a microhematocrit centrifuge. Modern electronic cell counters calculate the HCT using the measured RBC count and mean cell volume (MCV). The RBC count, MCV, and HCT are accurate if measured using an electronic cell counter that has been adjusted to accommodate the variably sized RBCs of animals. The Hb content is measured spectrophotometrically using the cyanmethemoglobin method.

Microhematocrit Tube

The HCT determined by centrifugation of blood in a microhematocrit tube may be 1 to 3 percentage points higher than the electronically calculated value due to trapped plasma. The capacity of the spleen to expand and contract can result in substantial changes in the HCT, especially in horses and dogs. Excitement or exercise immediately before sampling can result in 30, 40, and 50% increases in the HCT of cats, dogs, and horses, respectively. Conversely, anesthesia (especially with barbiturates) can cause splenic enlargement and the HCT may drop below the reference range.

Other information can be gained from the microhematocrit tube in addition to the HCT. The height of the buffy coat roughly correlates with the total leukocyte count, although it can also be increased when a marked thrombocytosis is present. The buffy coat may appear reddish due to the presence of a marked reticulocytosis.

The plasma in the microhematocrit tube is normally clear and colorless in dogs, cats, pigs, and sheep. It is clear and light yellow in horses because plasma bilirubin concentration is higher in horses than in other domestic animal species. Plasma may appear light yellow in cattle eating green plants containing carotenoids. Hyperbilirubinemia occurs in fasting horses, imparting a deeper yellow coloration to plasma. In other species, yellow plasma with a normal HCT suggests hyperbilirubinemia secondary to liver disease. Hyperbilirubinemia associated with a marked decrease in HCT suggests an increased destruction of RBCs.

Lipemia is indicated if the plasma appears white and cloudy. A layer of lipid may also be seen at the top of the plasma column if due to hyperchylomicronemia. The presence of lipemia is frequently the result of a recent meal (postprandial lipemia), but diseases including diabetes mellitus, pancreatitis, and hypothyroidism may result in lipemia in dogs. Hereditary causes include lipoprotein lipase deficiency in cats and dogs and idiopathic hyperlipidemia in miniature schnauzer dogs. Ponies (especially obese ones), miniature horses, and donkeys are susceptible to developing lipemia associated with pregnancy, lactation, and/or anorexia. These conditions result in the mobilization of unesterified fatty acids from adipose tissue and subsequent overproduction of very-low-density lipoproteins (VLDLs) by the liver.

The presence of Hb is indicated if the plasma appears red in color. The Hb in plasma can result from the lysis of RBCs during the collection and/or handling of blood samples or from true intravascular hemolysis. Some *in vitro* hemolysis is often observed in lipemic samples. The presence of hemoglobinuria indicates that intravascular hemolysis has occurred.

After the HCT is measured and the appearance of the plasma and buffy coat are noted, the microhematocrit capillary tube is broken just above the buffy coat and the plasma is placed in a refractometer for plasma protein determination. Plasma protein values in newborn animals (approximately 4.5 to 5.5 g/dL) are lower than adult values and increase to the adult range by 3 to 4 months of age. The presence of lipemia or hemolysis will falsely increase the measured plasma protein value.

Maximum information can be gained by interpretation of the HCT and plasma protein concentrations simultaneously. Various combinations of low, normal, or high HCT values may occur with low, normal, or high plasma protein concentrations. The various combinations and examples of how they can be interpreted are given in Table 3–1.

Abnormal Erythrocyte Morphology

Rouleaux. RBCs on blood films from healthy horses and cats often exhibit rouleaux (adhesion of RBCs together like a stack of coins) formation (Fig. 3–5). Increased concentrations of fibrinogen and globulin proteins potentiate rouleaux formation in association with inflammatory conditions. Prominent rouleaux formation in species other than horses and cats should be noted as an abnormal finding.

Agglutination. The aggregation or clumping of RBCs together in clusters (not chains like rouleaux) is termed agglutination (Fig. 3–5). It is caused by the occurrence of immunoglobulins bound to RBC surfaces. Because of their pentavalent nature, IgM immunoglobulins have the greatest propensity to produce agglutination. High-dose heparin treatment in horses also causes RBC agglutination by an undefined mechanism.

TABLE 3–1. Concomitant Interpretation of Hematocrit (HCT) and Total Plasma Protein (TPP) Concentration

Normal HCT With:
    Low TPP—Gastrointestinal protein loss, proteinuria, severe liver disease
    Normal TPP—Normal
    High TPP—Increased globulin synthesis, dehydration-masked anemia
High HCT With:
    Low TPP—Protein loss with splenic contraction
    Normal TPP—Splenic contraction, primary or secondary erythrocytosis, dehydration-masked hypoproteinemia
    High TPP—Dehydration
Low HCT With:
    Low TPP—Substantial ongoing or recent blood loss, overhydration
    Normal TPP—Increased erythrocyte destruction, decreased erythrocyte production, chronic blood loss
    High TPP—Anemia of chronic disease, multiple myeloma, lymphoproliferative diseases

Anisocytosis. Variation in RBC diameters in stained blood films is called anisocytosis (Color Plate 2). It is greater in normal cattle than in other normal domestic animals. Anisocytosis is increased when different populations of cells are present. Increased anisocytosis is usually present in regenerative anemias, but may be present in some nonregenerative anemias as well.

Polychromasia. The presence of bluish red RBCs in stained blood films is called polychromasia (Color Plate 2). Polychromatophilic RBCs are reticulocytes that stain bluish red due to the combined presence of Hb (red-staining) and ribosomes (blue-staining). Low numbers of polychromatophilic RBCs are usually seen in blood from normal dogs and pigs because up to 1.5% reticulocytes may be present in dogs and up to 1% reticulocytes may be present in pigs even when the HCT is normal. Slight polychromasia may be present in normal cats, but many normal cats exhibit no polychromasia in stained blood films. There is a direct correlation between the degree of polychromasia and reticulocytosis in dogs (and presumably in the pig) and aggregate reticulocyte percentages in cats (see subsequent discussion of reticulocyte counts). Polychromasia is absent in stained blood films from normal cattle, sheep, goats, and horses because reticulocytes are not normally present in these species. The presence of increased polychromasia in anemic animals indicates an increased percentage of reticulocytes. Polychromasia is not present in regenerative anemias in horses, because horses rarely release reticulocytes from the bone marrow.

FIGURE 3–5. The pattern of RBC adhesion that occurs with rouleaux is compared to the pattern that occurs with agglutination.

 Rouleaux

 Agglutination

Hypochromasia.   The presence of RBCs with decreased Hb concentration and increased central pallor is called hypochromasia (Color Plate 2). Not only is the center of the cell paler than normal, but the diameter of the area of central pallor is increased relative to the red-staining periphery of the cell. True hypochromic RBCs must be differentiated from torocytes, which have colorless, punched-out centers, but wide, dense red-staining peripheries. Torocytes are generally artifacts. Hypochromasia is measured as a decrease in mean corpuscular hemoglobin concentration (MCHC) (discussed later). Increased hypochromasia is observed in iron deficiency anemia.

Poikilocytosis.   Poikilocytosis is a general term used to describe the presence of abnormally shaped RBCs (Fig. 3–6). Poikilocytosis may be present in

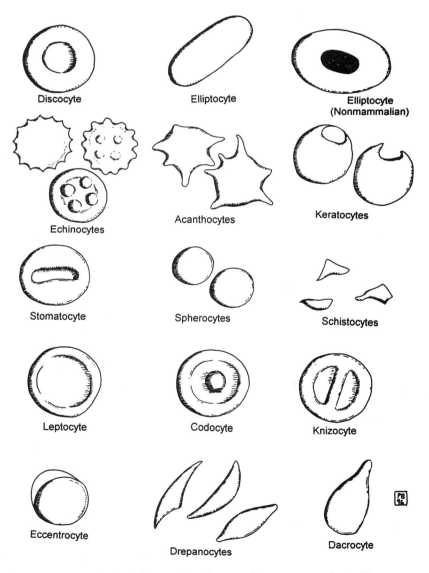

FIGURE 3–6.   RBC shapes. See the text for causes and significance.

clinically normal goats and young cattle. In some instances, these shapes appear to be related to the Hb types present. Severe iron deficiency anemia in dogs may exhibit pronounced poikilocytosis, the etiology of which is unknown. Poikilocytes can form when oxidant injury results in Heinz body formation and/or membrane injury. One or more blunt RBC surface projections may form as the membrane adheres to Heinz bodies bound to its internal surface. A variety of abnormal RBC shapes have been reported in dogs and cats with doxorubicin toxicity and in animals with dyserythropoiesis. More specific terminology is used for certain abnormal shapes.

Echinocytes (Crenated RBCs). Echinocytes are spiculated RBCs where the spicules are relatively evenly spaced and of similar size. Spicules may be sharp or blunt. Highly spiculated echinocytes have been called burr cells. When observed in stained blood films, echinocytosis is usually an artifact that results from excess ethylenediaminetetraacetic acid (EDTA), improper smear preparation, or prolonged sample storage before blood film preparation. They are common in normal pig blood smears, forming when RBCs contact glass surfaces. Echinocytes form when the surface area of the outer lipid monolayer increases relative to the inner monolayer. Echinocytic transformation occurs *in vitro* in the presence of fatty acids, lysophospholipids, and amphipathic drugs that distribute preferentially in the outer half of the lipid bilayer. Echinocytes also form when RBCs are dehydrated, pH is increased, RBC adenosine triphosphate (ATP) is depleted (*e.g.*, hypophosphatemia), and intracellular calcium is increased. Transient echinocytosis occurs in dogs following coral snake and rattlesnake envenomation, presumably secondary to the action of phospholipases present in venom. Echinocytes may occur in uremic animals, immediately after transfusion of stored blood, or in some pyruvate kinase–deficient dogs. They have also been reported in dogs with doxorubicin toxicity. Echinocytosis occurs in horses where total body depletion of cations has occurred (endurance exercise, furosemide treatment, systemic disease).

Acanthocytes. RBCs with irregularly spaced, variably sized spicules are called acanthocytes. They form when RBC membranes contain excess cholesterol compared to phospholipids. Alterations in RBC membrane lipids can result from increased blood cholesterol content or the presence of abnormal plasma lipoprotein composition. Acanthocytes have been recognized in animals with liver disease, possibly due to alterations in plasma lipid composition, which can alter RBC lipid composition. They have also been reported in dogs with disorders such as hemangiosarcoma, disseminated intravascular coagulation, and glomerulonephritis that result in RBC fragmentation.

Keratocytes. RBCs containing what appears to be one or more intact or ruptured "vesicles" are called keratocytes. These nonstaining areas appear to be circular areas of apposed and sealed membrane rather than true vesicles. Removal or rupture of this area results in the formation of one or two projections. Keratocytes have been recognized in various disorders including iron deficiency anemia, liver disorders and doxorubicin toxicity in cats, and hemangiosarcoma in dogs. Keratocyte formation is potentiated by storage of cat blood collected with EDTA.

Stomatocytes. Cup-shaped RBCs that have oval or elongated areas of central pallor when viewed in stained blood films are called stomatocytes. They most often occur as artifacts in thick blood film preparations. Stomatocytes form when RBC water content is increased as occurs in hereditary stomatocytosis in dogs. Stomatocytes also form when amphipathic drugs are present that distribute preferentially in the inner half of the lipid bilayer.

Spherocytes. Spherical RBCs that result from cell swelling and/or loss of cell membrane are referred to as spherocytes. They lack central pallor and have smaller diameters than normal on stained blood films. Spherocytes occur most frequently in association with immune-mediated hemolytic anemia in the dog. Other potential causes of spherocyte formation include coral snake bites, zinc toxicity, RBC parasites, and transfusion of stored blood. Since RBCs from other common domestic animals exhibit less central pallor than those of dogs, it is difficult to be certain when spherocytes are present in these species.

Schistocytes (Schizocytes). RBC fragments with two or three pointed extremities are called schistocytes. They are smaller than normal discocytes. Schistocytes may be seen in dogs with microangiopathic hemolytic anemia associated with disseminated intravascular coagulation (DIC). Schistocytes are not typically seen in cats and horses with DIC, possibly because the RBCs of these species are smaller and less likely to be split by fibrin strands in the circulation. They can also occur in the absence of DIC in conditions such as severe iron deficiency anemia, myelofibrosis, liver disease, and hemophago-cytic histiocytic disorders.

Leptocytes. These cells are thin, flat hypochromic-appearing RBCs with increased membrane to volume ratios. Some leptocytes appear folded, some appear as triconcave knizocytes that give the impression that the RBC has a central bar of Hb, and others appear as codocytes. Codocytes (target cells) are bell-shaped cells that exhibit a central density or "bull's-eye" in stained blood films. Small numbers of codocytes are often seen in normal dog blood. Leptocytes may be seen in iron deficiency anemia and rarely in hepatic insuffi-ciency that result in a balanced accumulation of membrane phospholipids and cholesterol. Polychromatophilic RBCs can sometimes appear as leptocytes.

Eccentrocytes (Hemighosts). An RBC in which the Hb is localized to part of the cell, leaving an Hb-poor area visible in the remaining part of the cell, is termed an eccentrocyte. They are formed by the adhesion of opposing areas of the cytoplasmic face of the RBC membrane. Eccentrocytes have been seen in animals ingesting or receiving oxidants and in a horse with glucose-6-phosphate dehydrogenase (G6PD) deficiency.

Elliptocytes (Ovalocytes). RBCs from nonmammals and animals in the Camellidae family normally have RBCs that are elliptical or oval in shape. Abnormal elliptocytes have been recognized in cats with bone marrow ab-normalities (myeloproliferative disorders and acute lymphocytic leukemia), hepatic lipidosis, portosystemic shunts, and doxorubicin toxicity, and in a dog with myelofibrosis. Hereditary elliptocytosis has been reported in a dog with a membrane protein 4.1 deficiency.

Drepanocytes (Sickle Cells). These fusiform or spindle-shaped RBCs are often observed in blood from normal deer. Drepanocyte formation in deer depends on the Hb types present. It is an *in vitro* phenomenon that occurs when oxygen tension is high and pH is between 7.6 and 7.8. Hb polymerization occurs in some normal Angora goats, resulting in spindle-shaped or fusiform RBCs that have been termed acuminocytes by some others.

Dacrocytes. These RBCs are teardrop-shaped with single elongated or pointed extremities. Dacrocytes have been seen in dogs and cats with myeloproliferative disorders, dogs with myelofibrosis, and a dog with hypersplenism.

Nucleated RBCs.   Rubricytes and metarubricytes are seldom present in the blood of normal adult mammals, although low numbers may occur in miniature schnauzers and dachshunds with no evidence of underlying disease. Nucleated RBCs are often seen in blood in association with regenerative anemias (Color Plate 2); however, their presence does not necessarily indicate a regenerative response is present. Nucleated RBCs may be seen in lead poisoning in which there is minimal or no anemia, in conditions where bone marrow is damaged (such as endotoxic shock), in association with hematopoietic neoplasia, nonhematopoietic neoplasia, and in inherited dyserythropoietic disorders. Low numbers of nucleated RBCs are seen in a wide variety of disorders in dogs including cardiovascular disease, trauma, hyperadrenocorticism, and various inflammatory conditions.

Howell-Jolly Bodies.   These small, spherical nuclear remnants (Color Plate 2) form in the bone marrow and are removed by "pitting" action of the spleen. They may be present in low numbers in RBCs of normal cats and horses. They are often present following splenectomy or in association with regenerative anemias in other species.

Heinz Bodies.   These inclusions are large aggregates of oxidized, precipitated Hb that are attached to the internal surfaces of RBC membranes. In contrast to Howell-Jolly bodies, which stain dark blue, they stain red to pale pink with Romanowsky-type stains. Heinz bodies appear light blue with reticulocyte stains (Color Plate 2). They can also be visualized as dark, refractile inclusions in new methylene blue "wet" preparations (Fig. 3–7). In contrast to other domestic animal species, normal cats may have 5 to 10% Heinz bodies within their RBCs. Not only is cat Hb more susceptible to denaturation by endogenous oxidants, but the cat spleen is less efficient in the removal (pitting) of Heinz bodies from RBCs than are spleens of other species. Increased numbers of Heinz bodies may occur with minimal anemia in cats with spontaneous diseases, such as diabetes mellitus, hyperthyroidism, and lymphoma. Small Heinz bodies are seen in other species following splenectomy.

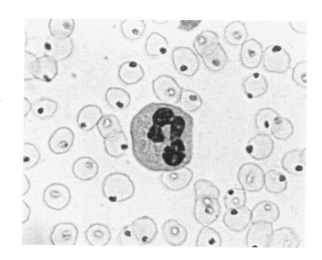

FIGURE 3–7. The new methylene blue wet-mount staining procedure was used to demonstrate Heinz bodies in cat RBCs. A neutrophil is also present.

Dietary causes of Heinz body hemolytic anemia include consumption of onions in small and large animals, consumption of kale and other *Brassica* species by ruminants, consumption of lush winter rye by cattle, and consumption of red maple leaves by horses. Heinz bodies have been recognized in RBCs from selenium-deficient Florida cattle grazing on St. Augustine grass pastures and in postparturient New Zealand cattle grazing primarily on perennial ryegrass. Copper toxicity results in Heinz body formation in sheep. Heinz body formation has been reported in some dogs ingesting zinc-containing objects (*e.g.*, U.S. pennies minted after 1982). Naphthalene ingestion may have caused Heinz body formation in a dog. Heinz body hemolytic anemias have occurred following the administration of a variety of drugs including acetaminophen and methylene blue in cats and dogs, methionine and phenazopyridine in cats, menadione (vitamin K_3) in dogs, and phenothiazine in horses. Ingestion of crude oil has resulted in Heinz body hemolytic anemia in marine birds.

Basophilic Stippling. This term is used to describe blue-staining punctate inclusions in RBCs stained with routine Romanowsky-type blood stains. Basophilic stippling commonly occurs in regenerative anemias in ruminants (Color Plate 2) and rarely occurs in regenerative anemias in other species. Basophilic stippling may be prominent in any species with lead poisoning.

Siderotic Inclusions. These inclusions contain iron. They often appear as focal basophilic stippling when present in routinely stained blood films (Fig. 3–8). A Prussian blue staining procedure is used to verify the presence of iron-positive material. RBCs containing these inclusions are called siderocytes. Siderocytes are rare or absent in blood of normal animals, but may occur with lead poisoning, hemolytic anemia, dyserythropoiesis, myeloproliferative diseases, chloramphenicol therapy, and experimental pyridoxine deficiency in pigs.

Infectious Agents. A number of infectious organisms are recognized to occur in/on RBCs. *Babesia* spp. (Fig. 3–9), *Theileria* spp., and *Cytauxzoon felis* (Fig. 3–10) are intracellular protozoa. *Anaplasma* spp. (Color Plate 2) are intracellular rickettsial organisms that infect ruminant RBCs. *Haemobartonella* spp. (Figs. 3–11 and 3–12) and *Eperythrozoon* spp. (Color Plate 2) are rickettsial organisms that attach to the outside (epicellular) of RBCs. Dis-

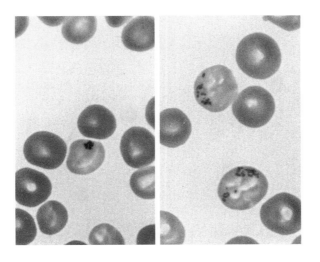

FIGURE 3–8. Wright-Giemsa–stained blood from a dog treated with chloramphenicol. The RBCs containing focal basophilic stippling were classified as siderocytes based on positive Prussian blue staining. (From Harvey JW, Wolfsheimer KJ, Simpson CF, et al: Pathologic sideroblasts and siderocytes associated with chloramphenicol therapy in a dog. Vet Clin Pathol 1985;14[1]:36, with permission.)

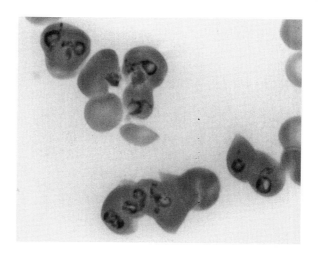

FIGURE 3–9. Dog RBCs containing *Babesia canis* organisms (Wright-Giemsa stain).

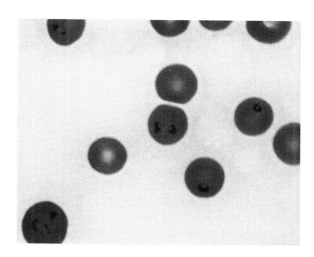

FIGURE 3–10. Cat RBCs containing *Cytauxzoon felis* organisms (Wright-Giemsa stain).

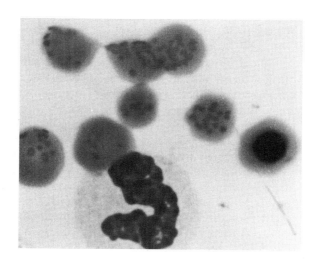

FIGURE 3–11. Cat RBCs parasitized by *Haemobartonella felis* organisms. A nucleate RBC and neutrophil are present (Wright-Giemsa stain).

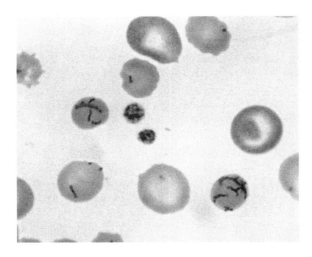

FIGURE 3–12. Dog RBCs parasitized by *Haemobartonella canis* organisms (Wright-Giemsa stain).

temper inclusions may also be seen in dog RBCs (Color Plate 3). It is important to differentiate these infectious agents from stain artifacts, Howell-Jolly bodies, and platelets overlying RBCs.

Reticulocyte Counts

Reticulocyte stains are commercially available. After incubation of blood and stain together, blood films are made and reticulocyte counts are done by examining 500 to 1000 RBCs and determining the percentage that are reticulocytes. The blue-staining reticulum seen in reticulocytes (Color Plate 2) does not occur as such in living cells, but results from the precipitation of ribosomes in immature RBCs during the staining process. As a reticulocyte matures, the number of ribosomes decreases until only small punctate (dot-like) inclusions are observed in RBCs (punctate reticulocytes) within the reticulocyte stain. To reduce the chance that a cell with a staining artifact is counted as a punctate reticulocyte, it is recommended that at least two discrete blue inclusions be visible in a cell without requiring fine-focus adjustment of the microscope. These inclusions should be away from the cell margin to avoid confusion with *Haemobartonella* organisms or small Heinz bodies.

In healthy cats, as well as cats with regenerative anemia, the number of punctate reticulocytes is much greater than that seen in other species. This apparently occurs because the maturation (loss of ribosomes) of reticulocytes in cats is slower than that in other species. Consequently, reticulocytes in cats are classified as aggregate (if coarse clumping is observed) or punctate (if small individual inclusions are present). Percentages of both types should be reported separately. Normal cats have from 0 to 0.4% aggregate and 1 to 10% punctate reticulocytes. Percentages of aggregate reticulocytes correlate directly with percentages of polychromatophilic RBCs observed in blood films stained with Wright-Giemsa stain. Aggregate reticulocytes in the circulation mature to punctate reticulocytes in a day or less. A week or more is required for maturation (total disappearance of ribosomes) of punctate reticulocytes. In contrast to those of the cat, most reticulocytes in other species are of the aggregate type. Consequently, no attempt is made to differentiate stages of reticulocytes except in cats.

Except for horses, increased numbers of reticulocytes are released in response to anemia, with better responses to hemolytic anemias than to hemorrhage. When the degree of anemia is severe, basophilic macroreticulocytes or so-called stress reticulocytes may be released into blood. It is proposed that one less mitotic division occurs during production and immature reticulocytes, twice the normal size, are released. Increased erythropoietin (EPO) results in a diminution in the adventitial cell and endothelial cell barrier separating marrow hematopoietic cells from the sinus, thereby potentiating the premature release of stress reticulocytes from the marrow. Although a portion of these macroreticulocytes apparently are rapidly removed from the circulation, it appears from studies in cats that some can mature into macrocytic RBCs with relatively normal life spans.

Inasmuch as reticulocyte counts are given as a percentage of total RBCs, the reticulocyte count would be higher in an anemic animal than in a normal animal even if the absolute number of reticulocytes in the circulation was the same. Consequently, it has been recommended that the reticulocyte count be corrected by dividing the patient's HCT by the mean normal HCT for the species, and multiplying this value times the original reticulocyte count to obtain a corrected reticulocyte count.

$$\text{Corrected reticulocyte count (\%)} = \frac{\text{patient's HCT}}{\text{species mean HCT}}$$
$$\times \text{ uncorrected reticulocyte count (\%).}$$

An even better way of evaluating the reticulocyte response is by determining the absolute reticulocyte count. This is done by multiplying the percentage of reticulocytes counted by the total RBC count.

$$\text{Absolute reticulocyte count (cells/}\mu\text{L)} = \text{RBC count (cells/}\mu\text{L)}$$
$$\times \text{ uncorrected reticulocyte count (\%).}$$

Reticulocyte counts above $80,000/\mu$L are considered to be increased in dogs. Normal cats have between 0 and $30,000/\mu$L aggregate reticulocytes, but punctate reticulocytes may be as high as $500,000/\mu$L.

The reticulocyte response to blood loss anemia in the cat is shown (Fig. 3–13). As in other species, about 4 days are required for maximal aggregate reticulocyte response to anemia, because of the time required for the production of aggregate reticulocytes from progenitor cells. The maximal punctate response occurs considerably later, primarily because of the long time required for punctate reticulocytes to mature to RBCs. As can be seen in Figure 3–13, punctate reticulocyte release from bone marrow continues after the HCT begins to increase and aggregate reticulocyte release has ceased. Consequently, cats with mild anemia may have increased punctate reticulocyte counts and normal aggregate reticulocyte counts.

Erythrocyte Indices

Determination of RBC indices can assist in the differential diagnosis of anemia. Of the parameters routinely determined or calculated, the mean cell volume is the most useful.

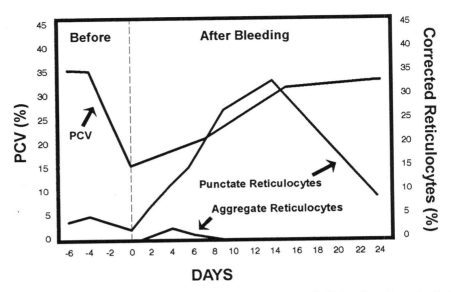

FIGURE 3–13. Reticulocyte response following controlled bleeding in cats. Reticulocyte counts have been corrected using HCT values. (The graph used data from Alsaker RD, Laber J, Stevens JB, et al: A comparison of polychromasia and reticulocyte counts in assessing erthrocyte regenerative response in the cat. J Am Vet Med Assoc 1977;170:39.)

Mean Cell Volume. The MCV represents the average volume of a single RBC in femtoliters (10^{-15} L). The MCV is determined most accurately by direct measurement with electronic cell counters. It can be determined indirectly by dividing the HCT (as a percentage) by the RBC count (in millions of cells per microliter) and multiplying by 10, but is less accurate because two separate measurements are required. The MCV varies greatly depending on species. Mammals have smaller RBCs than do birds, reptiles, or amphibians. Species with larger RBCs have lower RBC counts, resulting in similar HCTs in mammals and birds.

High MCV values are usually associated with regenerative anemias, although macrocytosis (without anemia or reticulocytosis) occurs in some apparently healthy toy and miniature poodle dogs. In addition, dogs with hereditary stomatocytosis may have high MCVs with normal or only slightly increased reticulocyte count, because the stomatocytes are swollen with increased intracellular water. High MCVs may occur in animals with myeloproliferative disorders, and macrocytosis is often seen in feline leukemia virus (FeLV)–positive cats with nonregenerative anemias. Folate deficiency has been reported as a cause of macrocytic nonregenerative anemia in a cat fed tuna (intended for human consumption) for 4 years. High MCVs may occur as an artifact secondary to agglutination of RBCs as can occur in immune-mediated disorders or following heparin administration to horses. Macrocytic anemia has been reported in Hereford calves with congenital dyserythropoiesis. Many nucleated RBCs are present in blood, but reticulocyte counts are only slightly increased.

Macrocytosis is more likely to occur in response to hemolytic anemia than in response to hemorrhage, at least in part, because serum iron concentration is increased in animals with hemolytic anemia. While iron does not stimulate erythropoiesis, decreased iron availability may limit the erythropoietic response following hemorrhage. Reticulocytes, especially those produced in response to severe anemia (stress reticulocytes), are larger than mature RBCs. A week or more is required before macrocytosis occurs. Although the bone marrow normally contains some reticulocytes undergoing maturation, most reticulocytes released from the bone marrow in response to anemia must be formed *de novo*. Four or 5 days are required for a peak reticulocyte response to occur, and then the newly produced, larger cells must compromise a high enough percentage of the total RBCs present to increase the MCV above the reference range. Although there is a reduction in size as reticulocytes mature into RBCs, larger than normal reticulocytes produce larger than normal RBCs.

The RBCs produced in the fetus are larger than those produced in adults. There is a gradual decrease in MCV during fetal development. The MCV is within adult reference ranges in horses and cattle at birth, but still above adult reference ranges in dogs and cats at birth. It declines as the larger RBCs formed in the fetus are replaced by smaller RBCs produced after birth.

Microcytic anemias usually indicate the presence of iron deficiency. Microcytic iron deficiency anemia in adult animals is almost always due to chronic hemorrhage. Depending on the initial MCV and magnitude of ongoing blood loss, 1 or more months are required before the MCV decreases below the reference range. Body iron stores must be depleted and then the microcytes formed must comprise a high enough percentage of the total RBCs present to decrease the MCV below the reference range. Microcytic anemia rarely occurs as a result of a dietary iron deficiency in adult animals. However, iron deficiency without blood loss is common in nursing animals, because milk is low in iron and there is increased demand for iron in these rapidly growing animals. Although microcytes are often formed in nursing animals, the MCV may not be reduced in dogs and cats because of the persistence of macrocytes formed before birth. Copper is needed for optimal iron absorption and release from body iron stores. Consequently, prolonged copper deficiency results in microcytic anemia in some species. Pyridoxine, vitamin B_6, is required for the first step in heme synthesis. Although natural cases of pyridoxine deficiency have not been documented in domestic animals, microcytic anemias with high serum iron values have been produced experimentally in dogs, cats, and pigs with dietary pyridoxine deficiency.

The MCV may be slightly decreased in association with the anemia of chronic disease, but the MCV is at the low end of the reference range in most cases. Microcytosis is common in dogs with portosystemic shunts. The MCV is seldom more than 6 fL below the reference range and the HCT is within the reference range or only a slight anemia is present. A nonregenerative microcytic anemia with many circulating nucleated RBCs has been reported in three related English springer spaniels with dyserythropoiesis, polymyopathy, and heart disease. Japanese Akita dogs normally have MCV below the reference range established for other breeds of dogs.

Mean Cell Hemoglobin Concentration. The MCHC represents the average Hb concentration within RBCs. It is calculated by dividing the Hb value (in grams per deciliter) by the HCT (as a percentage) and multiplying by 100. The MCHC is expressed as grams per deciliter of RBCs. (Note: Hb values in blood are expressed as grams per deciliter whole blood.) Reference ranges established using HCT values determined by electronic cell counters tend to be slightly higher than those determined using HCT values measured by centrifugation, because of the presence of small amounts of trapped plasma in centrifuged samples.

High MCHC values are artifacts. They may result from *in vivo* or *in vitro* hemolysis, lipemia, or presence of Heinz bodies. In the case of hemolysis, some Hb is free in plasma, but the formula used to calculate the MCHC assumes that all Hb is contained within RBCs. Lipemia and Heinz bodies cause turbidity in the spectrophotometric assay for Hb, thereby giving erroneously elevated Hb values. A high MCHC may also occur if agglutination of RBCs occurs when assayed in an electronic cell counter as may occur with cold-acting autoantibodies or following heparin therapy in some horses. Large aggregates are too large to be considered RBCs; consequently, cell counters are programmed to exclude them from RBC measurements. This results in erroneously low HCT values. Agglutination should not interfere with HCT values determined by centrifugation, so long as blood samples are well mixed before hematocrit tubes are filled. The MCHC will not be falsely elevated by the above factors if it is determined by density measurement (*e.g.*, VetAutoread Hematology System, IDEXX, Inc.).

MCHC values may be decreased in animals with regenerative anemias, especially those with high percentages of stress reticulocytes. Hb synthesis is not complete until late in reticulocyte maturation; consequently, it is less complete in stress reticulocytes, because these cells are released from the bone marrow earlier than normally occurs.

Low MCHC values may also occur in animals with chronic iron deficiency. When determined using electronic cell counters, the MCHC is usually normal in animals with slight microcytosis, but is usually low when the MCV is markedly reduced. The MCHC is low in iron deficiency because iron is not adequate for synthesis of normal amounts of Hb. Low MCHC values occur in dogs with hereditary stomatocytosis, because the increased intracellular water, which occurs in this condition, dilutes the Hb concentration within the cells.

Mean Cell Hemoglobin.   The mean cell hemoglobin (MCH) is calculated by dividing the Hb value (in grams per deciliter) by the RBC count (in millions per microliter) and multiplying by 10. The MCH provides no added value, because it depends on the MCV and MCHC. It usually correlates directly with the MCV, except in animals with macrocytic hypochromic RBCs.

Red Cell Distribution Width.   The red cell distribution width (RDW) is an electronic measure of anisocytosis or RBC volume heterogeneity. A histogram plot of the volume of individual RBCs reveals a curve that approximates a gaussian distribution. Consequently, one can calculate the degree of size variation by determining the standard deviation (SD) of RBC volumes. However, the SD depends on the size of the cells, as well as the degree of size variation around the MCV. To provide a measure of size variation that does not depend on how large the cells are, the coefficient of variation of RBC volume is calculated by dividing the SD by the MCV and then multiplying by 100. In short, the RDW is the SD of RBC volumes expressed as a percentage of the mean.

Reference values vary depending on the instrument used to measure the RDW. Cattle and horses normally have higher RDW values than cats and dogs. One need only refer to the upper limit of a reference range when examining data from a patient, because there is no pathologic state where RBCs have greater volume homogeneity than normal.

The utility of the RDW has not been extensively evaluated in veterinary medicine. It is expected to be increased in cases where the degree of anisocytosis (as estimated on the stained blood film) is increased. It is often increased in regenerative anemias, because reticulocytes and young RBCs are larger than mature RBCs. Like the MCV, the number of large RBCs in blood must reach a certain level before the RDW of a given patient exceeds the reference range. In some animals, the RDW will be increased before the MCV exceeds the reference range. As an animal responds to anemia and young RBCs become the predominant population, the RDW will begin to decline and may return to the reference range, even though the MCV is still above normal.

The RDW is also expected to increase in iron deficiency where smaller than normal RBCs are produced. Like regenerative anemias, the increase is most likely to be seen during the phase of disease where there are a significant number of normal and abnormal sized cells present. In severe chronic iron deficiency the RDW might decrease toward normal because the whole population of RBCs is small. The RDW may increase again following iron therapy, as normal sized cells are produced.

Other causes of increased RDW include conditions where substantial fragmentation of RBCs is occurring and following blood transfusion, if the MCV of donor blood is substantially different from that of the recipient. The RDW is also increased in dogs with hereditary stomatocytosis. Animals with non-regenerative anemias will have normal RDW values unless significant dyserythropoiesis is present.

Direct Antiglobulin Test

A direct antiglobulin (Coombs') test is done when autoagglutination is absent, but immune-mediated hemolytic anemia is still suspected. Species-specific antisera against IgG, IgM, and the third component of complement (C_3) are used to detect the presence of one or more of these factors on the surface of RBCs. This test is discussed in greater detail in Chapter 6.

Serum Iron Assays

Serum iron concentration is increased in animals with hemolytic anemias and in dogs and horses following the administration of glucocorticoid steroids. Serum iron is decreased following glucocorticoid administration to cattle. It is low in both iron deficiency and the anemia of chronic disease. The total iron-binding capacity (TIBC) of serum is a measure of serum transferrin concentration because insignificant amounts of circulating iron are bound to other proteins. Serum TIBC is low-normal or decreased in the anemia of chronic disease and increased in some species with iron deficiency. The TIBC is normal in dogs with chronic iron deficiency anemia.

These disorders can usually be differentiated by examination of bone marrow for stainable iron, which is minimal or absent in iron deficiency and normal or high in the anemia of chronic disease. Stainable iron is not present in the bone marrow of normal cats; consequently, a lack of stainable iron does not suggest iron deficiency in this species.

Serum ferritin concentration correlates with tissue iron stores in domestic animals, including cats. Consequently, serum ferritin concentration can help differentiate true iron deficiency (serum ferritin is low) from the anemia of chronic disease (serum ferritin is normal or high), but commercial assay kits for ferritin are not available except for humans. Serum ferritin is an acute-phase protein; consequently, increased values are expected in inflammatory conditions. Increased serum ferritin occurs in chronic hemolytic anemias (*e.g.*, pyruvate kinase deficiency) and in canine malignant histiocytosis.

Methemoglobin Determination

Methemoglobin differs from Hb in that the iron moiety of heme groups has been oxidized from the ferrous (+2) to the ferric (+3) state. Methemoglobinemia refers to methemoglobin content in blood above 1.5% of total Hb. Clinical signs associated with methemoglobinemia are the result of hypoxia because methemoglobin cannot bind O_2. Both low blood oxygen tension and methemoglobinemia can result in cyanotic-appearing mucous membranes and dark-colored blood samples. Hypoxemia is documented by measuring a low Po_2 of an arterial blood sample. Methemoglobinemia is suspected when arterial blood with normal or increased Po_2 is dark colored. Methemoglobin is quantified spectrophotometrically, but a spot test can be used to determine whether clinically significant levels of methemoglobin are present. One drop of blood from the patient is placed on a piece of absorbent white paper and a drop of normal control blood is placed next to it. If the methemoglobin content is 10% or greater the patient's blood should have noticeably brown coloration. Methemoglobinemia results from either increased production of methemoglobin by oxidants or decreased reduction of methemoglobin associated with a deficiency in the RBC methemoglobin reductase enzyme. Methemoglobinemia and mild to moderate hemolytic anemia were reported in a trotter mare and her dam. The cause of this presumably familial abnormality was not determined.

Toxic Methemoglobinemia. Significant methemoglobinemia has been associated with clinical cases of benzocaine, acetaminophen, and phenazopyridine toxicities in cats and/or dogs, copper toxicity in sheep, and red maple toxicity in horses. These oxidants can also produce Heinz body hemolytic anemias. Nitrite produces methemoglobinemia without Heinz body formation or development of anemia. Methemoglobinemia occurs in ruminants eating nitrate-accumulating plants, especially when the plants have been fertilized with nitrogenous compounds. Nitrate is relatively nontoxic, but it is reduced to nitrite by ruminal microorganisms.

Methemoglobin Reductase Deficiency. Persistent methemoglobinemia resulting from RBC methemoglobin reductase (cytochrome-b_5 reductase) deficiency has been recognized in Chihuahua, borzoi, English setter, terrier-mix, cockapoo, poodle, Welsh corgi, Pomeranian, and toy American Eskimo dogs, and recently in a domestic short-haired cat. In contrast to methemoglobinemia produced by oxidant drugs and compounds, animals with methemoglobin reductase deficiency usually exhibit no clinical signs of illness. The diagnosis of this deficiency is made by measuring enzyme activity within RBCs.

Erythropoietin Assay

EPO is a glycoprotein hormone that stimulates erythropoiesis in a number of ways. Serum EPO is increased in response to various anemias, except the anemia of chronic renal disease, in which EPO production is decreased. The EPO assay has received limited use in veterinary medicine. It is useful in differentiating polycythemia vera (where EPO values are normal or low) from secondary polycythemias (where values are high). Animal studies have utilized bioassays in the past, but they are generally not sensitive enough to measure EPO in healthy animals. Radioimmunoassays show considerable promise, but commercial tests developed for human assays may not always cross-react sufficiently for use in other species. Individual radioimmunoassays require validation for each species to be assayed before they can be used clinically.

DIFFERENTIAL DIAGNOSIS OF ANEMIA

True or absolute anemia is defined as a decrease in RBC mass within the body. HCT, Hb, and RBC count values are usually below their reference ranges; however, the anemia can sometimes be masked by concomitant dehydration. Low RBC parameters may also be present in blood when the total body RBC mass is normal (relative anemia). This can result from overhydration, resulting in RBC dilution, and from splenic sequestration of RBCs as occurs with splenic relaxation during anesthesia, heparin-induced RBC agglutination in horses, and various causes of splenomegaly.

Anemia is a problem, not a diagnosis. Anemia is classified in various ways to assist in determining the specific cause of the anemia so that effective therapy can be given. In addition to laboratory findings, past history, presenting complaints, and results of other test procedures such as radiology are important in reaching a final diagnosis.

Anemia may occur following blood loss, increased RBC destruction, or decreased RBC production. Factors that can be useful in categorizing anemia into these broad causes (and often into more specific causes) include reticulocyte counts, RBC indices, RBC morphology on stained blood films, the appearance of the plasma, plasma protein concentration, serum iron measurements, serum bilirubin determination, direct antiglobulin test, and bone marrow evaluation.

Anemia may also develop as a result of the expansion of the vascular space faster than the expansion of the total body RBC mass. This hemodilution contributes to the anemia of the neonate (to be discussed later) and to a mild anemia that develops during pregnancy in most domestic animals, the horse being an exception.

Regenerative *Versus* Nonregenerative Anemia

The most useful approach in the classification of anemia is to determine whether or not evidence of a bone marrow response to the anemia is present in blood. For all species except the horse, this involves determining whether absolute reticulocyte numbers are increased in blood. Horses rarely release reticulocytes from the bone marrow even when an increased production of RBCs occurs. MCV and/or RDW values are increased in some horses responding to anemia, but others recover from anemia without these parameters exceeding reference ranges. Consequently, bone marrow evaluation is often needed to determine if an appropriate response to anemia is present in a horse. Myeloid to erythroid (M:E) ratios below 0.5 and the bone marrow reticulocyte counts above 5% suggest a regenerative response to anemia.

Increased polychromasia is usually present in regenerative anemias because many reticulocytes stain bluish red with routine blood stains. Cats with mild anemias may not release aggregate reticulocytes from the marrow, but will release punctate reticulocytes. Because punctate reticulocytes do not contain sufficient numbers of ribosomes within them to impart a bluish color to the cytoplasm, mild regenerative anemias in cats may lack polychromasia in stained blood films. Increased anisocytosis is often present in regenerative anemias because of the presence of large immature RBCs, although anisocytosis may be marked in some nonregenerative anemias as well.

Some nucleated RBCs (rubricytes and metarubricytes) are often seen on blood films in association with regenerative anemia (except in horses); however, their presence is a much less useful indicator of a regenerative response than is the degree of reticulocytosis. Nucleated RBCs may be present in anemic and nonanemic disorders with minimal or no reticulocytosis.

Howell-Jolly bodies are often present with RBCs in regenerative anemias, but they also occur in normal cats and horses and in splenectomized animals of other species. Basophilic stippling occurs in regenerative anemias in ruminants, but rarely in other species. Basophilic stippling can also occur in RBCs of any species with lead toxicity whether anemia is present or absent.

The presence of compensatory reticulocytosis indicates that the anemia has resulted from either blood loss or increased RBC destruction. Several factors should be kept in mind when interpreting the magnitude of a reticulocyte response. In regenerative anemias, animals with lower HCT should have higher reticulocyte percentages for three reasons. First, severe anemia will evoke a greater stimulus for increased RBC production. Second, animals with more severe anemias have lower RBC counts. Inasmuch as reticulocyte counts are measured as a percentage of total RBCs, the reticulocyte percentage would be higher in an anemic animal than in a normal animal even if the absolute number of reticulocytes in the circulation was the same. Consequently, it has been recommended that the absolute reticulocyte count be determined or that the reticulocyte count be corrected for the HCT relative to the mean reference value for the species (see previous reticulocyte count section). Lastly, in severe anemia, reticulocytes can be released from the marrow earlier in their development than normally occurs. These large "stress" reticulocytes apparently remain in the circulation longer than other reticulocytes before maturation is complete. Factors have been utilized in an attempt to correct for this longer reticulocyte circulation time in people and some veterinary authors have empirically applied these same factors to anemic dogs to calculate what has been called the reticulocyte index. This approach has not been validated in dogs and its use has recently been questioned in people.

Hemolytic anemia usually elicits a more dramatic regenerative response than hemorrhagic anemia, at least in part due to greater availability of iron. There are also species differences in the ability to increase RBC production.

Dogs respond more dramatically with higher reticulocyte counts, more polychromasia, and more rapid return of HCT toward normal than do cats in similar disease situations. The return of the HCT to normal is slower in cattle than in cats and slower yet in horses.

Anemias with no increase or low numbers of reticulocytes are classified as poorly regenerative or nonregenerative, respectively. The lack of a reticulocyte response in nonequine species generally indicates that the anemia results from insufficient RBC production in the marrow. A minimal reticulocyte response may be present if the anemia develops acutely following hemorrhage or hemolysis, because about 4 days are required for a substantial reticulocyte response to occur.

Classification of Anemia Using Erythrocyte Indices

An anemia can also be classified using the MCV and MCHC values to assist in determining the cause of the anemia. The terms used for size are macrocytic (increased MCV), normocytic (normal MCV), and microcytic (decreased MCV). Terms used to describe MCHC values are normochromic (normal MCHC) and hypochromic (decreased MCHC). Anemias are not classified as hyperchromic because high MCHC values are artifacts. A comparison of RBC indices and causes of anemia is given in Table 3–2.

HEMOLYTIC ANEMIAS

Hemolytic anemias occur as a result of increased RBC destruction within the body. Causes of hemolytic anemia in animals are given in Table 3–3. RBCs may be lysed within the circulation (intravascular hemolysis), but more frequently they are lysed following phagocytosis by cells of the mononuclear phagocyte system (extravascular hemolysis).

Hemolytic anemias are regenerative if sufficient time has elapsed for a bone marrow response to the anemia. They are often macrocytic hypochromic or macrocytic normochromic, but may be normocytic normochromic if sufficient time has not elapsed for bone marrow release of significant numbers of large reticulocytes. Macrocytic hypochromic RBCs may also occur in hereditary stomatocytosis in dogs as a result of membrane abnormalities and RBC swelling. An example of a hemolytic anemia that is consistently nonregenerative and normocytic normochromic is cytauxzoonosis in cats. Animals die before there is time for a regenerative response to the anemia to occur. Increased erythrocyte phagocytosis occurs in animals with malignant histiocytosis and in animals with the hemophagocytic syndrome, but the anemia may not be regenerative if histiocyte proliferation within the marrow or the associated release of inflammatory mediators interferes with normal erythropoiesis.

An increase in the plasma bilirubin concentration imparts a yellow color to the plasma. Hyperbilirubinemia associated with a substantial decrease in the HCT suggests increased phagocytosis of RBCs.

If substantial intravascular hemolysis occurs rapidly, hemoglobinemia, and subsequently hemoglobinuria, may be observed. Disorders where significant intravascular hemolysis sometimes occurs include immune-mediated he-

TABLE 3–2. Comparison of Classification of Anemias by RBC Indices and Etiology

Normocytic Normochromic
1. Acute hemolysis before sufficient time has elapsed for significant reticulocyte response
2. Acute hemorrhage before sufficient time has elapsed for significant reticulocyte response or mild hemorrhage that does not stimulate substantial reticulocyte response
3. Early iron deficiency before microcytes predominate
4. Chronic inflammation and neoplasia (sometimes slightly microcytic)
5. Chronic renal disease
6. Endocrine deficiencies
7. Selective erythroid aplasia
8. Aplastic and hypoplastic bone marrows
9. Lead toxicity (may not be anemic)
10. Vitamin B_{12} deficiency

Macrocytic Hypochromic
1. Regenerative anemias with marked reticulocytosis
2. Hereditary stomatocytosis in dogs

Macrocytic Normochromic
1. Regenerative anemias (decreased MCHC is not always present)
2. FeLV infections with no reticulocytosis
3. Folate deficiency (rare)
4. Congenital dyserythropoiesis of Hereford calves
5. Erythroleukemia or AML-M6 and myelodysplastic syndromes
6. Poodle macrocytosis (healthy miniature poodles with no anemia)

Microcytic Normochromic/Hypochromic[a]
1. Chronic iron deficiency (months in adults, weeks in nursing animals)
2. Anemia of chronic disease (usually normocytic)
3. Portosystemic shunts in dogs (often not anemic)
4. Copper deficiency (rare)
5. Pyridoxine deficiency (experimental in pigs)
6. Familial dyserythropoiesis of English springer spaniel dogs
7. Normal Akita dogs (not anemic)

[a]The presence of low MCHC along with low MCV strongly suggests iron deficiency anemia.

molytic anemia, oxidant chemical and plant toxicities, severe hypophosphatemia, leptospiral and clostridial infections, coral snake venom, zinc toxicity, copper toxicity, babesiosis, hypoosmolality, vena caval syndrome of dirofilariasis in dogs, hepatic failure in horses, phosphofructokinase deficiency in dogs, postparturient cattle without hypophosphatemia, and splenic torsion in dogs. In most of these disorders, however, RBC destruction occurs primarily by increased phagocytosis.

BLOOD LOSS ANEMIAS

Causes of blood loss anemia are given in Table 3–4. In some cases, the diagnosis of blood loss anemia and its cause is apparent from the history and/or physical findings. In other cases, hemorrhage is apparent, but its cause must be determined. Finally, blood loss anemia and its cause may not be recognized until laboratory tests and other diagnostic tests are done. The gastrointestinal tract and urogenital tracts are common sites of occult hemorrhage. Tests that may assist in the diagnosis of gastrointestinal hemorrhage

TABLE 3–3. Causes of Hemolytic Anemias in Domestic Animals

1. **Immune-mediated RBC destruction**—Autoimmune hemolytic anemia (primarily dogs); neonatal isoerythrolysis (primarily horses and cats); lupus erythematosus (primarily dogs); incompatible blood transfusions; drugs including propylthiouracil (cats), penicillin, and cephalosporins.
2. **RBC parasites (may have an immune-mediated component)**—*Anaplasma* spp. (ruminants), *Haemobartonella* spp. (cats and dogs), *Eperythrozoon* spp. (pigs and sheep), *Babesia* spp., *Cytauxzoon felis*, *Theileria* spp. (ruminants, clinical disease outside the United States)
3. **Other infectious agents (may have an immune-mediated component)**—*Leptospira* and *Clostridium* spp. (primarily ruminants), feline leukemia virus (at times), equine infectious anemia virus, *Sarcocystis* spp. (cattle and sheep), *Trypanosoma* spp. (primarily outside the United States)
4. **Chemicals and plants (most are oxidants)**—Onions, red maple (horses), *Brassica* spp. (ruminants), lush winter rye (cattle), copper (sheep), phenothiazine (horses), acetaminophen (cats and dogs), methylene blue (cats and dogs), benzocaine (cats and dogs), phenazopyridine (cats), methionine (cats), vitamin K (dogs), propylene glycol (cats), naphthalene (dogs?), zinc (dogs and ruminants), indole (experimental in cattle and horses), tryptophan (experimental in horses), crude oil (marine birds), and snake venoms
5. **Fragmentation**—Disseminated intravascular coagulation (primarily dogs), dirofilariasis (especially vena caval syndrome) in dogs, hemangiosarcoma (dogs), vasculitis, hemolytic uremia syndrome
6. **Hypo-osmolality**—Hypotonic fluid administration (primarily in large animals), water intoxication (primarily in cattle)
7. **Hypophosphatemia**—Postparturient hemoglobinuria (cattle), ketoacidotic diabetic animals following insulin therapy (cats and dogs), hepatic lipidosis (cats), hyperalimentation (small animals)
8. **Hereditary RBC defects**—Pyruvate kinase deficiency (dogs and cats), phosphofructokinase deficiency (dogs), glucose-6-phosphate dehydrogenase deficiency (horses), hereditary stomatocytosis (mild anemia in dogs), erythropoietic porphyria (cattle), hereditary nonspherocytic hemolytic anemias of unknown etiology (poodle and beagle dogs and trotter horses with accompanying methemoglobinemia)
9. **Miscellaneous**—Liver failure (horses), hypersplenism, splenic torsion (dogs), selenium deficiency in cattle grazing on St. Augustine grass, postparturient hemoglobinuria in cattle not associated with hypophosphatemia

TABLE 3–4. Causes of Blood Loss Anemias in Domestic Animals

1. **Trauma and surgery**
2. **Parasites**—Hookworms, fleas, blood-sucking lice, *Haemonchus* spp., *Coccidia* spp.
3. **Coagulation disorders**—Vitamin K deficiency, sweet clover (dicoumarol) toxicity (cattle), rodenticide toxicity, bracken fern toxicity (cattle), disseminated intravascular coagulation, inherited coagulation factor deficiencies (see Chapter 5)
4. **Platelet disorders**—Thrombocytopenia and inherited platelet function defects (see Chapter 5)
5. **Neoplasia**—Gastric tumors including carcinomas and leiomyosarcomas, transitional cell carcinoma of the bladder (dogs), and hemangiosarcoma with bleeding into body cavities and tissues (dogs)
6. **Gastrointestinal ulcers**

include the occult blood test in feces, fecal examination for parasite ova, and radiographic procedures to identify tumors or ulcers. Urinalysis and radiographic evaluation of the urinary system may assist in the diagnosis of renal or bladder hemorrhage.

External Hemorrhage

Although total blood volume is decreased, HCT and plasma protein concentration are normal immediately after substantial acute blood loss has occurred because there is a balanced loss of RBCs and plasma. The HCT may even be increased shortly after acute blood loss in horses because splenic contraction occurs which releases blood with a higher HCT into the general circulation. After several hours the HCT and plasma protein concentration decrease as the animal drinks and as fluid moves from extravascular spaces into the circulation to return the blood volume toward normal. If no further hemorrhage occurs, the plasma protein concentration will return to normal within 5 to 7 days. Consequently, the occurrence of a low plasma protein concentration in association with anemia suggests the presence of recent or ongoing hemorrhage. Considerably more time is required for the HCT to return to normal than is required for the plasma protein concentration to return to normal. Following blood loss that reduces the HCT in half, the HCT increases about 0.4, 0.8, and 1.6% units per day in horses, cats, and dogs, respectively.

The anemia appears nonregenerative shortly after blood loss, because 3 or 4 days are required for production of reticulocytes by the marrow. The MCV may not be increased following blood loss in animals, because the reticulocyte response may not be of sufficient magnitude to result in a high MCV. Few reticulocytes are released from the marrow in response to blood loss anemia in cattle and no reticulocytes are released following hemorrhage in horses.

Chronic external blood loss can result in iron deficiency. Iron deficiency anemia is common in adult dogs and ruminants, but seldom occurs in adult cats and horses because parasitism causing significant blood loss is uncommon in these species. If iron deficiency persists for several weeks, the anemia can become microcytic and hypochromic. Reticulocyte counts may be slightly to moderately increased in early iron deficiency anemia in dogs; however, as iron deficiency becomes more severe, minimal regenerative response is present (see discussion of iron deficiency in next section).

Internal Hemorrhage

Hemorrhage may occur into body cavities or tissues. This internal hemorrhage can share some characteristics of hemolytic anemias. Iron is conserved so that hypoferremia does not occur. Some plasma proteins and RBCs may be reabsorbed when hemorrhage occurs in body cavities. Consequently, total plasma protein concentration may be only transiently decreased. Slight hyperbilirubinemia may occur from phagocytosis and degradation of RBCs at the site of hemorrhage.

DECREASED ERYTHROCYTE PRODUCTION ANEMIAS

Anemias resulting from decreased RBC production lack evidence of bone marrow response to the anemia (*e.g.*, the absolute reticulocyte count in blood is not increased or only minimally raised for the degree of anemia). Nonregenerative anemias result from reduced or defective erythropoiesis (Table 3–5). They are usually normocytic. Exceptions include microcytic anemia associated with chronic iron deficiency, copper deficiency, pyridoxine deficiency, and dyserythropoiesis in English springer spaniel dogs and macrocytic anemia associated with folate deficiency, FeLV infection in cats, erythroleukemia, some myelodysplastic disorders, and dyserythropoiesis in polled Hereford calves. Bone marrow biopsies are often required to delineate the nature of nonregenerative anemias.

Nonregenerative Anemias Without Leukopenia or Thrombocytopenia

A nonregenerative anemia without an accompanying leukopenia or thrombocytopenia in blood suggests a bone marrow abnormality affecting only erythroid cells. Mild to moderate anemia of this type may occur in association with chronic renal disease, endocrine deficiencies, and the anemia of chronic disease. Erythroid production is reduced in these disorders, but often not enough to result in an M:E ratio in the marrow that is increased above the reference range.

Hormone Deficiencies. Because the kidney is the major site of EPO production in the body, chronic renal disease can result in a mild to moderate

---

TABLE 3–5. Anemias Resulting from Decreased Erythrocyte Production in Domestic Animals

Reduced Erythropoiesis
1. **Chronic renal disease**—Primarily lack of erythropoietin
2. **Endocrine deficiencies**—Hypothyroidism, hypoadrenocorticism, hypopituitarism, hypoandrogenism
3. **Chronic disease**—Inflammation and neoplasia
4. **Cytotoxic damage to the marrow**—Bracken fern poisoning (cattle), cytotoxic anticancer drugs, estrogen toxicity (dogs and ferrets), chloramphenicol (cats, usually not anemic), phenylbutazone (dogs), trimethoprim-sulfadiazine (dogs), trichloroethylene (cattle), radiation
5. **Infectious agents**—*Ehrlichia* spp. (dogs, horses, and cats), FeLV, nonbloodsucking trichostrongyloid parasites (ruminants)
6. **Immune-mediated**—Selective erythroid aplasia (dogs), idiopathic aplastic anemia?
7. **Myelophthisis**—Myelogenous leukemias, lymphoid leukemias, myelodysplastic syndromes, multiple myeloma, myelofibrosis, osteosclerosis, metastatic lymphomas, and mast cell tumors

Defective Erythropoiesis
1. **Disorders of heme synthesis**—Iron, copper, and pyridoxine deficiency
2. **Disorders of nucleic acid synthesis**—Folate and vitamin B_{12} deficiency
3. **Abnormal maturation**—Erythroleukemia or AML-M6 (cats), myelodysplastic syndromes with erythroid predominance (MDS-Er), inherited dyserythropoiesis of Hereford calves, inherited dyserythropoiesis of English springer spaniels

nonregenerative anemia secondary to reduced EPO production. Disorders such as hypopituitarism, hypoadrenocorticism, hypothyroidism, and hypoandrogenism may result in mild nonregenerative anemia because these hormones apparently increase the number of erythroid colonies formed, possibly by modulating the fraction of erythroid progenitor cells that will enter terminal differentiation at a given EPO concentration.

Anemia of Chronic Disease. A mild to moderate nonregenerative anemia often accompanies chronic inflammatory and neoplastic disorders. The cause of the anemia is multifactorial and only partially understood. Abnormalities that can contribute to the anemia include low serum iron, the production of inflammatory mediators that can inhibit erythropoiesis, and shortened RBC life spans, presumably secondary to membrane damage caused by endogenous oxidants generated during inflammation.

Disorders of Nucleic Acid Synthesis. Anemias resulting from folate deficiency are rarely reported in animals. Macrocytic anemia has been produced experimentally in pigs and a case has been recognized in a cat eating canned tuna for 4 years. Vitamin B_{12} (cobalamin) deficiency in people causes hematologic abnormalities similar to folate deficiency because vitamin B_{12} is necessary for normal folate metabolism in humans. In contrast, vitamin B_{12} deficiency does not cause macrocytic anemia in any animal species. Anemia has been reported in some experimental animal studies, but RBCs were of normal size. Cobalamin deficiency occurs secondarily to an inherited malabsorption of cobalamin in giant schnauzer dogs. Affected animals have normocytic, nonregenerative anemia with increased anisocytosis. Additional findings include neutropenia with hypersegmented neutrophils and giant platelets. A normocytic nonregenerative anemia was also present in a cobalamin-deficient cat that probably had an inherited disorder of cobalamin absorption.

Abnormalities in Heme Synthesis. Iron deficiency in adult domestic animals usually results from blood loss. The absolute reticulocyte count may be increased early in response to hemorrhage, but as iron deficiency becomes more severe, minimal regenerative response is present. Microcytic RBCs form when iron becomes limiting because erythroid cells undergo additional divisions resulting in smaller than normal cells. If sufficient time has elapsed for these small cells to account for a substantial portion of the total RBC population, the MCV will decrease below the normal reference range. When the MCV is only slightly decreased, the MCHC is usually normal. When the MCV is substantially below normal, the MCHC will also be decreased (hypochromic). RBCs in these microcytic hypochromic anemias will appear hypochromic (pale cells with prominent areas of central pallor) on stained blood films. Hematologic aspects of iron deficiency are compared to the anemia of chronic disease in Table 3–6.

Milk contains little iron; consequently, nursing animals can deplete body iron stores as they grow. Microcytic RBCs are produced in response to iron deficiency but a low MCV may not develop postnatally in species where the MCV is above adult values at birth. The potential for development of severe iron deficiency in young animals appears to be less in species that begin to eat food at an early age. Piglets are especially susceptible to the development of iron deficiency when not raised on dirt. Thus, the practice of iron injections of piglets raised on slatted floors.

Prolonged copper deficiency usually results in anemia in mammals. Because copper is required for normal iron metabolism, the anemia that de-

TABLE 3–6. Laboratory Findings in Chronic Iron Deficiency Anemia *Versus* the Anemia of Chronic Disease

Parameter	Chronic Iron Deficiency	Anemia Chronic Disease
HCT	Slight to marked decrease	Slight to moderate decrease
MCV	Slight to marked decrease	Normal to slight decrease
Serum iron	Slight to marked decrease	Slight to moderate decrease
Serum TIBC	Normal to increased	Normal to decreased
Serum ferritin	Decreased	Normal to increased
Marrow hemosiderin	Decreased or absent	Normal to increased

TIBC, total iron-binding capacity.

velops is generally microcytic, but it may be normocytic. Pyridoxine, vitamin B$_6$, is required for the first step in heme synthesis. While natural cases of pyridoxine deficiency have not been documented in domestic animals, microcytic anemias with high serum iron values have been produced experimentally in dogs, cats, and pigs with dietary pyridoxine deficiency.

Selective Erythroid Aplasia. Pure red cell aplasia can result in severe anemia in dogs and cats. Most cases appear to be acquired, but congenital erythroid aplasia may occur in dogs. Some cases in adult dogs appear to be immune mediated. Erythroid hypoplasia or dysplasia is also reported to be a rare sequela to vaccination against parvovirus in dogs. Selective erythroid aplasia occurs in cats infected with FeLV subgroup C, but not in cats infected only with subgroups A or B. High doses of chloramphenicol cause reversible erythroid hypoplasia in some dogs and erythroid aplasia in cats.

Dyserythropoiesis. Abnormal RBC maturation occurs as a component of inherited disorders in Hereford calves and English springer spaniel dogs. Megaloblastic erythroid cells are often seen in the bone marrow of animals (especially cats) with erythroleukemia and myelodysplastic syndromes with erythroid predominance, but other cytopenias are usually also present.

Nonregenerative Anemias With Leukopenia and/or Thrombocytopenia

This pattern suggests that either the marrow is hypocellular or high numbers of abnormal cells have replaced the normal hematopoietic precursers (myelophthisis). Pancytopenia may occasionally be present in blood in disorders other than marrow hypoplasia or aplasia and myelophthisis. Examples include the terminal stage of cytauxzoonosis in cats and anemic animals that develop septicemia. These disorders involve the peripheral utilization/destruction of blood cells.

Aplastic Anemia. This term is used to describe an anemia where granulocytic, megakaryocytic, and erythrocytic cell lines are markedly reduced in the bone marrow. When only the erythroid cell line is reduced or absent, terms such as pure red cell aplasia or selective erythroid aplasia or hypoplasia are used. These anemias can result from insufficient numbers of stem cells, abnormalities in the hematopoietic microenvironment, or abnormal humoral or cellular control of hematopoiesis. The above factors are interrelated and the exact defect in a given disorder is usually unknown.

Drug-induced causes of aplastic anemia or generalized marrow hypoplasia in animals include estrogen toxicity in dogs and ferrets, phenylbutazone toxicity in dogs, trimethoprim-sulfadiazine administration in dogs, bracken fern poisoning in cattle and sheep, trichloroethylene-extracted soybean meal in cattle, and various cancer chemotherapeutic agents and radiation. Thiacetarsamide, meclofenamic acid, and quinidine have also been incriminated as potential causes of aplastic anemia in dogs, as has griseofulvin in a cat.

Although some degree of marrow hypoplasia and/or dysplasia often occurs in cats with FeLV infections, true aplastic anemia is not a well-documented sequela. Anemia is a common finding in ill cats infected with feline immunodeficiency virus (FIV). It does not appear to result from a direct action(s) of the virus on erythroid progenitor cells, but generally occurs secondarily to inflammation, dysplasia, or neoplasia. Dogs that enter the chronic stage of ehrlichiosis generally have some degree of marrow hypoplasia and in severe cases can develop aplastic anemias.

Parvovirus infections can cause severe erythroid hypoplasia, as well as myeloid hypoplasia in canine pups, but animals usually do not become anemic because of the long life spans of RBCs. Either affected pups die acutely or the bone marrow returns rapidly to normal before anemia can develop. In contrast to its effects in pups, parvovirus is reported to have a minimal effect on erythroid progenitors in adult dogs. Parvovirus inhibits colony formation of both myeloid and erythroid progenitor cells in feline bone marrow cultures, but only myeloid hypoplasia was reported during histologic examination of bone marrow from viremic cats. Idiopathic aplastic anemias have also been reported in dogs and horses.

Myelophthisic Disorders.   Myelophthisic disorders are characterized by the replacement of normal hematopoietic cells with abnormal ones. Examples include myelogenous leukemias; lymphoid leukemias; multiple myeloma; myelodysplastic syndromes; myelofibrosis; osteosclerosis; and metastasis of lymphomas, carcinomas, and mast cell tumors. Myelophthisic disorders do not simply "crowd out" normal cells, but also alter the marrow microenvironment so that normal hematopoiesis is compromised. In the case of myelodysplastic syndromes, increased apoptosis (programmed cell death) probably accounts for the ineffective hematopoiesis that is present.

Physiologic Anemia of Neonatal Animals

HCT and Hb values increase during fetal development, reaching values near those of adult animals at birth (Fig. 3–14). Following birth, there is a rapid decrease in these parameters during the first few weeks of life that is followed by a gradual increase to adult values by 4 months of age in most species (Fig. 3–15). Factors involved in the development of the anemia of the neonate include absorption of colostral proteins during the first day of life (increases plasma volume through an osmotic effect), decreased RBC production during the early neonatal period, shortened life span of RBCs formed *in utero*, and rapid growth with hemodilution resulting from expansion of total plasma volumes more rapidly than total RBC mass.

In some species, production of RBCs is decreased because of low EPO concentrations at birth. The decreased stimulus for EPO production at birth may occur as a result of a placental blood transfusion that increases RBC

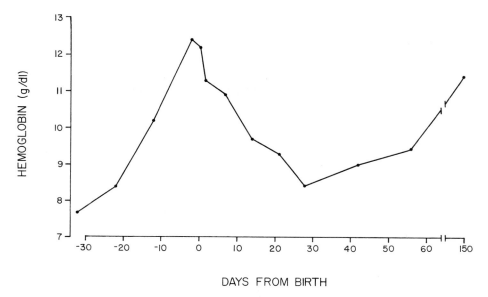

FIGURE 3–14. Blood hemoglobin values in prenatal and postnatal cats. (The graph used data from Windle WF, Sweet M, Whitehead WH: Some aspects of prenatal and postnatal development of the blood of cats. Anat Rec 1940;78:321.)

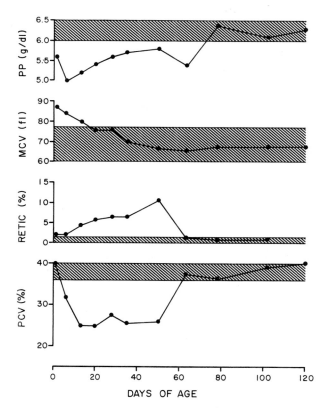

FIGURE 3–15. Age-related changes in total plasma protein (PP) concentration, mean cell volume (MCV), reticulocyte (RETIC) count, and packed cell volume (PCV) in blood from a basenji dog.

mass immediately after birth, a rapid increase in Po_2 associated with breathing air, and a decrease in Hb oxygen affinity resulting from an increase in RBC 2,3-DPG content after birth. Although not involved in the early, rapid decrease in HCT, iron availability may limit the response to anemia in some rapidly growing animals.

ERYTHROCYTOSIS (POLYCYTHEMIA)

Erythrocytosis refers to an increase in HCT, Hb, and RBC count above the normal reference range. The reference range can sometimes vary by breed as well as by species. The HCTs of hot-blooded horses (*e.g.*, thoroughbreds, quarter horses, and Arabians) are usually higher than those of draft horses, because of much larger spleens in the hot-blooded group. The reference range for the HCT in greyhound dogs (49 to 65%) is higher than that of other breeds. In addition, slightly increased HCTs are occasionally measured in individuals from certain breeds of dogs (*i.e.*, poodle, German shepherd, boxer, beagle, dachshund, and Chihuahua). These higher values are believed to result from splenic contraction in animals with a high normal RBC mass.

Relative Erythrocytosis

Erythrocytosis is either relative (spurious) or absolute (Table 3–7). A relative erythrocytosis is one in which the HCT is high, but the total RBC mass is normal. It is caused by splenic contraction or dehydration. Splenic contraction is stimulated by epinephrine release as occurs with excitement, fear, pain, or exercise. The HCT measured in blood from peripheral veins increases because the HCT in the spleen is considerably higher than that in the general circulation. Increases in HCT are pronounced in hot-blooded horses, which have especially large contractile spleens.

Dehydration results from increased water loss (diarrhea, vomiting, excessive diuresis, or sweating), or from water deprivation. The plasma protein concentration is also usually increased. The HCT may also be high when increased vascular permeability results in protein and water loss from the circulation into the tissues, as occurs in endotoxic shock.

TABLE 3–7. Erythrocytosis (Polycythemia) in Domestic Animals

Relative Erythrocytosis
1. **Splenic contraction**—Excitement, exercise, pain (primarily in horses, dogs, and cats)
2. **Dehydration**—Water loss, water deprivation, shock with fluid shift into tissues

Absolute Erythrocytosis
1. **Polycythemia vera**—A myeloproliferative disorder in adult dogs and cats
2. **Familial erythrocytosis in young cattle**—Etiology unknown
3. **Hypoxemia with compensatory increased erythropoietin production**—High altitude, chronic lung disease, heart disease with right-to-left shunting of blood, chronic methemoglobinemia (rare in dogs and cats)
4. **Inappropriate erythropoietin production**—Renal tumors, renal cysts, hydronephrosis (rare), nonrenal erythropoietin-secreting tumors (rare)

Absolute Erythrocytosis

An absolute erythrocytosis is one in which the HCT is high because the total RBC mass in the body is increased. Absolute erythrocytosis may occur secondary to increased EPO production (secondary erythrocytosis) or in disorders where increased RBC proliferation occurs in the presence of normal or low blood EPO values (primary erythrocytosis). Causes of secondary erythrocytosis include chronic hypoxemia (heart defects with right-to-left shunting of blood, chronic lung disease, high altitude, methemoglobinemia), renal disorders causing local tissue hypoxia (renal tumors, renal cysts, hydronephrosis), and EPO-secreting tumors.

Primary erthrocytosis in adult dogs and cats is generally called polycythemia vera. It results from an autonomous (EPO-independent) proliferation of erythroid precursor cells; consequently, polycythemia vera is considered a myeloproliferative disorder.

Familial erythrocytosis (HCTs of 60 to 80%) has been described in calves from a highly inbred Jersey herd. The cause of this defect was not determined. Affected calves had normal Hb types and arterial blood gas values, and lacked measured EPO in plasma. The majority of affected calves died by 6 months of age. HCTs of surviving animals returned slowly to normal by maturity.

Differential Diagnosis of Erythrocytosis

Splenic contraction is considered a likely cause of erythrocytosis when the HCT is slightly to moderately increased in the absence of evidence of dehydration. A slight to moderate increase in these values with increased plasma protein concentration suggests that dehydration is present. This interpretation is confirmed by finding evidence of dehydration on physical examination.

The persistence of a moderate or marked increase in HCT suggests that an absolute erythrocytosis is present. Tests that may help determine the cause of the absolute erythrocytosis include arterial blood gas measurements, diagnostic imaging, a methemoglobin screening test, and a validated EPO test. The cytologic examination of bone marrow is not useful. When present, methemoglobinemia is easily recognized using a simple spot test (see previous methemoglobinemia section). The presence of low arterial Po_2 suggests that either a heart defect (with right-to-left shunting of blood) or chronic lung disease is present. Diagnostic imaging procedures are used to differentiate heart and lung disease and examine for renal lesions. Plasma EPO values should be increased when hypoxemia, renal lesions, or EPO-secreting tumors cause the erythrocytosis, but low when polycythemia vera is present. A diagnosis of polycythemia vera is reached after ruling out other potential causes of persistent erythrocytosis.

References

Adams LG, Hardy RM, Weiss DJ, et al: Hypophosphatemia and hemolytic anemia associated with diabetes mellitus and hepatic lipidosis in cats. J Vet Intern Med 1993;7:266.

Andrews GA, Chavey PS, Smith JE: Enzyme-linked immunosorbent assay to measure serum ferritin and the relationship between serum ferritin and nonheme iron stores in cats. Vet Pathol 1994;31:674.

Brown DE, Meyer DJ, Wingfield WE, et al: Echinocytosis associated with rattlesnake envenomation in dogs. Vet Pathol 1994;31:654.

Bunch SE, Jordan HL, Sellon RK, et al: Characterization of iron status in young dogs with portosystemic shunt. Am J Vet Res 1995;56:853.

Callan MB, Jones LT, Giger U: Hemolytic transfusion reactions in a dog with an alloantibody to a common antigen. J Vet Intern Med 1995;9:277.

Cavill I: The rejected reticulocyte. Br J Haematol 1993;84:563.

Christopher MM, Broussard JD, Peterson ME: Heinz body formation associated with ketoacidosis in diabetic cats. J Vet Intern Med 1995;9:24.

Christopher MM, Harvey JW: Specialized hematology tests. Semin Vet Med Surg Small Anim 1992;7:301.

Christopher MM, Lee SE: Red cell morphologic alterations in cats with hepatic disease. Vet Clin Pathol 1994;23:7.

Cook SM, Lothrop CD Jr: Serum erythropoietin concentrations measured by radio-immunoassay in normal, polycythemic and anemic dogs and cats. J Vet Intern Med 1994;8:18.

Cotter SM: Autoimmune hemolytic anemia in dogs. Comp Contin Educ Pract Vet 1992;14:53.

Crow SE, Allen DP, Murphy CJ, et al: Concurrent renal adenocarcinoma and polycythemia in a dog. J Am Anim Hosp Assoc 1995;31:29.

Crystal MA, Cotter SM: Acute hemorrhage: A hematologic emergency in dogs. Comp Contin Educ Pract Vet 1992;14:60.

De Waal DT: Equine piroplasmosis: A review. Br Vet J 1992;148:6.

Desnoyers M, Hebert P: Heinz body anemia in a dog following possible naphthalene ingestion. Vet Clin Pathol 1995;24:124.

Durando MM, Alleman AR, Harvey JW: Myelodysplastic syndrome in a quarter horse gelding. Equine Vet J 1994;26:83.

Erslev AJ: Anemia of chronic disease. In Beutler E, Lichtman MA, Coller BS, Kipps TJ (eds): Williams Hematology, 5th ed. New York, McGraw-Hill, 1995, p 518.

Evans LM, Caylor KB: Polycythemia vera in a cat and management with hydroxyurea. J Am Anim Hosp Assoc 1995;31:434.

Fox LE, Ford S, Alleman AR, et al: Aplastic anemia associated with prolonged high-dose trimethoprim-sulfadiazine administration in two dogs. Vet Clin Pathol 1993;22:89.

Freeman MJ, Kirby BM, Panciera DL, et al: Hypotensive shock syndrome associated with acute Babesia canis infection in a dog. J Am Vet Med Assoc 1994;204:94.

Garner MM, Lung NP, Citino S, et al: Fatal cytauxzoonosis in a captive-reared white tiger (Panthera tigris). Vet Pathol 1996;33:82.

Geor RJ, Lund EM, Weiss DJ: Echinocytosis in horses: 54 cases (1990). J Am Vet Med Assoc 1993;202:976.

Giger U: Erythropoietin and its clinical use. Comp Contin Educ Pract Vet 1992;14:25.

Harvey JW: Methemoglobinemia and Heinz-body hemolytic anemia. In Bonagura JD (ed): Kirk's Current Veterinary Therapy XII. Small Animal Practice. Philadelphia, WB Saunders Co, 1995, p 443.

Harvey JW: Congenital erythrocyte enzyme deficiencies. Vet Clin North Am Small Anim Pract 1996;26:1003.

Harvey JW: The erythrocyte: Physiology, metabolism and biochemical disorders. In Kaneko JJ, Bruss ML, Harvey JW (eds): Clinical Biochemistry of Domestic Animals, 5th ed. San Diego, Academic Press, 1997 (in press).

Harvey JW: Haemobartonellosis. In Greene CE (ed): Infectious Diseases of the Dog and Cat, 2nd ed. Philadelphia, WB Saunders Co, 1997 (in press).

Holloway S, Senior D, Roth L, et al: Hemolytic uremic syndrome in dogs. J Vet Intern Med 1993;7:220.

Hoover JP, Walker DB, Hedges JD: Cytauxzoonosis in cats: Eight cases (1985–1992). J Am Vet Med Assoc 1994;205:455.

Houston DM, Myers SL: A review of Heinz-body anemia in the dog induced by toxins. Vet Hum Toxicol 1993;35:158.

Jain NC: Essentials of Veterinary Hematology. Philadelphia, Lea & Febiger, 1993.

Kaplan AJ: Onion powder in baby food may induce anemia in cats. J Am Vet Med Assoc 1995;207:1405.

King LG, Giger U, Diserens D, et al: Anemia of chronic renal failure in dogs. J Vet Intern Med 1992;6:264.

Klag AR, Giger U, Shofer FS: Idiopathic immune-mediated hemolytic anemia in dogs: 42 Cases (1986–1990). J Am Vet Med Assoc 1993;202:783.

Mandell CP, Jain NC, Farver TB: The significance of normoblastemia and leuko-erythroblastic reaction in the dog. J Am Anim Hosp Assoc 1989;25:665.

McConnico RS, Roberts MC, Tompkins M: Penicillin-induced immune-mediated hemolytic anemia in a horse. J Am Vet Med Assoc 1992;201:1402.

Meyer DJ, Harvey JW: Hematologic changes associated with serum and hepatic iron alterations in dogs with congenital portosystemic vascular abnormalities. J Vet Intern Med 1994;8:55.

Meyers S, Wiks K, Giger U: Macrocytic anemia caused by naturally occurring folate-deficiency in the cat. Vet Clin Pathol 1996;25:30.

Mogg TD, Palmer JE: Hyperlipidemia, hyperlipemia, and hepatic lipidosis in American miniature horses: 23 cases (1990–1994). J Am Vet Med Assoc 1995;207:604.

Morin DE, Garry FB, Weiser MG, et al: Hematologic features of iron deficiency anemia in llamas. Vet Pathol 1992;29:400.

Nash AS, Bobade PA: Haemobartonellosis. In Woldehiwet Z, Ristic M (eds): Rickettsial and Chlamydial Diseases of Domestic Animals. New York, Pergamon Press, 1993, p 89.

Newlands CE, Houston DM, Vasconcelos DY: Hyperferritinemia associated with malignant histiocytosis in a dog. J Am Vet Med Assoc 1994;205:849.

O'Keefe DA, Schaeffer DJ: Hematologic toxicosis associated with doxorubicin administration in cats. J Vet Intern Med 1992;6:276.

Perkins PC, Grindem CB: Evaluation of six cytometric methods for reticulocyte enumeration and differentiation in the cat. Vet Clin Pathol 1995;24:37.

Perkins PC, Grindem CB, Cullins LD: Flow cytometric analysis of punctate and aggregate reticulocyte responses in phlebotomized cats. Am J Vet Res 1995;56:1564.

Prache S: Haemolytic anaemia in ruminants fed forage brassicas: A review. Vet Res 1994;25:497.

Reagan WJ, Carter C, Turek J: Eccentrocytosis in equine red maple leaf toxicosis. Vet Clin Pathol 1994;23:123.

Schlesinger DP: Methemoglobinemia and anemia in a dog with acetaminophen toxicity. Can Vet J 1995;36:515.

Scott GR, Woldehiwet Z: Eperythrozoonoses. In Woldehiwet Z, Ristic M (eds): Rickettsial and Chlamydial Diseases of Domestic Animals. New York, Pergamon Press, 1993, p 111.

Sellon DC, Fuller FJ, McGuire TC: The immunopathogenesis of equine infectious anemia virus. Virus Res 1994;32:111.

Skikne BS, Cook JD: Effect of enhanced erythropoiesis on iron absorption. J Lab Clin Med 1992;120:746.

Skinner JG, Roberts L: Haptoglobin as an indicator of infection in sheep. Vet Rec 1994;134:33.

Sparkes AH, Hopper CD, Millard WG, et al: Feline immunodeficiency virus infection. Clinicopathologic findings in 90 naturally occurring cases. J Vet Intern Med 1993; 7:85.

Steffen DJ, Elliott GS, Leipold HW, et al: Congenital dyserythropoiesis and progressive alopecia in polled Hereford calves: Hematologic, biochemical, bone marrow cytologic, electrophoretic, and flow cytometric findings. J Vet Diagn Invest 1992;4:31.

Stockham SL, Harvey JW, Kinden DA: Equine glucose-6-phosphate dehydrogenase deficiency. Vet Pathol 1994;31:518.

Tyler RD, Cowell RL: Classification and diagnosis of anemia. Comp Haematol Int 1996;6:1.

Vaden SL, Wood PA, Ledley FD, et al: Cobalamin deficiency associated with methylmalonic acidemia in a cat. J Am Vet Med Assoc 1992;200:1101.

Walker DB, Cowell RL: Survival of a domestic cat with naturally acquired cytauxzoonosis. J Am Vet Med Assoc 1995;206:1363.

Walton RM, Modiano JF, Thrall MA, et al: Bone marrow cytological findings in 4 dogs and a cat with hemophagocytic syndrome. J Vet Intern Med 1996;10:7.

Wanduragala L, Ristic M: Anaplasmosis. In Woldehiwet Z, Ristic M (eds): Rickettsial and Chlamydial Diseases of Domestic Animals. New York, Pergamon Press, 1993, p 65.

Watson TDG: Lipoprotein metabolism in dogs and cats. Comp Haematol Int 1996; 6:17.

Weiss DJ, Geor RJ: Clinical and rheological implications of echinocytosis in the horse: A review. Comp Haematol Int 1993;3:185.

Weiss DJ, Kristensen A, Papenfuss N: Quantitative evaluation of irregularly spiculated red blood cells in the dog. Vet Clin Pathol 1993;22:117.

Whitney MS: Evaluation of hyperlipidemia in dogs and cats. Semin Vet Med Surg Small Anim 1992;7:292.

4

Evaluation of Leukocytic Disorders

NORMAL LEUKOCYTES

Classification and Numbers in Blood

Mammalian leukocytes or white blood cells (WBCs) have been classified as either polymorphonuclear (PMN) or mononuclear leukocytes. The polymorphonuclear leukocytes have condensed, segmented nuclei. They are commonly referred to as granulocytes because they contain large numbers of cytoplasmic granules. The term granulocyte is preferred in veterinary medicine because nuclear segmentation does not occur in the granulocytes of most reptiles, and it is not as prominent in birds as it is in mammals. The granules in these cells are lysosomes containing hydrolytic enzymes, antibacterial agents, and other compounds. Primary granules are synthesized in the cytoplasm of late myeloblasts or early promyelocytes. They appear azurophilic (reddish purple) when stained with routine blood stains such as Wright-Giemsa. Secondary (specific) granules appear at the myelocyte stage of development in the bone marrow. Three types of granulocytes (neutrophils, eosinophils, basophils) are identified by the staining characteristics of their secondary granules (Color Plate 3).

In most mammalian species, neutrophil granules either do not stain or appear light pink with routine blood stains. In birds, reptiles, and some mammalian species (e.g., rabbits, guinea pigs, and manatees), the granules of these cells stain red and the cells are called heterophils. They must be differentiated from eosinophils, which also have red-staining granules. The granule shape can often help differentiate these cells. Heterophils usually have rod-shaped or oval granules and eosinophils usually have round granules. Eosinophils are so named because their granules have an affinity for eosin, the red dye in routine blood stains (Color Plate 3). Eosinophils from domestic cats have rod-shaped granules, but they are easily differentiated from neutrophils in this species. Eosinophils from dogs often exhibit cytoplasmic vacuoles. Eosinophils from greyhound dogs appear highly vacuolated and may be mistaken for vacuolated neutrophils by inexperienced observers. Iguanas and psittacine birds have WBCs with green-staining granules that are believed to be eosinophils. Basophil granules are acidic and consequently have an affinity for the basic (blue) dyes in routine blood stains (Color Plate 3). The basophils of domestic cats are distinctive. Their primary granules are dark blue and their secondary granules are light lavender in color. Often only the light lavender granules are observed in basophils present in blood smears.

Mononuclear leukocytes in blood are classified as either lymphocytes or monocytes (Color Plate 3). These cells are not devoid of granules, but rather have lower numbers of cytoplasmic granules than do granulocytes. T- and B-lymphocytes cannot be differentiated from one another based on morphology in stained blood films. Lymphocytes have high nuclear to cytoplasmic ratios. Their nuclei have coarsely clumped chromatin. Nuclei are usually round, but may be oval or slightly indented. Most lymphocytes in the blood of domestic animals are small to medium in size. Lymphocytes in cattle are often larger with more abundant cytoplasm than is seen in other species, sometimes making these cells difficult to differentiate from monocytes. Monocytes are usually larger than lymphocytes, have nuclei with finer chromatin clumping that are more variable in shape (round-, kidney-, or band-shaped) and have nuclear to cytoplasmic ratios of 1 or less. Monocytes often exhibit cytoplasmic vacuoles in films prepared from blood collected with an anticoagulant. A low percentage of lymphocytes in blood have focal accumulations of red- or purple-staining granules within the cytoplasm (Color Plate 4). Many of these granular lymphocytes appear to be natural killer (NK) cells. Dust-like red- or purple-staining granules may also be seen dispersed within the cytoplasm of monocytes.

The total number of WBCs varies considerably by species. Of common domestic animals, the mean WBC count is highest in pigs (16,000/μL) and lowest in cattle and sheep (8000/μL). Neutrophils and lymphocytes are the most numerous WBC types present in blood of healthy domestic mammals. Dogs, cats, and horses usually have more neutrophils in blood than lymphocytes. In contrast, lymphocytes are usually most numerous in pigs, cattle, sheep, and goats. Numbers of neutrophils and lymphocytes change with age after birth. The neutrophil to lymphocyte ratio tends to be higher at birth than in later life, in part because of increased blood cortisol concentrations at birth. Cortisol causes circulating neutrophil numbers to increase and circulating lymphocyte numbers to decrease. Ruminants have neutrophil to lymphocyte ratios above 1.0 at birth due to neutrophil numbers above and lymphocyte numbers below those of adults. Within 24 hours, the number of neutrophils decreases and the number of lymphocytes increases, with lymphocytes exceeding neutrophils during the first week of life. Low numbers of monocytes, eosinophils, and basophils are present in normal mammals. Basophil numbers are especially low in dogs and cats, with none being seen in blood from many normal animals.

Leukocyte Kinetics

In contrast to erythrocytes, WBCs do not exhibit a life span in blood, but rather leave blood randomly in response to chemotactic stimuli. Following release from bone marrow, neutrophils are normally present in blood for only a few hours before egress into the tissues. Neutrophils occur in circulating and marginal pools in blood, with 50% or less of the total blood neutrophil pool being present in the circulating pool (Fig. 4–1). The circulating neutrophil pool (CNP) is assessed by routine blood sample collection procedures. Much of the marginal neutrophil pool (MNP) is present within lung capillaries. The MNP consists primarily of neutrophils that transiently stop moving in capillaries. Lesser numbers of marginating neutrophils are rolling along arteriolar and venular endothelial surfaces. A net movement of neutrophils from the MNP to the CNP increases the circulating blood neutrophil count. A net movement in the opposite direction results in a decreased circulating blood neutrophil count. Eosinophils, basophils, and monocytes are also present in blood for a short time (less than a day) before randomly leaving the blood and entering the tissues.

Except for certain lymphocyte populations, leukocytes do not reenter the circulation after migration into the tissues. Neutrophils, eosinophils, and basophils appear to survive no more than a few days in tissues and their survival is much shorter in sites of inflammation. In contrast, monocytes develop into macrophages in the tissues where, under normal conditions, they survive weeks to months.

Most lymphocytes reside within lymphoid organs (lymph nodes, thymus, spleen, and bone marrow). A small number of lymphocytes circulate in blood. Most lymphocytes in blood have come from peripheral lymphoid organs (primarily lymph nodes). Depending on the species and individual variability, about 50 to 75% of blood lymphocytes are T-lymphocytes and about 20 to 35% are B-lymphocytes. NK cells appear as large granular lymphocytes in most species and account for 5 to 10% of blood lymphocytes. Many blood lymphocytes are memory cells, which are thought to be antigen-primed and in a resting state. They naturally express levels of adhesion molecules that

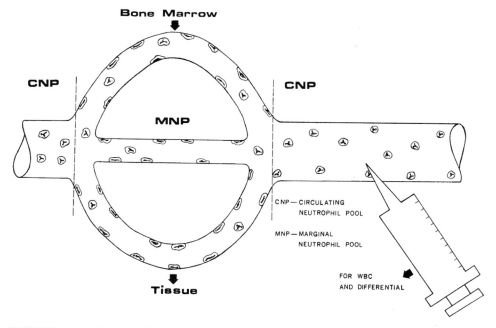

FIGURE 4–1. Neutrophil distribution in blood. Neutrophils occur in the circulating neutrophil pool (CNP) and marginal neutrophil pool (MNP), with 50% or less of the total blood neutrophil pool being present in the CNP.

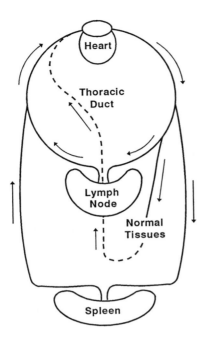

FIGURE 4–2. Circulation routes for lymphocytes. Solid lines represent blood vessels and dashed lines represent lymphatic vessels.

allow them to circulate from blood, through tissue, and then back into blood. It is estimated that recirculating lymphocytes enter a new lymphoid organ or tissue every 1 to 2 days. This allows the full repertoire of lymphocytes to be available for immune reactions throughout the body. Most of the blood lymphocytes migrate into lymph nodes through high endothelial venules (HEVs), exit the lymph nodes in the efferent lymphatics, traverse the thoracic duct, and reenter the blood (Fig. 4–2). Low numbers of blood lymphocytes enter tissues such as skin and intestinal mucosa through vessels with activated endothelial cells, are picked up by peripheral lymphatics, and carried to lymph nodes where they exit by efferent lymphatics, traverse the thoracic duct, and reenter the blood. Recirculating lymphocytes bind to and traverse HEVs and vessels with activated endothelial cells because these cell types have adhesion molecules on their surfaces that recognize complementary adhesion molecules expressed on lymphocyte surfaces. Lymphocytes that have been exposed to an antigen in a given tissue tend to develop adhesion molecules that favor its return to that tissue. Plasma cells and proliferating lymphocytes such as occur in germinal centers do not express the adhesion molecules necessary for migration.

Lymphocytes generally survive much longer than granulocytes. T-lymphocytes generally survive several years. Memory B-lymphocytes are also long-lived. Survival of other B-lymphocytes is shorter, often lasting only a few days. NK cell life spans have not been well characterized, with values from a few days to several months being reported in laboratory animals.

Leukocyte Functions

Neutrophil Functions. Neutrophils are essential in the defense against invading microorganisms, primarily bacteria. To be effective, they must recognize inflammatory signals, leave the blood, migrate through tissue to a site where bacteria are present, and then neutralize them. Neutrophils display glycoprotein adhesion molecules on their surfaces that are needed for various adhesion-dependent functions including adhesion to endothelium and subendothelial structures, spreading, chemotaxis, and phagocytosis. Unless activated, neutrophils and endothelial cells exhibit little tendency to adhere to each other. When endothelial cells are activated by inflammatory mediators such as histamine, interleukin-1 (IL-1), and tumor necrosis factor (TNF), they rapidly express P-selectin (from storage granules) and E-selectin adhesion molecules on their surface. The expression of these oligosaccharide-binding glycoproteins, acting in concert with the L-selectin adhesion molecule expressed on the surface neutrophils, results in the initial adhesion of unstimulated neutrophils to activated endothelial cells (Fig. 4–3). As a result, the velocity of neutrophils in the circulation is markedly decreased and they are seen to roll along endothelium.

Activated endothelial cells produce factors including interleukin-8 (IL-8) and platelet activating factor (PAF) (a biologically active phospholipid) that result in neutrophil activation. Other mediators that can activate neutrophils include opsonized particles, immune complexes, granulocyte-macrophage colony-stimulating factor (GM-CSF), granulocyte colony-stimulating factor (G-CSF), and chemotactic factors produced during inflammation. Neutrophil activation results in increased expression and enhanced binding affinity of β_2 integrin adhesion molecules, but shedding of L-selectin molecules. β_2 integrins (CD11a,b,c/CD18) are heterodimers that bind to varying degrees to intercellular adhesion molecules (ICAMs). The tight binding of β_2 integrins to ICAMs (which are up-regulated on activated endothelial cells) results in firm adhesion of neutrophils to endothelial cells. Adherent (activated) neutrophils

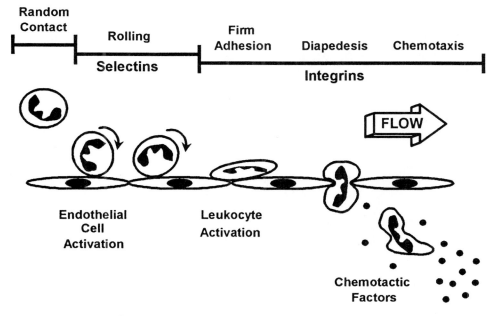

FIGURE 4–3. Endothelial cell activation, neutrophil rolling along vessel walls, tight adhesion between neutrophils and endothelial cells, diapedesis, and chemotaxis.

spread and exhibit pseudopod formation. Neutrophil activation also promotes degranulation, superoxide generation, and production of arachidonate metabolites to be discussed later.

In addition to increased β_2 integrins, activated neutrophils have increased numbers of receptors and/or enhanced receptor affinity for chemotactic agents on their surfaces. These receptors are also found in granules, suggesting that they are mobilized to the cell surface during neutrophil activation. When exposed to a chemoattractant, neutrophils penetrate the vessel wall by moving between endothelial cells. Neutrophils crawl toward the source of the chemoattractant in a "treadmill" pattern of motion by apposition of new β_2 integrin adhesion molecules to their respective receptors on cells or within the extracellular matrix. This directional active migration of neutrophils toward a point of greatest concentrations of chemoattractants is called chemotaxis. A wide variety of substances can function as chemoattractants. They include plasma protein fragments (C5a complement fragment and kallikrein), leukotriene B_4 (a product of arachidonic acid metabolism via the lipoxygenase pathway), lymphokines and monokines (including various colony-stimulating factors), PAF (1-0-alkyl-2-acetyl sn-glyceryl phosphorylcholine), and bacterial products (*e.g.*, N-formyl-methionyl oligopeptides).

For phagocytosis to occur, neutrophils must be able to first bind invading bacteria to their surfaces (Fig. 4–4). This adherence is greatly potentiated if bacteria have been opsonized (have antibodies and complement components bound to their surfaces) because neutrophils have immunoglobulin Fc (CD32) and C3b (CD35) receptors on their surfaces. Following binding, bacteria are engulfed by extending cytoplasmic processes around the organisms.

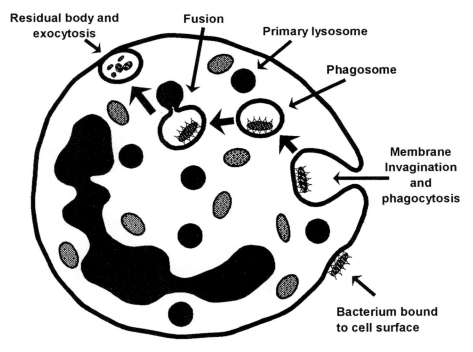

FIGURE 4–4. Basic events involved in the phagocytosis, killing, and discharge of killed bacteria and degraded bacterial products.

The membrane that surrounds the phagocytic vacuole that is formed came from the plasma membrane of the neutrophil.

Bacterial killing involves a multiplicity of mechanisms that are set into motion by two cellular events: initiation of the respiratory burst and degranulation. The respiratory burst is initiated by the activation of an NADPH oxidase enzyme (Fig. 4–5). This enzyme is normally "inactive" in resting (unstimulated phagocytes). Enzyme activation depends on the assembly of multiple components, some of which are already membrane-bound and others must be translocated from the cytoplasm to the membrane. Activated NADPH oxidase is located in plasma membrane and becomes incorporated into the phagocytic vacuole. It catalyzes the one-step reduction of O_2 to form superoxide (O_2^-). The NADPH needed to generate superoxide is formed in the pentose phosphate pathway. The superoxide formed undergoes dismutation to form hydrogen peroxide as shown below.

$$2O_2 + NADPH \rightarrow 2O_2^- + NADP^+ + H^+ (oxidation)$$

$$2O_2^- + 2H^+ \rightarrow O_2 + H_2O_2 \ (dismutation).$$

Hydrogen peroxide and superoxide can diffuse from the phagocytic vacuole into the cytoplasm of the cell. Activated neutrophils utilize the superoxide dismutase and glutathione peroxidase reactions to protect themselves from these oxidants. The latter reaction requires that additional NADPH be generated to maintain glutathione in the reduced form. Activation of the respiratory burst requires neither phagocytosis nor degranulation to occur. In addition to opsonized particles, soluble factors such as C5a can activate the respiratory burst.

Superoxide, other free radicals (e.g., hydroxyl radical), and H_2O_2 may be involved directly in the killing of bacteria, but killing is potentiated by degranulation, which results in the fusion and release of contents of lysosomal

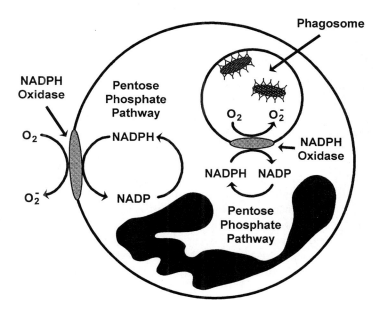

FIGURE 4–5. Generation of superoxide free radicals by the membrane-associated NADPH oxidase enzyme.

granules into the phagocytic vacuole (Fig. 4–4). Myeloperoxidase is an iron-containing enzyme located in the primary granules of neutrophils. The myeloperoxidase reaction greatly enhances the bactericidal potency of H_2O_2. This reaction apparently catalyzes oxidation of chloride to hypochlorous acid, resulting in halogenation of bacterial cell walls (see below) and loss of integrity.

$$Cl^- + H_2O_2 + H^+ \rightarrow HOCl + H_2O$$

$$R\text{-}NH_2 + HOCl \rightarrow R\text{-}NHCl + H_2O.$$

Other enzymes are also present in primary and secondary granules. These include collagenase, acid and neutral hydrolases, and lysozyme which hydrolyzes glycosidic linkages in cell walls of certain bacteria. These enzymes are probably more important in digestion than in killing. Nonenzymatic agents are also involved in neutrophil defense. Definsins are small antimicrobial peptides (4000 MW) within primary granules that act against bacteria and other microorganisms by altering their membrane permeability. They are inserted into the lipid bilayer, disrupting interaction between lipid molecules. Lactoferrin occurs within secondary granules. It chelates iron required for microbial growth.

Following killing and digestion of bacteria, the phagocytic vacuole fuses with the plasma membrane and discharges killed bacteria, products of degraded bacteria, and contents of granules to the outside of the cell in a process called exocytosis (Fig. 4–4). Discharge of granules can also occur following activation of neutrophils in the absence of phagocytosis. Considerable tissue injury occurs in areas where neutrophils are activated because of the oxidants they produce and the granule contents they release.

Eosinophil Functions. Functions of eosinophils are not completely defined. They have limited phagocytic abilities and provide poor host defense against bacterial or viral agents. Eosinophils are active in killing metazoan parasites (flukes and tissue stages of helminths) that have antibodies and/or complement bound to their surfaces. Eosinophils release substances that inhibit some of the inflammatory effects of mast cell degranulation. However, activated eosinophils also generate inflammatory mediators, which can result in tissue injury.

Metazoan parasites stimulate both humoral and cellular immunity. B-lymphocytes produce IgG antibodies that may bind to parasites and activate complement, thereby inflicting damage to the parasite and initiating an inflammatory reaction. Specific IgE antibodies may also be produced that bind to mast cells. The binding of parasite antigens to these antibodies results in mast cell activation and degranulation and release of inflammatory mediators and potent chemoattractants for eosinophils. These chemoattractants include histamine, leukotriene C_4 (a product of the lipoxygenase pathway of arachidonic metabolism), tetrapeptides, and intermediate molecular weight peptides. Other factors such as the C5a component of complement, PAF, and leukotriene B_4 also function as chemoattractants, but these factors are not specific for eosinophils. T-lymphocytes activated by parasite antigens produce factors (IL-5, IL-3, and GM-CSF) that not only stimulate the production and release of eosinophils but also activate them and promote their survival.

Similar to neutrophil adhesive processes, selectins and β_2 integrins are involved in eosinophil adhesion to activated endothelial cells. In addition, endothelial cells activated by IL-4 express vascular cell adhesion molecule-1

(VCAM-1) which binds to very late antigen-4 (VLA-4) on the surface of eosinophils. This integrin is not expressed on neutrophils and presumably helps provide specificity for eosinophil localization.

Eosinophils accumulate in the tissues in response to chemoattractants generated in response to parasites. They bind to the opsonized parasites via their surface receptors to IgG and complement. The parasites are much too large for eosinophils to ingest, but when activated, eosinophils exhibit dramatic NADPH oxidase activity which generates oxidants. They also exocytose their granules in the area of the invading parasite. Eosinophil peroxidase released from granules interacts with hydrogen peroxidase generated from the respiratory burst and halide ions. This complex, other oxygen metabolites, and the major basic protein (MBP) released from secondary granules are primarily involved in the killing of metazoan parasites.

Basophil Functions. Basophils generally occur in low numbers in the circulation. They contain most of the histamine measured in blood. Histamine in granules is bound to polyanions (including heparin) and these polyanions are responsible for the metachromatic staining (purple color with blue dyes) of the granules. Basophils have biochemical characteristics similar to mast cells and probably share a common progenitor cell with mast cells in bone marrow, but they are clearly different cell types. Basophils have segmented nuclei and mast cells have round nuclei. Mast cells usually have more cytoplasmic granules than basophils. In cats, both primary and secondary granules in basophils are morphologically different from mast cell granules.

The functions of basophils are unclear, but they may be similar to mast cells once they migrate into tissues. As discussed previously, mast cell activation and degranulation result in inflammation that may help expel metazoan parasites and recruit eosinophils that kill these parasites. Basophils and mast cells are involved in allergic conditions. Following binding of an antigen to a specific surface-bound IgE antibody, these cells degranulate and release histamine and other mediators that account for the inflammation present in immediate hypersensitivity reactions. Other foreign material (physical or chemical agents) can also cause degranulation of these cells. In some instances, this reaction may help expel the foreign material.

Monocyte/Macrophage Functions. M-CSF not only stimulates monocyte production but also stimulates the transformation of monocytes into macrophages. Although most tissue macrophages are of blood monocyte origin, some proliferation of macrophages can be stimulated by growth factors in tissues during inflammation. The development of monocytes into macrophages is associated with a five- to ten-fold increase in size, an increase in granules (lysosomes), an increase in size and number of mitochondria, and an increase in phagocytic capacity. Macrophage function is augmented by various cytokines, the most potent of which is reported to be gamma interferon. M-CSF and GM-CSF also enhance macrophage function. The mononuclear phagocyte system consists of "fixed" macrophages (Kupffer cells in the liver, littoral cells in spleen, and nurse cells in marrow), mobile phagocytic cells (monocytes, peritoneal and pleural macrophages, and alveolar macrophages), and multinucleated giant cells that may form during chronic inflammatory conditions from a fusion of other mononuclear phagocytes.

Macrophages move more slowly and are less potent in killing bacteria, but are notably more active in fungal and viral infections than are neutrophils. Macrophages can synthesize new membrane material and replace expended lysosomes. Therefore, they have more staying power in combating infections than do neutrophils, which have limited synthetic abilities.

Antimicrobial properties of macrophages are less well understood than neutrophils. Lactoferrin is absent, but NADPH oxidase and myeloperoxidase activities are present, although the activity of the latter is considerably less than in neutrophils. Lysozyme is present, but few organisms are sensitive to it in their native states. Nitric oxide, a free radical generated from L-arginine, appears to be important in microbial killing by macrophages.

Macrophages demonstrate necrotaxis and necrophagocytosis (phagocytosis of devitalized tissue). Opsonization of necrotic tissue is not required for necrophagocytosis to occur. Consequently, they serve an important function in cleaning up necrotic tissue and other debris within the body.

Macrophages have other important functions in immunity including antigen processing; killing of tumor cells after sensitization by T-lymphocytes; and synthesis of CSFs, interleukins, complement components, interferon, and TNF. Macrophages remove aged or damaged erythrocytes and store the iron from these cells in the form of ferritin and hemosiderin.

Lymphocyte and NK Cell Functions. A thorough discussion of lymphocyte and NK cell functions is beyond the scope of this text; consequently, the reader is referred to current immunology textbooks for more detailed information. The production and location of lymphocyte types are discussed in Chapter 2. Although bone marrow and thymus seed other lymphoid organs with B- and T-lymphocytes, respectively, it should be noted that local proliferation of lymphocytes occurs in lymphoid organs in response to specific antigens.

B-lymphocytes are primarily responsible for humoral immunity; however, immunoglobulin production also requires the participation of T-lymphocytes and macrophages. Macrophages bind foreign antigens and process them so that they become highly immunogenic. A processed antigen is presented to virgin T-lymphocytes and B-lymphocytes. Interactions between T-lymphocytes, B-lymphocytes, and the processed antigen result in a clonal proliferation of both cell types. When these antigen-specific cells recognize the same antigen at a later date, they undergo a secondary heightened proliferative response. Antigen activation of B-lymphocytes may also occur independent of T-lymphocytes if the antigen is a high-molecular-weight polymer. Following activation, B-lymphocytes are transformed into immunoglobulin-producing immunocytes and plasma cells. IgM is initially produced by these cells, but with continued antigenic stimulation IgG becomes the predominant antibody type produced. Clonal amplification of these cells results in the production of greater amounts of antibody against the foreign antigen. In addition to immunoglobulin production, B-lymphocytes produce a limited number of cytokines that may influence the proliferation and/or function of other blood cell types.

T-lymphocytes are largely responsible for cellular immunity. In contrast to B-lymphocytes, which produce immunoglobulins that are carried to the site of a foreign antigen, T-lymphocytes can migrate to the site of a foreign antigen. T-lymphocytes are involved in immune regulation, cytotoxicity, delayed-type hypersensitivity, and graft-*versus*-host reactions. They are also actively involved in the control of hematopoiesis. To produce these effects, different subpopulations produce a large number of cytokines with diverse biologic activities. Normal immune regulation requires a balanced participation of T-helper (CD4+CD8−) and T-suppressor (CD4−CD8+) lymphocytes. Altered T-lymphocyte function may result in the development of autoimmune diseases. Cytotoxic T-lymphocytes are antigen-dependent cells that can destroy target cells (*e.g.*, neoplastic cells) by a contact-dependent, major histocompatibility (MHC) −dependent, nonphagocytic process.

NK cells appear as granular lymphocytes in most species. These cytotoxic cells lyse target cells without deliberate prior sensitization and without restriction by MHC antigens.

DIFFERENTIAL LEUKOCYTE COUNTS

Blood films are generally examined following methanol fixation and staining with Romanowsky-type stains such as Wright or Wright-Giemsa stains. As a quality-control measure, the number of leukocytes present should be estimated to ensure that the number present on the slide is consistent with the total leukocyte count measured using manual or automated methods. The leukocyte count in blood (cells/μL) may be estimated by multiplying the number of leukocytes seen per field using a 10X objective by 100 to 150 and the number of leukocytes seen per field using a 20X objective by 400 to 600. Total leukocyte counts may be falsely decreased if clumped or lysed leukocytes are present. Total leukocyte counts may be falsely increased if abnormally large platelets, clumps of platelets, or large Heinz bodies are present. These falsely increased total leukocyte counts occur most often in cats. When present, nucleated RBCs in blood are counted as part of the WBC count when manual methods or automated impedance cell counters are used; consequently, the total WBC counts will be too high if nucleated RBCs are present. Lastly, the total WBC counts may be too high if the erythrocyte-lysing agent used in an automated machine does not cause complete lysis of erythrocytes prior to performing the leukocyte count.

A differential leukocyte count is done by identifying 200 consecutive leukocytes using a 40X or 50X objective, and the percentage of each leukocyte type present is multiplied by the total leukocyte count to get the absolute number of each cell type present per microliter of blood. It is the absolute number of each leukocyte type that is important. Relative values (percentages) can be misleading when the total leukocyte count is abnormal. Consider two dogs, one with 7% lymphocytes and a total leukocyte count of 40,000/μL, and the other with 70% lymphocytes and a total leukocyte count of 4000/μL. The first case would be said to have a "relative" lymphopenia and the second case would be said to have a "relative" lymphocytosis. Both cases, in fact, have the same normal absolute lymphocyte count (2800/μL).

Nucleated RBCs (NRBCs) are counted along with WBCs when WBC counts are done using manual methods or automated impedance cell counters. When encountered during blood film examination, the number of nucleated RBCs per 100 leukocytes should be tabulated and the total leukocyte count should be corrected for the number of NRBCs present (see formula below) prior to calculating the absolute cell counts for each blood cell type.

$$\text{Corrected WBC count} = (\text{measured WBC} \times 100)/(100 + \text{NRBC}).$$

If WBC counts are done using automated cell counters that use technology which can differentiate NRBCs from WBCs (*e.g.*, morphologic characteristics of cells are determined using a laser beam), the above calculation will not be necessary. However, the number of NRBCs present should still be recorded.

ABNORMAL NEUTROPHIL MORPHOLOGY

Toxic Cytoplasm

The cytoplasm of neutrophils from common domestic animals is nearly colorless. When the cytoplasm is basophilic, has foamy vacuolation, and/or contains Doehle bodies, it is said to be toxic (Color Plate 4). These morphologic abnormalities develop in neutrophilic cells within the bone marrow prior to their release into the circulation. Foamy basophilia often occurs with severe bacterial infections, but can occur with other causes of toxemia.

Doehle Bodies.   Doehle bodies are bluish angular cytoplasmic inclusions of neutrophils composed of retained aggregates of rough endoplasmic reticulum (Color Plate 4). By themselves, these inclusions represent mild evidence of toxicity and are sometimes seen in neutrophils of cats that do not exhibit signs of illness. Doehle bodies must be differentiated from distemper inclusions in dogs and granules present in neutrophils from cats with inherited Chediak-Higashi syndrome.

Toxic Granulation.   Toxic granulation refers to the presence of purple-staining cytoplasmic granules. These granules consist of primary granules that have retained the staining intensity normally observed in promyelocytes in the bone marrow. Toxic granulation suggests severe toxemia and occurs most frequently in horses. Toxic granulation must be differentiated from other conditions where cytoplasmic granules are observed. It should not be confused with the pink staining of secondary granules that is not a sign of toxicity. Purple granules are often seen in neutrophils from foals without other evidence of cytoplasmic toxicity, the clinical significance of which is unclear. Toxic granulation must be differentiated from the granules present in some Birman cats and in animals with certain lysosomal storage disorders.

Inherited Disorders.   Chediak-Higashi syndrome is a disorder characterized by enlarged cytoplasmic granules in many types of granule-containing cells. Neutrophils from affected cats and cattle contain large pink to red granules. Small reddish granules have been reported as an inherited anomaly in Birman cats without evidence of illness. Basophilic granulation occurs in the cytoplasm of neutrophils from cats and dogs with certain lysosomal storage disorders including mucopolysaccharidosis type VI, mucopolysaccharidosis VII, and GM_2 gangliosidosis (Color Plate 4).

Infectious Agents.   Distemper inclusions are formed in bone marrow precursor cells and may be present in blood cells during the acute viremic stage of the disease. These viral inclusions can be difficult to visualize in the cytoplasm of neutrophils in Wright- or Giemsa-stained blood films, but can easily be seen as homogeneous round, oval, or irregularly shaped 1- to 4-μm red inclusions when stained with Diff-Quik (Color Plate 3). Morulae of *Ehrlichia* species that infect neutrophils (*e.g.*, *E. equi* and *E. ewingii*) may be found in neutrophils during the acute stage of infection (Fig. 4–6). These morulae appear as tightly packed basophilic clusters of organisms within the cytoplasm. Gametocytes of the protozoal organism *Hepatozoon canis* may be

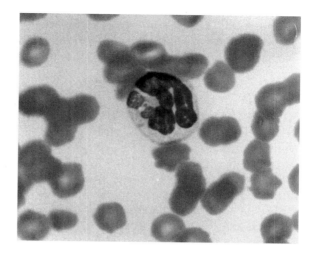

FIGURE 4–6. Horse blood neutrophil containing two *Ehrlichia equi* morulae. Wright-Giemsa stain.

seen in the cytoplasm of circulating neutrophils. These appear as large oblong structures. The nucleus of a gametocyte usually stains poorly with routine blood stains.

Left Shifts

When increased numbers of immature neutrophils are present in blood, their presence is referred to as a left shift (Color Plate 4). The magnitude of a left shift can vary from slightly increased numbers of bands to severe left shifts with metamyelocytes, myelocytes, and rarely even promyelocytes present in blood. The term regenerative left shift is used when a neutrophilia with a left shift is present and the mature neutrophils predominate. The term degenerative left shift is used when the immature neutrophils outnumber mature neutrophils and the total neutrophil count is normal or low. The term leukemoid response is used when an inflammation-induced neutrophilia with a left shift is so marked that it must be differentiated from chronic myelogenous leukemia.

The term hyposegmentation refers to a left shift with condensed nuclear chromatin without nuclear constrictions. It occurs as an inherited trait in the Pelger-Huet anomaly in dogs and cats. Eosinophils and basophils may also be affected. No clinical signs are associated with animals that are heterozygous for this disorder. A pseudo–Pelger-Huet anomaly may occur transiently with chronic infections or rarely with the administration of certain drugs.

Hypersegmentation

Hypersegmentation refers to the presence of five or more distinct nuclear lobes within neutrophils (Color Plate 4). It occurs as a normal aging process and may reflect prolonged transit time in blood as can occur with resolving chronic inflammation, with glucocorticoid administration, or with hyperadrenocorticism. Hypersegmentation may be present in myeloproliferative disorders. Idiopathic hypersegmentation has been reported as a rare occurrence in horses without evidence of clinical disease. It has also been described in dogs with an inherited defect in cobalamin absorption.

NEUTROPHILIA

Neutrophilia may develop as a result of increased neutrophil production and/or release from the bone marrow, decreased movement of neutrophils from blood into the tissues, or net movement of neutrophils from the marginal neutrophil pool (MNP) to the circulating neutrophil pool (CNP) as shown in Figure 4–7. Neutrophilia develops rapidly in blood following epinephrine release, as occurs with exercise, fear, or excitement (physiologic leukocytosis). This results from a shift of neutrophils from the MNP to the CNP. The cell count usually does not increase above twice normal and no left shift occurs (Table 4–1). The epinephrine effect is more commonly seen in young animals. Some animals (e.g., cats and horses) may exhibit an accompanying

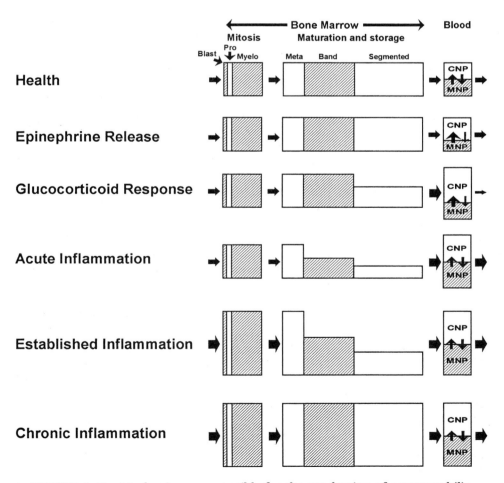

FIGURE 4–7. Mechanisms responsible for the production of a neutrophilia.

TABLE 4–1. Expected Findings in Different Types of Neutrophilias

Type	Lymphocytes Count	Left Shift
Physiologic (epinephrine)	Normal or increased	None
Stress (glucocorticoids)	Usually decreased	None or slight
Inflammation	Often decreased	Often present

lymphocytosis. Leukogram effects should return to normal within 30 minutes of removal of the stimulus.

The increased endogenous release or exogenous administration of glucocorticoid steroids has profound effects on circulating blood cell numbers within a few hours after administration (stress leukogram). Potential causes of increased endogenous release of glucocorticoids include pain, prolonged emotional stress, abnormal body temperature, and hyperadrenocorticism. The duration of effects depends on the nature of the glucocorticoid given (long-acting or short-acting). Neutrophilia occurs because glucocorticoids cause increased release of mature neutrophils from bone marrow stores and decreased egress of neutrophils from blood into tissues. A higher percentage of neutrophils is also present in the CNP compared to the MNP, but the size of the MNP may not actually be decreased because the total blood neutrophil pool is increased. The absolute number of neutrophils seldom increases above twice normal and a left shift is usually not present. Glucocorticoids also cause lymphopenia and eosinopenia in all domestic animals (Table 4–1). Monocytosis is commonly observed in dogs and occasionally in cats. The magnitude of the neutrophilia decreases with time, but the lymphopenia and eosinopenia persist as long as plasma glucocorticoid concentrations are increased. For example, most dogs with Cushing's disease have lymphopenia and eosinopenia with normal neutrophil counts.

Neutrophilia without a significant left shift may also be present in association with hemorrhage, hemolysis, necrosis, chemical and drug toxicities, malignancy, mild inflammation, and some chronic inflammatory conditions. The mechanism(s) causing neutrophilia in these disorders is not always clear. Various conditions can result in increased concentrations of hematopoietic growth factors in the circulation that result in increased neutrophil production and release. In mild inflammatory conditions and some chronic inflammatory conditions, the increased peripheral demand for neutrophils is met by increased production and release of mature neutrophils from the marrow.

Prominent left shifts are usually associated with inflammatory conditions (Table 4–1). These inflammatory conditions are not always infectious. For example, a regenerative left shift is common in some immune-mediated disorders. The presence of a significant left shift indicates that the stimulus for release of neutrophils from bone marrow is greater than can be accommodated by release from mature neutrophil stores alone. Regenerative left shifts are generally viewed as an adequate marrow response at that moment. The presence of significant cytoplasmic toxicity requires a more guarded prognosis. When a leukemoid response is present (total leukocyte count of 50,000 to 100,000/μL and left shift to include at least myelocytes), a localized purulent inflammatory condition such as pyometra is suspected. Animals with chronic myelogenous leukemia (CML) have persistent marked neutrophilia with pronounced left shift that may extend to myeloblasts. This diagnosis is usually reached by ruling out inflammatory causes and documenting the concomitant occurrence of additional proliferative abnormalities in blood and bone marrow. CML is a common disorder in people, but has rarely been reported in domestic animals, being most often recognized in dogs.

Neutrophilia with or without a modest left shift is usually present in some animals with inherited neutrophil dysfunctions. The neutrophilia may be marked in dogs and cattle with deficiencies in β_2 integrin adhesion molecules. Inherited neutrophil dysfunctions should be included in the differential diagnosis when unexplained, recurrent bacterial infections occur in a young animal.

NEUTROPENIA

Neutropenia can develop from decreased release of neutrophils from bone marrow, increased egress of neutrophils from blood, destruction of neutrophils within the blood, or a shift of neutrophils from the CNP to the MNP (Fig. 4–8). Decreased release from bone marrow can result from decreased progenitor cells or from dysgranulopoiesis. Conditions in which granulocyte

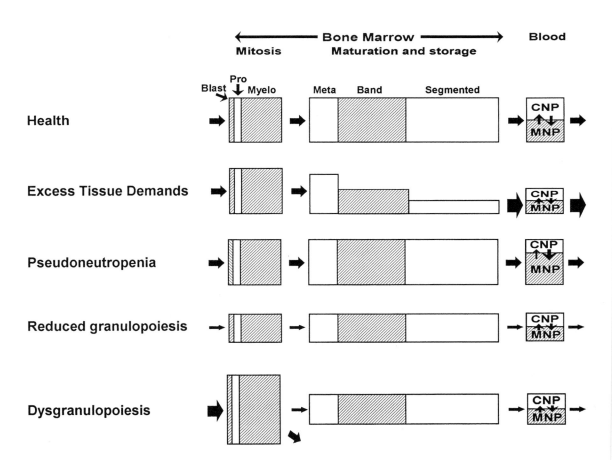

FIGURE 4–8. Mechanisms responsible for the production of a neutropenia.

precursors are present in normal or increased numbers in bone marrow but the release of mature neutrophils into blood is decreased include acute myeloid leukemias, myelodysplastic syndromes, feline leukemia virus (FeLV) infections, and feline immunodeficiency virus (FIV) infections.

Conditions associated with decreased numbers of normal progenitor cells in the marrow include idiosyncratic drug reactions (*e.g.*, phenylbutazone, trimethoprim/sulfadiazine, griseofulvin, and cephalosporins), estrogen toxicity (exogenous or endogenous) in dogs and ferrets, cytotoxic chemotherapy drugs, viral diseases such as parvovirus and some FeLV infections, rickettsial diseases such as ehrlichiosis, myelophthisic disorders, and inherited disorders including cyclic hematopoiesis in gray collie dogs and some cats with Chediak-Higashi syndrome. Lithium carbonate stimulates neutrophil production in dogs and people, but it causes a bone marrow neutrophilic maturation arrest and neutropenia in cats. The long-term use of a recombinant G-CSF from one species in a second species can result in a persistent neutropenia in the second species when antibodies made against the recombinant G-CSF also neutralize the endogenous G-CSF of the species receiving treatment.

Neutropenia can develop in acute inflammatory conditions where the demand for neutrophils depletes the bone marrow storage pool and insufficient time has elapsed for increased granulopoiesis to occur. Neutropenia is common in overwhelming septic conditions (*e.g.*, septicemia) and secondary to endotoxemia. Degenerative left shifts are often present in these disorders. A common example of this type of presentation is acute salmonellosis in horses. Although not well documented in animals, neutropenia may also develop as a result of immune-mediated phagocytosis or hypersplenism. Finally, neutropenia can occur following the net movement of neutrophils from the circulating to the marginal neutrophil pool as occurs during shock.

INHERITED NEUTROPHIL DEFECTS

Chediak-Higashi Syndrome

The Chediak-Higashi syndrome has been reported in cattle, Persian cats, Aleutian mink, the beige mouse, and a killer whale, as well as in humans. This disorder is characterized by partial oculocutaneous albinism, increased susceptibility to infections, hemorrhagic tendencies, and the presence of enlarged membrane-bound granules in many cell types including blood leukocytes. The giant granules may arise from unregulated fusion of primary lysosomes during cell development. Neutrophils from affected animals exhibit reduced mobility and defective phagocytic and/or bactericidal responses, explaining the increased susceptibility to bacterial infections that is present. Neutropenia is a common finding in cats with the Chediak-Higashi syndrome.

β_2 Integrin Adhesion Molecule Deficiencies

An autosomal recessive deficiency in leukocyte surface adhesion glycoproteins (β_2 integrins), resulting from a defect in the CD18 β subunit, has been recognized in Irish setter dogs and Holstein cattle. This defect results in decreased neutrophil adhesion, impaired chemotaxis and aggregation, and minimal bactericidal activity. Similar defects also occur in monocytes. As a result, animals have recurrent bacterial infections. Clinical signs include gingivitis, oral ulcers, periodontitis, chronic pneumonia, poor wound healing, and stunted growth. Marked neutrophilia with or without a modest left shift is usually present. Increased numbers of other blood leukocyte types may also occur at times. Mild to moderate nonregenerative anemia and a polyclonal hyperglobulinemia may be present.

Unknown Neutrophil Function Defects

A less well-defined defect in neutrophils has been reported in Doberman pinscher dogs. Neutrophil chemotaxis and phagocytosis are normal, but these cells have reduced bactericidal ability. The bactericidal defect appears to be the result of inadequate generation of superoxide radicals following stimulation. An inadequate oxidant burst may also occur in young Weimaraner dogs that present with recurrent infections.

Cyclic Hematopoiesis

Cyclic hematopoiesis (previously termed cyclic neutropenia) is transmitted as an autosomal recessive trait in gray collie dogs. The "gray collie syndrome" is associated with several distinct abnormalities (abnormal hair pigmentation, bilateral scleral ectasia, enteropathy, and gonadal hypoplasia) in addition to cyclic hematopoieses. The specific cause of the disorder is unknown, but it may involve a G-CSF postreceptor signal transduction defect in stem cells. Blood neutrophil, monocyte, eosinophil, reticulocyte, and platelet counts exhibit 11- to 13-day cyclic fluctuations, with neutrophil fluctuations being most dramatic. Neutrophils may be completely absent in blood during neutropenic episodes, which last 2 to 4 days. A neutrophilia may follow the neutropenic period. Affected pups are susceptible to bacterial and fungal infections during the neutropenic episodes. They usually die by 6 months of age.

ABNORMAL LYMPHOCYTE MORPHOLOGY

Antigenic Stimulation

Lymphocytes are stimulated to proliferate in response to antigenic stimulation. They increase in size, have less dense nuclear chromatin, and exhibit increased cytoplasmic basophilia (Color Plate 3). Most of these antigenically stimulated cells remain in peripheral lymphoid tissues, but some may enter the circulation, although usually in low numbers. Various terms including reactive lymphocytes, transformed lymphocytes, and immunocytes have been used to describe them. Some reactive lymphocytes are large with pleomorphic nuclei and others are plasmacytoid (plasma cell-like) in appearance. Plasma cells are present in lymphoid organs, but they are rarely observed in blood even when plasma cell neoplasia (*e.g.*, multiple myeloma) is present (Color Plate 4). Plasma cells have a lower nucleus to cytoplasm ratio and greater cytoplasmic basophilia than resting lymphocytes. The presence of prominent Golgi may create a pale perinuclear area in the cytoplasm. They typically have eccentrically located nuclei with coarse chromatin clumping in a mosaic pattern. When it is not possible to decide whether basophilic lymphocytes are reactive or neoplastic, the term atypical lymphocytes is sometimes used.

Lymphoblasts

Basophilic lymphoid cells are called lymphoblasts when a nucleolus or multiple nucleoli are present in the nucleus. Rare lymphoblasts may be observed in disorders with increased antigenic stimulation, but when several of these cells are found during a differential count, lymphoid neoplasia is suspected.

Cytoplasmic Granules and Vacuoles

A low percentage of lymphocytes in blood from normal animals contains cytoplasmic granules (Color Plate 4). Many of these granular lymphocytes appear to be NK cells. Increased numbers of granular lymphocytes have been seen in both neoplastic and nonneoplastic conditions.

Basophilic granules may be seen in the lymphocytes from animals with certain lysosomal storage diseases including mucopolysaccharidosis I, VI, and VII in dogs and/or cats and GM_2 gangliosidosis in pigs. Discrete vacuoles may occur in the cytoplasm of lymphocytes from animals with inherited lysosomal storage diseases including mucopolysaccharidosis VII (cats), GM_2 gangliosidosis (cats), GM_1 gangliosidosis (cats and dogs), α-mannosidosis (cats), Niemann-Pick type C disease (cats), and fucosidosis (dogs). Basophilic granules and vacuoles may not become apparent in some lysosomal disorders until the affected animal reaches adulthood.

LYMPHOCYTOSIS

Lymphocyte numbers in blood vary with age, being higher than adults in young animals of some species (*e.g.*, cats) and lower than adults in young animals of other species (*e.g.*, horses). Lymphocytosis sometimes occurs with epinephrine release in animals (especially horses and cats), presumably because of transiently increased lymphatic flow associated with increased muscular contractions. Although increased proliferation of lymphocytes is common in lymph nodes in response to foreign antigens, evidence of this reaction is often not present in blood. In some cases, reactive lymphocytes account for a substantial proportion of total lymphocytes present in blood, but an absolute lymphocytosis is uncommon. An example where reactive lymphocytosis may be present is as a vaccination reaction in young dogs. Lymphocytosis is sometimes present in animals with chronic inflammatory conditions. Persistent lymphocytosis often occurs in cattle infected with the bovine leukemia virus (BLV), a B-lymphotrophic retrovirus. Persistent lymphocytosis is a subclinical condition in cattle, but some animals will subsequently develop lymphoma. Marked lymphocytosis is always present in animals with chronic lymphocytic leukemia. A lymphocytosis often occurs in animals with acute lymphocytic leukemia and occasionally occurs in animals with lymphoma (see lymphoproliferative disorders section). Granular lymphocytes may be increased in response to infectious agents (*e.g.*, *Ehrlichia* spp.) or in association with neoplastic disorders involving these cells.

LYMPHOPENIA

Lymphocytes are sequestered in bone marrow, lymph nodes, and spleen following endogenous or exogenous glucocorticoid steroids. Glucocorticoids can also potentiate apoptosis of sensitive lymphocytes (*e.g.*, transformed lymphocytes or neoplastic lymphocytes). Lymphopenia often accompanies severe systemic bacterial and viral infections because of the endogenous release of glucocorticoids. It often occurs following the use of immunosuppressive drugs and irradiation that result from lymphocyte destruction.

Lymphocytes are present in afferent lymph from gastrointestinal and bronchial lymphoid tissues and efferent lymph from lymph nodes. The loss of lymphocyte-rich afferent lymph (*e.g.*, lymphangiectasia) or efferent lymph (*e.g.*, thoracic duct rupture) results in lymphopenia because most blood lymphocytes recirculate through lymphoid tissues. Lymphopenia can also occur when lymph node architecture is disrupted (*e.g.*, multicentric lymphoma or generalized granulomatous inflammation), preventing the normal recirculation of lymphocytes.

Lymphopenia occurs with hereditary T-lymphocyte deficiency or combined T- and B-lymphocyte deficiency because the T-lymphocyte accounts for a majority of lymphocytes normally present in the circulation. Profound lymphopenia occurs in Arabian foals with severe combined immunodeficiency that affects both the T- and B-lymphocyte lineages.

ABNORMAL MONOCYTE MORPHOLOGY

Cytoplasmic vacuoles have been reported in some animals with lysosomal storage disorders, but monocytes from normal individuals often exhibit cytoplasmic vacuoles in films prepared from blood collected with an anticoagulant. Transformation of monocytes into macrophages typically occurs in the tissues, but macrophages are sometimes seen in blood (Fig. 4–9). In addition to other blood cell types, canine monocytes may also contain distemper inclusions, and monocytes from animals with Chediak-Higashi syndrome may have one or more enlarged eosinophilic granules in the cytoplasm. Morulae of *Ehrlichia* species that infect mononuclear phagocytes (*e.g.*, *E. canis* and *E. risticii*) can rarely be found in blood monocytes or macrophages during the acute stage of infection (Fig. 4–9). These morulae appear as tightly packed basophilic clusters of organisms within the cytoplasm.

MONOCYTOSIS

Monocytosis may occur in conditions that also cause a neutrophilia. It may be present in both acute and chronic inflammation. Glucocorticoid steroids

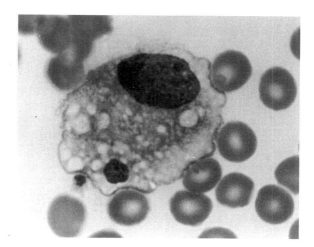

FIGURE 4–9. Dog blood macrophage containing an *Ehrlichia canis* morula. Wright-Giemsa stain.

can induce monocytosis in dogs. Normal domestic animals may have few or no monocytes in blood; consequently, the term monocytopenia is not usually used. Monocytosis may occur in animals with monocytic or myelomonocytic leukemias. In contrast to other causes of monocytosis, high numbers of monoblasts will be present in bone marrow (and often in blood) in animals with these leukemias.

EOSINOPHILIA

Eosinophilia may accompany parasitic diseases, especially those caused by nematodes and flukes. Eosinophilia is more likely present when intestinal nematodes are migrating within the body than when they are only located within the intestine. Eosinophilia may occur in association with inflammatory conditions of organs such as skin, lung, intestine, and uterus that normally contain numerous mast cells. It may be present in animals with IgE-mediated allergic hypersensitivity reactions such as flea-bite allergies and feline asthma. Although not usually present, eosinophilia may occur in animals with mast cell tumors and rarely in animals with other tumor types. Eosinophilia occurs in some animals with eosinophilic granulomas and it is consistently present in animals with the hypereosinophilic syndrome, a heterogenous group of disorders that can be difficult to differentiate from eosinophilic leukemia.

EOSINOPENIA

The absolute eosinophil count may be zero in some normal animals, making eosinopenia of limited significance. Glucocorticoids rapidly produce eosinopenia secondary to the sequestration of eosinophils within the bone marrow. Long-term glucocorticoid therapy may decrease eosinophil production by decreasing the production of growth factors from T-lymphocytes. Glucocorticoids also potentiate apoptosis of eosinophils in the tissues.

BASOPHILIA

Basophilia is generally associated with IgE-mediated disorders. When present, basophilia usually accompanies eosinophilia. Basophilia may occur in some animals with mast cell tumors (primarily noncutaneous types). It has been reported in animals with altered lipoprotein metabolism (*e.g.*, hypothyroidism). Basophilia has rarely been reported in association with basophilic leukemia in animals. Basophilic leukemia must be differentiated from mast cell neoplasia with mastocytemia (sometimes called mast cell leukemia). Mast cells have round nuclei and basophils have segmented nuclei.

MASTOCYTEMIA

Mastocytemia occurs in association with noncutaneous and metastatic cutaneous mast cell tumors. Low numbers of mast cells may also be present in blood of animals with inflammatory diseases.

HEMATOPOIETIC NEOPLASMS

Hematopoietic neoplasms arise from bone marrow, lymph nodes, spleen, or thymus. They are classified as either lymphoproliferative disorders or myeloproliferative disorders. The term leukemia is used when neoplastic cells are seen in blood and/or bone marrow. An exception is the neoplastic proliferation of plasma cells in bone marrow (multiple myeloma), which is not referred to as a leukemia. True leukemias are of bone marrow origin and neoplastic cells are usually present in blood. Leukocyte counts may be low, normal, or high in animals with leukemias. The term acute is used to describe leukemias in which a predominance of blast cells occurs in the bone marrow, and the term chronic is used for leukemias in which there is a predominance of well-differentiated cells in blood and bone marrow. The progression of disease is usually rapid (weeks to months) in acute leukemias and slow (months to years) in chronic leukemias.

Lymphoproliferative Disorders

The term lymphoma denotes a neoplastic condition of lymphocytes originating from a peripheral lymphoid tissue and the term lymphocytic leukemia indicates a neoplastic condition of lymphocytes originating from bone marrow. When neoplastic cells are present in blood in an animal with a lymphoma, the terms "lymphoma with leukemia" or "lymphosarcoma cell leukemia" have been used. Metastasis from bone marrow to lymphoid tissues and from lymphoid tissues to bone marrow is common. Consequently, it may be difficult to differentiate true leukemia from lymphoma with leukemia in animals with advanced stages of disease.

Chronic Lymphocytic Leukemia. Chronic lymphocytic leukemia (CLL) is rare, being reported most often in old animals. A marked lymphocytosis, involving normal-appearing small- to medium-sized lymphocytes, is always present. Bone marrow examination also reveals increased numbers of normal-appearing lymphocytes.

Acute Lymphocytic (Lymphoblastic) Leukemia. Neoplastic lymphocytes present in bone marrow of animals with acute lymphocytic leukemia (ALL) exhibit decreased nuclear chromatin condensation and increased cytoplasmic basophilia. Other abnormalities including increased anisocytosis, anisokaryosis, prominent nucleoli, and nuclear pleomorphism may also be present. Neoplastic cells are also usually present in blood and a lymphocytosis commonly occurs.

Lymphoma. Lymphomas are classified in various ways. They may be classified by anatomic site involved (*e.g.*, alimentary, thymic, cutaneous), by cell morphology (*e.g.*, small noncleaved, lymphoblastic, immunoblastic), and by cell type (*e.g.*, B-cell, T-cell, granular lymphocyte). Neoplastic cells are recognized in blood in less than half of the animals presenting with lymphoma.

Multiple Myeloma. Multiple myeloma (plasma cell myeloma) is a B-cell tumor of bone marrow that is manifested as a proliferation of plasma cells. A monoclonal immunoglobulin is usually secreted by the tumor, resulting in a monoclonal hyperglobulinemia. Extramedullary plasma cell tumors (plasmacytomas) rarely have an associated monoclonal hyperglobulinemia.

Myeloproliferative Disorders

Myeloproliferative disorders are characterized by the purposeless proliferation of one or more of the nonlymphoid marrow cell lines (granulocytic, monocytic, erythrocytic, or megakaryocytic). Myeloproliferative disorders are generally considered to be benign or malignant neoplastic diseases, but some hematologists also consider the myelodysplastic syndrome (MDS) to be a myeloproliferative disorder because MDS may precede the development of neoplasia. The unitary concept of myeloproliferative disorders was developed because all nonlymphoid blood cells are derived from a common myeloid stem cell and neoplastic transformations in these disorders usually occur in pluripotent progenitor cells. Although the proliferation of one cell type may predominate, a marrow cell line is seldom singly affected. Morphologic or functional disorders of other cell lines can usually be detected. In addition, some of these disorders appear to evolve into one another. For example, cats with MDS with excessive proliferation of nucleated RBCs (MDS-Er) may evolve into erythroleukemia and eventually myeloblastic leukemia. Cats with myeloproliferative disorders are generally infected with FeLV and/or FIV viruses. Myeloproliferative disorders are uncommon in other domestic animal species and the causes are unknown. Irradiation has been experimentally shown to cause myeloproliferative disorders in dogs.

Myelodysplastic Syndromes. The bone marrow in MDS is usually normocellular or hypercellular, but cytopenias are present in blood. This apparent ineffective hematopoiesis appears to result from extensive apoptosis. Apoptosis or programmed cell death is a physiologic mechanism of gene-directed cellular self-destruction in which intracellular endonucleases initially cut DNA into fragments. Recognizable apoptotic cells with fragmented nuclei exist for only 10 to 15 minutes before removal by phagocytic cells.

Proliferative abnormalities that may be present in bone marrow include erythroid hyperplasia with minimal reticulocyte production, megaloblastic erythroid precursors, maturation arrest in the granulocytic series at the myelocyte-metamyelocyte stage, abnormal megakaryocyte morphology including dwarf megakaryocytes, and increased numbers (5 to 29%) of blast cells. A nonregenerative anemia is nearly always present, with leukopenia and/or thrombocytopenias also commonly present. Additional abnormalities that may be present in blood include anisocytosis, poikilocytosis, nucleated RBCs out of proportion to the degree of reticulocytosis, large bizarre platelets, immature granulocytes, and abnormal granulocyte morphology (large size, hyposegmentation, hypersegmentation).

Several types of MDS have been described in animals. Cases with refractory anemia, with or without other refractory cytopenias, may be described as myelodysplastic syndrome–refractory cytopenia (MDS-RC). MDS with erythroid predominance in the bone marrow (M:E less than 1) may be classified as MDS-Er. When myeloblasts are increased (5 to 29% of bone marrow nucleated cells), the term myelodysplastic syndrome–excess blast (MDS-EB) may be used.

Acute Myeloid Leukemias. Acute myeloid leukemias (AML) are diagnosed when the percentage of blast cells in the bone marrow equals or exceed 30% of all nucleated cells, excluding lymphocytes, macrophages, plasma cells, and mast cells. Several types of AML have been recognized in animals. Myeloblastic leukemia without maturation is designated AML-M1 and myeloblastic leukemia with differentiation is designated AML-M2. When both myeloblasts and monoblasts are increased, the term acute myelomonocytic leukemia (AML-M4) may be used. When only monoblasts are increased the disorder is classified as acute monocytic leukemia (AML-M5). Erythroleukemia (AML-M6) has increased numbers of rubriblasts and myeloblasts. Megakaryoblastic leukemia (AML-M7) has increased numbers of megakaryoblasts in bone marrow. Additional subdivisions of AML are possible. The reader is referred to the article by Dr. Raskin in the reference list for more information concerning classification of AML. Cytochemistry, immunocytochemistry, and electron microscopy may be used to help identify the type(s) of blast cells present. When the blast cells cannot be identified with certainty, the term acute undifferentiated leukemia (AUL) may be used.

Chronic Myeloproliferative Disorders. Chronic myeloproliferative disorders are neoplastic proliferations of hematopoietic cells resulting in high numbers of differentiated cells in blood. Like MDS, animals with chronic myeloproliferative disorders have less than 30% blast cells in the bone marrow with few or no blast cells in the blood. Dysplastic changes may be present in both disorders, but they tend to be more noticeable in MDS. The major difference between these disorders is that high numbers of one or more blood cell type occur in chronic myeloproliferative disorders and cytopenias frequently occur in MDS.

Chronic myelogenous leukemia (CML) presents with a high total leukocyte count (more than 50,000/μL) with marked neutrophilic left shift in blood. Increased numbers of monocytes, eosinophils, and/or basophils may also be present. Myeloblasts are either absent or present in low numbers in blood. They account for less than 30% of all nucleated cells in bone marrow. CML is a rare disorder in animals that must be differentiated from severe inflammatory leukemoid reactions. The presence of cytoplasmic toxicity, increased inflammatory plasma proteins, and physical evidence of inflammation suggest a leukemoid reaction is present. Eosinophilic leukemia and basophilic leukemia are variants of CML where eosinophilic cells and basophilic cells, respectively, predominate in blood and marrow. Differentiation of eosinophilic leukemia and the hypereosinophilic syndrome in cats can be difficult. The hypereosinophilic syndrome is characterized by a mature eosinophilia with frequent involvement of the intestines.

Polycythemia vera and primary thrombocythemia are chronic myeloproliferative disorders characterized by high numbers of mature erythrocytes and platelets, respectively. These disorders are discussed in Chapters 3 and 5, respectively.

References

Avalos BR, Broudy VC, Ceselski SK, et al: Abnormal response to granulocyte colony-stimulating factor (G-CSF) in canine cyclic hematopoiesis is not caused by altered G-CSF receptor expression. Blood 1994;84:789.

Babior BM, Golde DW: Production, distribution, and fate of neutrophils. In Beutler E, Lichtman MA, Coller BS, Kipps TJ (eds): Williams Hematology, 5th edition. New York, McGraw-Hill, 1995, p 773.

Beale KM, Altman D, Clemmons RR, et al: Systemic toxicosis associated with azathioprine administration in domestic cats. Am J Vet Res 1992;53:1236.

Beutler E: Metabolism of neutrophils. In Beutler E, Lichtman MA, Coller BS, Kipps TJ (eds): Williams Hematology, 5th edition. New York, McGraw-Hill, 1995, p 767.

Bookbinder PF, Butt MT, Harvey HJ: Determination of the number of mast cells in lymph node, bone marrow, and buffy coat cytologic specimens from dogs. J Am Vet Med Assoc 1992;200:1648.

Brown DE, Thrall MA, Walkley SU, et al: Feline Niemann-Pick disease type C. Am J Pathol 1994;144:1412.

Burns AR, Simon SI, Kukielka GL, et al: Chemotactic factors stimulate CD18-dependent canine neutrophil adherence and motility on lung fibroblasts. J Immunol 1996;156:3389.

Campbell TW: Hematology of exotic animals. Comp Contin Educ Pract Vet 1991;13:950.

Carlos TM, Harlan JM: Leukocyte-endothelial adhesion molecules. Blood 1994;84:2068.

Cayatte SM, McManus PM, Miller WH, Jr, et al: Identification of mast cells in buffy coat preparations from dogs with inflammatory skin diseases. J Am Vet Med Assoc 1995;206:325.

Colgan SP, Gasper PW, Thrall MA, et al: Neutrophil function in normal and Chediak-Higashi syndrome cats following administration of recombinant canine granulocyte colony-stimulating factor. Exp Hematol 1992;20:1229.

Corcoran BM, Foster DJ, Fuentes VL: Feline asthma syndrome: A retrospective study of the clinical presentation in 29 cats. J Small Anim Pract 1995;36:481.

Dale DC: Neutropenia. In Beutler E, Lichtman MA, Coller BS, Kipps TJ (eds): Williams Hematology, 5th edition. New York, McGraw-Hill, 1995, p 815.

Dale DC: Neutrophilia. In Beutler E, Lichtman MA, Coller BS, Kipps TJ (eds): Williams Hematology, 5th edition. New York, McGraw-Hill, 1995, p 824.

Dial SM, Mitchell TW, LeCouteur RA, et al: GM_1-gangliosidosis (type II) in three cats. J Am Anim Hosp Assoc 1994;30:355.

Dieringer TM, Brown SA, Rogers KS, et al: Effects of lithium carbonate administration to healthy cats. Am J Vet Res 1992;53:721.

Doré M, Korthuis RJ, Granger DN, et al: P-selectin mediates spontaneous leukocyte rolling in vivo. Blood 1993;82:1308.

Duncan JR, Prasse KW, Mahaffey EA: Veterinary Laboratory Medicine. Clinical Pathology, 3rd edition. Ames, Iowa State University Press, 1994.

Felsburg PJ, Somberg RL, Perryman LE: Domestic animal models of severe combined immunodeficiency: Canine x-linked severe combined immunodeficiency and severe combined immunodeficiency in horses. Immunodef Rev 1992;3:277.

Foster AP, Lees P, Cunningham FM: Platelet activating factor is a mediator of equine neutrophil and eosinophil migration *in vitro*. Res Vet Sci 1992;53:223.

Galli SJ, Dvorak AM: Production, biochemistry, and function of basophils and mast cells. In Beutler E, Lichtman MA, Coller BS, Kipps TJ (eds): Williams Hematology, 5th edition. New York, McGraw-Hill, 1995, p 805.

Gebb SA, Graham JA, Hanger CC, et al: Sites of leukocyte sequestration in the pulmonary microcirculation. J Appl Physiol 1995;79:493.

Gilbert RO, Rebhun WC, Kim CA, et al: Clinical manifestations of leukocyte adhesion deficiency in cattle: 14 cases (1977–1991). J Am Vet Med Assoc 1993;202:445.

Gitzelmann R, Bosshard NU, Superti-Furga A, et al: Feline mucopolysaccharidosis VII due to β-glucuronidase deficiency. Vet Pathol 1994;31:435.

Huibregtse BA, Turner JL: Hypereosinophilic syndrome and eosinophilic leukemia: A comparison of 22 hypereosinophilic cats. J Am Anim Hosp Assoc 1994;30:591.

Jain NC: Essentials of Veterinary Hematology. Philadelphia, Lea & Febiger, 1993.

Joffe DJ, Allen AL: Ulcerative eosinophilic stomatitis in three Cavalier King Charles spaniels. J Am Anim Hosp Assoc 1995;31:34.

Keller CB, Lamarre J: Inherited lysosomal storage disease in an English springer spaniel. J Am Vet Med Assoc 1992;200:194.

Knapp DW, Leibnitz RR, DeNicola DB, et al: Measurement of NK activity in effector cells purified from canine peripheral lymphocytes. Vet Immunol Immunopathol 1993;35:239.

Latimer KS, Bounous DI, Collatos C, et al: Extreme eosinophilia with disseminated eosinophilic granulomatous disease in a horse. Vet Clin Pathol 1996;25:23.

Lewis JH: Comparative hemostatis in vertebrates. New York, Plenum Press, 1996.

Lichtman MA: Monocytosis and monocytopenia. In Beutler E, Lichtman MA, Coller BS, Kipps TJ (eds): Williams Hematology, 5th edition. New York, McGraw-Hill, 1995, p 881.

Lichtman MA: Basophilopenia, basophilia, and mastocytosis. In Beutler E, Lichtman MA, Coller BS, Kipps TJ (eds): Williams Hematology, 5th edition. New York, McGraw-Hill, 1995, p 852.

Lichtman MA: Classification and clinical manifestations of neutrophil disorders. In Beutler E, Lichtman MA, Coller BS, Kipps TJ (eds): Williams Hematology, 5th edition. New York, McGraw-Hill, 1995, p 810.

McEntee MF, Horton S, Blue J, et al: Granulated round cell tumor of cats. Vet Pathol 1993;30:195.

Monteith CN, Cole D: Monocytic leukemia in a horse. Can Vet J 1995;36:765.

Müller KE, Bernadina WE, Kalsbeek HC, et al: Bovine leukocyte adhesion deficiency—clinical course and laboratory findings in eight affected animals. Vet Q 1994;16:65.

Nagahata H, Kehrli ME, Jr, Murata H, et al: Neutrophil function and pathologic findings in Holstein calves with leukocyte adhesion deficiency. Am J Vet Res 1994;55:40.

Nagahata H, Nochi H, Sanada Y, et al: Analysis of mononuclear cell functions in Holstein cattle with leukocyte adhesion deficiency. Am J Vet Res 1994;55:1101.

Neer TM, Dial SM, Pechman R, et al: Mucopolysaccharidosis VI in a miniature Pinscher. J Vet Intern Med 1995;9:429.

O'Keefe DA, Schaeffer DJ: Hematologic toxicosis associated with doxorubicin administration in cats. J Vet Intern Med 1992;6:276.

Pollack MJ, Flanders JA, Johnson RC: Disseminated malignant mastocytoma in a dog. J Am Anim Hosp Assoc 1991;27:435.

Prieur DJ, Collier LL: Neutropenia in cats with the Chediak-Higashi syndrome. Can J Vet Res 1987;51:407.

Raskin RE: Myelopoiesis and myeloproliferative disorders. Vet Clin North Am Small Anim Pract 1996;26:1023.

Reagan WJ, Murphy D, Battaglino M, et al: Antibodies to canine granulocyte colony-stimulating factor induce persistent neutropenia. Vet Pathol 1995;32:374.

Schleimer RP, Bochner BS: The effects of glucocorticoids on human eosinophils. J Allergy Clin Immunol 1994;94:1202.

Sellon RK, Rottman JB, Jordan HL, et al: Hypereosinophilia associated with transitional cell carcinoma in a cat. J Am Vet Med Assoc 1992;201:591.

Smolen JE, Boxer LA: Functions of neutrophils. In Beutler E, Lichtman MA, Coller BS, Kipps TJ (eds): Williams Hematology, 5th edition. New York, McGraw-Hill, 1995, p 779.

Somberg RL, Robinson JP, Felsburg PJ: T lymphocyte development and function in dogs with X-linked severe combined immunodeficiency. J Immunol 1994;153:4006.

Sparkes AH, Hopper CD, Millard WG, et al: Feline immunodeficiency virus infection. Clinicopathologic findings in 90 naturally occurring cases. J Vet Intern Med 1993; 7:85.

Tizard I: Veterinary Immunology. An Introduction, 4th edition. Philadelphia, WB Saunders Co, 1992.

Trowald-Wigh G, Håkansson L, Johannisson A, et al: Leucocyte adhesion protein deficiency in Irish setter dogs. Vet Immunol Immunopathol 1992;32:261.

Wardlaw AJ, Kay AB: Eosinophils: production, biochemistry and function. In Beutler E, Lichtman MA, Coller BS, Kipps TJ (eds): Williams Hematology, 5th edition. New York, McGraw-Hill, 1995, p 798.

Wardlaw AJ, Kay AB: Eosinopenia and eosinophilia. In Beutler E, Lichtman MA, Coller BS, Kipps TJ (eds): Williams Hematology, 5th edition. New York, McGraw-Hill, 1995, p 844.

Weiser MG, Thrall MA, Fulton R, et al: Granular lymphocytosis and hyperproteinemia in dogs with chronic ehrlichiosis. J Am Anim Hosp Assoc 1991;27:84.

Wellman ML, Hammer AS, DiBartola SP, et al: Lymphoma involving large granular lymphocytes in cats: 11 cases (1982–1991). J Am Vet Med Assoc 1992;201:1265.

5

Evaluation of Hemostasis: Coagulation and Platelet Disorders

Hemostasis depends on vascular integrity, platelet numbers and function, and coagulation. Vascular integrity is determined in large measure by the health of endothelial cells and their extracellular matrix. Damage to vessel walls can result in hemorrhage and/or the activation of platelets and coagulation. When arteries are severed, there is a transient reflex vasoconstriction which slows the loss of blood and allows some time for the commencement of platelet plug formation and coagulation, which eventually result in the formation of a stable thrombus.

BLOOD PLATELETS

Blood platelets (thrombocytes) in mammals are small, round to oval anucleated cell fragments that form from cylinders of megakaryocyte cytoplasm. Their cytoplasm appears light blue with many small reddish purple granules when visualized using routine blood stains. Unstimulated platelets appear as thin discs when examined by scanning electron microscopy. They have a life span of 5 to 10 days in most domestic animals. Normal platelet counts vary depending on the species, with minimal reference values as low as 100,000/μL in horses and maximal reference values as high as 800,000/μL in several domestic animal species. The numbers normally present in blood greatly exceed that needed for adequate hemostasis. The spleen stores about one-third of the total platelet mass. Platelets are released from the spleen with α-adrenergic stimulation as occurs during exercise.

Thrombocytes in nonmammalian species have nuclei and are much larger than those in mammals. They have a high nuclear to cytoplasmic ratio and are often oval or elongated in shape with light blue cytoplasm in stained blood films. Cytoplasmic vacuoles may be present at one or both ends of a cell. Granules are not apparent. When thrombocytes are more round in shape, they can be difficult to differentiate from lymphocytes. Like mammalian platelets, thrombocytes appear in clumps in blood films when activated. Thrombocyte counts are much lower in nonmammalian species than they are in mammals.

As in other blood cells, glucose is the major energy source for platelets. In contrast to anucleated red blood cells (RBCs), platelets have mitochondria and consequently the Krebs cycle and oxidative phosphorylation, but little of the pyruvate produced by glycolysis is metabolized through the Krebs cycle. Biochemically, platelets have often been compared to white skeletal muscle. They have active anaerobic glycolysis and synthesize and utilize large amounts of glycogen. Platelets have a dense tubular system that is analogous to the Ca^{++}-sequestering sarcoplasmic reticulum present in skeletal muscle (Fig. 5–1). Most domestic animal species have a well-developed canalicular system that is continuous with the surface membrane. Microtubules and microfilaments are present and composed of a variety of contractile proteins including actin, myosin, and related proteins. A major mediator of energy utilization in platelets is an actomyosin-like Ca^{++}- and Mg^{++}-dependent adenosine triphosphatase (ATPase).

Adenine nucleotides are present in approximately equal amounts in metabolic and storage pools. As in other cells, ATP accounts for most of the adenine nucleotide in the metabolic pool. The ATP in this pool provides energy for cell functions. In addition to energy needed for normal homoeostatic processes, platelets expend a large amount of energy during aggregation and the release reactions to be discussed later. Approximately 50% of the adenine nucleotides are present in platelet-dense bodies or δ-granules (storage pool). In addition to ATP, these dense bodies contain considerable

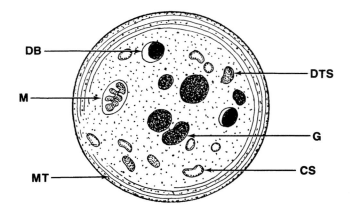

FIGURE 5–1. Platelet ultrastructure. DB, dense bodies; M, mitochondria; MT, microtubules; DTS, dense tubular system; G, granules; CS, canalicular system.

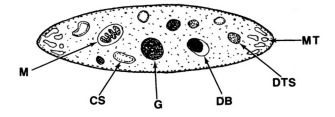

ADP, Ca^{++}, and serotonin that are secreted outside the platelets during the release reaction (degranulation). Other granules (α-granules) are also secreted when platelets are activated. Some of the contents of these α-granules are synthesized by megakaryocytes and others are taken up from the plasma. Granule contents vary by species. Contents that may be present include adhesive proteins (von Willebrand factor [vWF], fibrinogen, fibronectin, thrombospondin), coagulation factors V and XI, fibrinolytic inhibitors (plasminogen activator inhibitor, α_2-plasmin inhibitor), platelet factor 4 (PF-4) (a protein that neutralizes heparin-like molecules), P-selectin, and other components including leukotactic, mitogenic, and vascular permeability factors and the β-thromboglobulin family of proteins of unknown function.

Platelets express various glycoprotein molecules on their surfaces that are needed for normal adhesion (platelet to extracellular matrix) and aggregation (platelet-to-platelet binding) to occur. The glycoprotein (GP) complex Ib\IX\V is especially important for the adhesion of platelets to vWF that is bound to the subendothelial matrix. The GPIIb/IIIa complex ($\alpha_{IIb}\beta_3$ integrin) is especially important for normal platelet aggregation mediated by fibrinogen.

Platelets have three primary functions in hemostasis. The first is the formation of a platelet plug at the site of vessel injury. Formation of a platelet plug alone is sufficient to stop bleeding from a small vessel. Second, platelet activation results in the exposure of negatively charged phospholipids (platelet factor 3 [PF-3]) on the surface of platelets which binds certain coagulation factors in close proximity, thereby accelerating coagulation. Finally, the presence of platelets helps maintain normal vascular integrity in some way. Vascular endothelium is thin and more prone to disruption in animals with low platelet counts (thrombocytopenia).

PRIMARY HEMOSTASIS

Vascular Phase

Primary hemostasis consists of a vascular and a platelet phase (Fig. 5–2). Following the severing of vessels, a reflex vasoconstriction temporarily retards blood flow, allowing time for initiation of platelet plug formation and coagulation. The damage or removal of endothelial cells exposes the subcellular matrix, resulting in platelet adhesion and activation, as well as the activation of intrinsic coagulation. Endothelial cells and other damaged tissues release ADP and tissue thromboplastin, which promote platelet aggregation and extrinsic coagulation, respectively.

Platelet Phase

In response to vessel wall injury or exposure to foreign surfaces, platelets rapidly undergo the processes of adhesion, shape change, secretion, and aggregation through a complex series of coordinated processes that culminate in the formation of a precisely located platelet plug.

Platelet Adhesion. Optimal platelet adhesion requires binding of platelet surface GPIb of the GPIb/IX/V complex to vWF molecules that have been

PLATELET SYSTEM   VASCULAR SYSTEM   COAGULATION SYSTEM

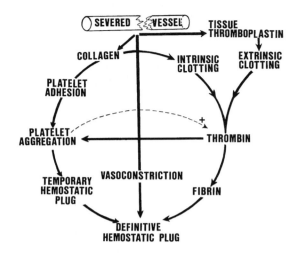

FIGURE 5–2. Overview of primary hemostasis.

deposited in the extracellular matrix, primarily associated with collagen in microfibrils (Fig. 5–3). vWF is a component of the factor VIII macromolecular complex. It is a large disulfide-bonded tetramer (MW 850,000) that circulates as large multimers (8 to 12 × 10^6 daltons) in blood. vWF multimers bind to factor VIII coagulant activity (VIII:C), a smaller protein (MW 250,000) that functions as a procoagulant in the intrinsic coagulation system. This binding of factor VIII:C to vWF appears to prolong its circulation time. These two factors are controlled by different genes and are synthesized independently. vWF, also referred to as factor VIII:R (related antigen), is autosomally controlled and synthesized by endothelial cells and megakaryocytes (in some species). VIII:C, also referred to as factor VIII:AHF (antihemophilic factor), is X-linked and synthesized by endothelial cells.

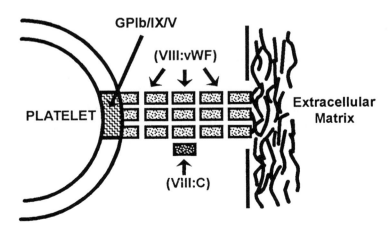

FIGURE 5–3. The von Willebrand factor (vWF) component of the factor VIII complex (VIII:vWF) is needed for optimal binding of platelets to subendothelial matrix. vWF binds to a glycoprotein complex GPIb\IX\V on the platelet surface. VIII:C, coagulant component of the factor VIII complex.

In addition to occurring in the circulation, vWF is present in platelet granules in some species (dog platelets contain little vWF) and is bound to the extracellular matrix of the vascular subendothelium, where it was secreted by endothelial cells. Platelets do not bind to circulating vWF, but GPIb on the platelet surface binds to vWF deposited in the extracellular matrix. It appears that the conformation of vWF changes upon binding to extracellular matrix components so that it readily binds to the GPIb receptor, especially when shear force is applied as occurs in flowing blood.

Platelet Activation. The adhesion of platelets to the extracellular matrix, and binding of collagen and other strong agonists (stimulators), such as high concentrations of thrombin and thromboxane A_2, result in the activation of phospholipase C (PLC) in the membrane (Fig. 5–4). PLC cleaves a unique membrane phospholipid phosphatidylinositol 4,5-bisphosphate (PIP_2) into inositol triphosphate (IP_3) and diacylglycerol (DG). IP_3 binds to a receptor in the dense tubular system causing the release of intracellular Ca^{++}, and DG potentiates the activation of protein kinase C. These reactions stimulate platelets in various ways and result in shape change, secretion, and aggregation.

Agonists such as adenosine diphosphate (ADP) and serotonin and low concentrations of thrombin activate phospholipase A_2, which stimulates the hydrolysis of phospholipids (especially phosphatidylcholine) with the release of arachidonic acid, which is subsequently metabolized to thromboxane A_2 (TxA_2) by the cyclooxygenase enzyme pathway (Fig. 5–5). Phospholipase A_2 (in conjunction with an acetyltransferase) is also involved in generating platelet-activating factor (PAF, 1-0-alkyl-2-0-acetyl sn-glyceryl-3-phosphoryl choline), another agonist causing platelet aggregation. PAF can be produced not only by activated platelets but also by activated endothelial cells and leukocytes.

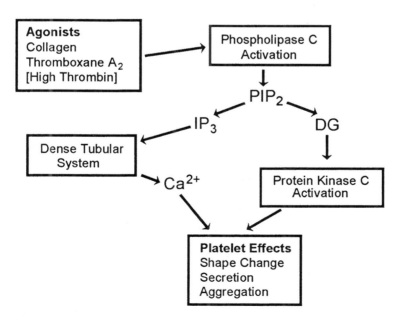

FIGURE 5–4. Activation of phospholipase C and the resultant platelet effects. PIP_2, phospholipid phosphatidylinositol 4,5-bisphosphate; IP_3, inositol triphosphate; DG, diacylglycerol; Ca^{2+}, calcium ions.

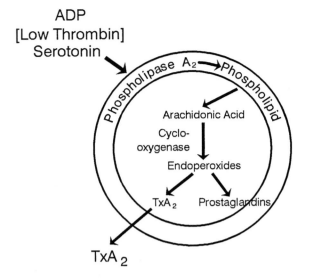

FIGURE 5-5. Activation of phospholipase A_2 and the generation of thromboxane A_2 (TxA$_2$).

Platelet activation is inhibited by prostacyclin (PGI$_2$). When stimulated by thrombin, endothelial cells produce PGI$_2$ as a product of arachidonic acid metabolism. The antagonist has an antiaggregatory effect on platelets by stimulating cyclic adenosine monophosphate (cAMP) synthesis in platelets. Agonists tend to counteract this effect by lowering platelet cAMP concentrations.

Shape Change. The discoid shape of resting platelets is maintained by circumferential bundles of microtubules beneath the platelet membrane and an extensive network of short actin filaments, forming a membrane skeleton. Following binding to vWF and extracellular matrix components, platelets are activated, the microtubular bundles depolymerize, and actin polymerization increases, resulting in platelet "spreading" with the formation of pseudopods. Platelet membrane phospholipids (PF-3) and glycoprotein receptors are also exposed. Platelets have surface receptors for various subendothelial components including collagen, fibronectin, laminin, and thrombospondin. The collagen receptor (GPIa/IIa) functions both for adhesion and as an agonist receptor. Most of these receptors are β_1-integrins.

Platelet Secretion. Platelet secretion (release or degranulation) requires energy-dependent contractile mechanisms. Dense bodies and granules are crushed together (fusion and dissolution) by a surrounding web of microtubules and microfilaments. The contents of dense bodies and granules are discharged into the open canalicular system that is continuous with the platelet surface. Bovine platelets have a minimal canalicular system and granules and dense bodies primarily discharge their contents by fusing with the external platelet membrane. Contraction of individual platelets and the platelet mass facilitates the discharge of material into surrounding plasma. ADP, serotonin, and calcium released from dense bodies promote platelet aggregation.

Platelet Aggregation. ADP, TxA$_2$, thrombin (a product of coagulation), and PAF consistently important agonists that promote platelet aggregation (binding of platelets together). Serotonin and epinephrine are also important agonists in some species. Optimal platelet aggregation requires fi-

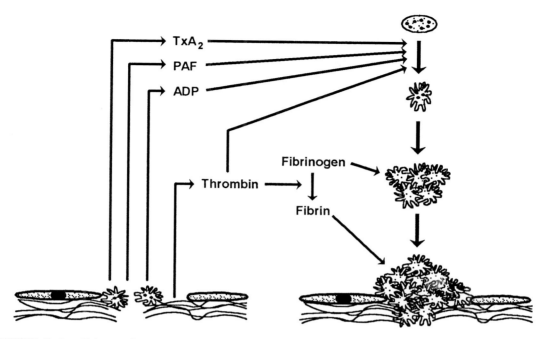

FIGURE 5–6. Primary factors involved in platelet aggregation. TxA$_2$, thromboxane A$_2$; PAF, platelet-activating factor; ADP, adenosine diphosphate.

brinogen and Ca^{++}. The actions of the above agonists result in the exposure/activation of a β_3-integrin platelet surface GPIIb/IIIa receptor that binds to fibrinogen (Fig. 5–6). Aggregation occurs when symmetric fibrinogen molecules bind to exposed receptors on adjacent platelets. vWF also promotes platelet aggregation when shear forces are large in flowing blood. The resultant platelet plug formed may be sufficient to stop bleeding from small vessels. As will be discussed later, the bleeding time test is dependent on platelet numbers and function. Avian thrombocytes differ from mammalian platelets in that ADP is not secreted following platelet activation and it is not an important agonist in the induction of platelet aggregation in birds. Serotonin appears to be an important agonist for avian thrombocytes.

SECONDARY HEMOSTASIS

Overview

Secondary hemostasis is composed of coagulation and consolidation of the temporary hemostatic platelet plug into a definitive hemostatic plug. Coagulation is an enzymatic process involving the conversion of proenzymes to active enzymes. Some activated coagulation factors are themselves enzymes and others combine together in physical complexes to generate specific enzymatic activities. A cascade effect of enzymatic activation results in an amplification of the original stimulus (Fig. 5–7). The final product of coagulation is the formation of cross-linked fibrin strands around and, to a lesser extent,

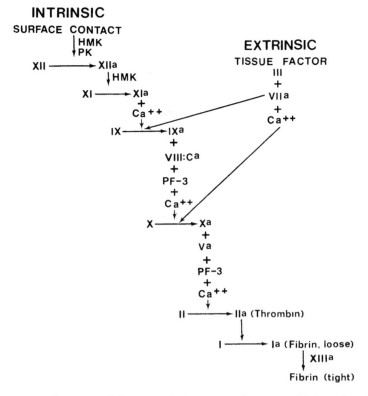

FIGURE 5–7. A diagram of the coagulation cascade. HMK, high-molecular-weight kininogen; PK, prekallikrein; PF-3, platelet factor 3; VIII:C, coagulant component of the factor VIII complex; Ca^{++}, calcium ions. Roman numerals refer to coagulation factors with these numbers and an associated "a" indicates the factor is activated.

through the platelet plug, making it stronger and decreasing the likelihood that rebleeding will occur.

Coagulation factors have been given one or more names, as well as being assigned a Roman numeral. Fibrinogen (factor I), prothrombin (factor II), tissue factor (factor III), and calcium (factor IV) are usually referred to by their names. Other factors are more often referred to by their numbers. There is no factor VI. All factors except Ca^{++} are proteins, most of which are synthesized in the liver. All factors except tissue factor are normally present in the circulation.

Vitamin K is required for the synthesis of functional factors II, VII, IX, and X. Following synthesis of the protein molecules in the liver, a vitamin K– dependent carboxylation of glutamic acid residues of these molecules is required for them to bind Ca^{++} and become functional.

Coagulation can be activated by two different mechanisms *in vitro*: (1) binding of factor VII to tissue factor extracted from tissue juice (extrinsic pathway) or (2) binding of factor XII to surfaces, resulting in "contact activation" (intrinsic pathway). Factor XII can be activated by binding to a wide variety of surfaces including collagen, basement membranes, skin, and many foreign surfaces including glass. These two activation pathways share a common pathway that generates thrombin, which not only converts fibrinogen to fibrin but also activates factors V, VIII, and XIII.

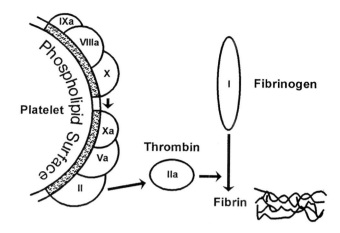

FIGURE 5–8. Assembly of coagulation factors on platelet surface phospholipids (platelet factor 3). Roman numerals refer to coagulation factors with these numbers and an associated "a" indicates the factor is activated.

The activation of platelets by agonists results in a translocation of negatively charged phospholipids from the internal to the external plasma membrane. These negatively charged surface phospholipids have been termed PF-3 or platelet coagulant activity (PCA). PF-3 greatly accelerates coagulation because positively charged calcium ions bind to the negatively charged phospholipid and carboxyl groups of coagulation factors. Binding of coagulation factors to platelets not only brings them together to enhance interactions but also helps protect them from inhibitors (Fig. 5–8).

Extrinsic Coagulation Pathway

It appears that coagulation *in vivo* is initiated by tissue factor (tissue thromboplastin). Tissue factor (TF) is a transmembrane glycoprotein with phospholipid-binding sites. It is not detected in undisturbed endothelial cells, but is present in the membrane of many other cell types that are not normally in contact with the circulation. When it is released from damaged cells, it binds to circulating factor VII. It is unclear how the initial activated factor VII (VIIa) is formed, but the TF-VIIa complex in the presence of phospholipid and Ca^{++} activates factors IX and X to IXa and Xa, respectively. The TF-VIIa complex and Xa provide positive feedback to activate more TF-VII. It appears that the extrinsic system functions *in vivo* to rapidly provide trace amounts of thrombin to activate factors XI, VIII, and V and cause platelets to aggregate, all of which accelerate intrinsic coagulation.

Intrinsic Coagulation Pathway

Contact activation of coagulation occurs when factor XII is bound to a negatively charged surface and interacts with prekallikrein (PK) that is also bound to the surface by high-molecular weight kininogen (HMK). Active factor XII (XIIa) and kallikrein are generated by reciprocal activation. Surface-bound XIIa activates factor XI that is bound to the surface by HMK. Both PK and factor XI circulate complexed with HMK. For many years this method of activation of coagulation was considered to be the major initiating pathway of coagulation. However, since people, cats, and dogs with factor XII deficiency exhibit no hemorrhagic tendencies and some animals (whales, birds, reptiles) naturally lack this factor, it is generally accepted that factor XII is not involved in normal hemostasis.

Factor XI deficiency does result in mild bleeding tendencies, but it is unclear how factor XI is activated *in vivo*. It has been suggested that feedback activation of factor XI may occur by small amounts of thrombin generated following the extrinsic activation of coagulation. Factor IX is activated by both XIa (in the presence of Ca^{++}) and the TF-VIIa complex (in the presence of phospholipid and Ca^{++}). Factor VIII:C is activated by a small amount of thrombin (and possibly Xa). Conversion of factor VIII:C to VIII:Ca requires the dissociation of this molecule from vWF. Factor VIII:Ca is not an enzyme, but it functions as a cofactor that combines with the enzyme IXa in the presence of PF-3 and Ca^{++} to form a complex that activates factor X.

Common Coagulation Pathway

Factor V is activated by minute amounts of thrombin to Va. It functions as a cofactor for Xa and forms a complex (prothrombinase) in the presence of PF-3 and Ca^{++} that converts prothrombin to thrombin. The thrombin formed converts fibrinogen to fibrin monomers which polymerize spontaneously by hydrogen bonding to form unstable non–cross-linked fibrin polymers around the platelet plug. The last step in fibrin polymerization involves the formation of covalent cross-links between fibrin monomers. Factor XIII (fibrin-stabilizing factor) is activated by thrombin. The XIIIa formed is a Ca^{++}-dependent transglutaminase that catalyzes the formation of covalent bonds between lysine and glutamine residues of different monomers. The cross-linked fibrin formed is an insoluble protein polymer that stabilizes the platelet plug.

Inhibitors of Thrombus Formation

Unstimulated platelets do not adhere to the surface of vascular endothelial cells because these endothelial cells possess thromboresistant properties. They synthesize and release PGI_2 and nitric oxide (NO), powerful vasodilators that inhibit platelet aggregation. They synthesize heparan sulfate proteoglycans, which are tightly associated with the endothelium and can accelerate the inactivation of coagulation factors by antithrombin III. Endothelial cells also express thrombomodulin. This cell surface glycoprotein inhibits thrombin's procoagulant activities and promotes protein C activation by thrombin (discussed later). Lastly, endothelial cells produce tissue plasminogen activator (tPA), which is integrally involved in fibrinolysis.

Antithrombin III is the major thrombin inhibitor. It also inhibits other serine proteases VIIa, IXa, Xa, and XIa. It requires the presence of glycosaminoglycans (*e.g.*, heparan sulfate on cell surfaces or in the intracellular matrix) for optimal activity.

α_1-Protease inhibitor (α_1-antitrypsin), C1-esterase inhibitor, and α_2-macroglobulin are less important inhibitors of thrombus formation. Factor Xa and the TF-VIIa complex are inhibited by the bivalent tissue factor pathway inhibitor (TFPI) formerly called the lipoprotein-associated coagulation inhibitor.

FIBRINOLYSIS

Thrombin binds to a protein receptor (thrombomodulin) on endothelial cells and this 1:1 complex activates protein C, a vitamin K–dependent plasma protein (Fig. 5–9). Thrombin that is bound to thrombomodulin no longer has significant procoagulant activity. Protein Ca (in the presence of a vitamin K–dependent protein S cofactor, a phospholipid surface, and Ca^{++}) also inhibits coagulation by proteolytically degrading factor Va and factor VIIIa. Protein Ca binds to an inhibitor of tPA and increases the release of tPA from endothelial cells. Plasminogen coprecipitates with fibrin as a thrombus forms. Conversion of plasminogen to plasmin by tPA is accelerated in the presence of fibrin (Fig. 5–10). Plasmin is not a highly specific enzyme, but its affinity for fibrin helps limit its action. Plasmin-catalyzed hydrolysis of fibrin results in the formation of fibrin degradation products (fibrin split products) that have antihemostatic properties.

Inhibitors of fibrinolysis also occur in plasma. α_2-Antiplasmin inhibits free plasmin, but plasmin bound to fibrin is protected. α_2-Macroglobulin inhibits protein Ca and may inhibit plasmin to some extent. It also inhibits some activated coagulation factors. Endothelial cells produce plasminogen activator inhibitor (PAI) that binds tPA in the circulation.

Fibrinolysis occurs more readily in capillaries than in the systemic circulation. A much higher density of endothelial cells occurs in capillaries. It is estimated that capillaries comprise greater than 99% of the endothelial surface area of the body. Consequently, thrombomodulin-mediated protein C

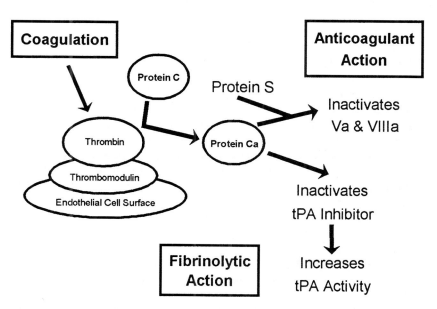

FIGURE 5–9. Actions involving protein C. tPA, tissue plasminogen activator. Roman numerals refer to coagulation factors with these numbers and an associated "a" indicates the factor is activated.

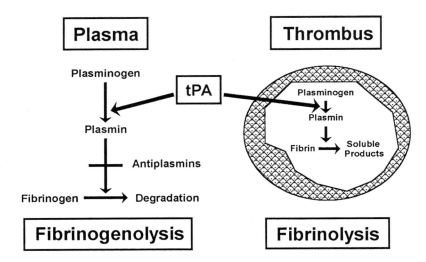

FIGURE 5–10. Actions of tissue plasminogen activator (tPA) and plasmin.

activation and thrombin clearance is greater in capillaries than in large vessels. In addition, tPA release is greater in capillaries and there may be less antiplasmin available to inhibit fibrinolysis. Rapid fibrinolysis of thrombi in large vessels could be life threatening, but fibrinolysis may be important in maintaining the integrity of capillary beds.

ANTICOAGULANTS

Coagulation is prevented in blood samples by using either calcium ion chelators (ethylenediaminetetraacetic acid [EDTA] and citrate) or heparin in blood collection tubes. EDTA is the preferred anticoagulant for complete blood count (CBC) determinations in most species. Minimal sample dilution occurs following mixing with EDTA, and blood films prepared using this anticoagulant exhibit optimal staining with routine blood stains. Unfortunately, blood from some birds and reptiles hemolyze when collected with EDTA. In those species, heparin is usually used as the anticoagulant. The disadvantage of heparin is that leukocytes do not stain as well and platelets clump more than they do in blood collected with EDTA.

Citrate is the preferred anticoagulant for collecting plasma for coagulation tests and for collecting platelets for platelet function tests. Samples collected in citrate solution are diluted by 10%. If platelet counts are done, they must be corrected for this dilution. Citrate is also the anticoagulant typically used in blood collection and storage for transfusions.

The binding of heparin to antithrombin III greatly accelerates the inhibition of thrombin by antithrombin III, thereby inhibiting coagulation. Coagulation factors VII, IXa, Xa, and XIa also appear to be inhibited by the antithrombin III–heparin complex. Heparin is used as an anticoagulant for CBCs in species where EDTA results in hemolysis. Lithium heparin is utilized as an anticoagulant when plasma (rather than serum) is used for clinical chemistry profiles. Heparin is often added to isotonic salt solutions used to flush intravenous lines and may be injected to inhibit blood coagulation *in vivo*.

SCREENING TESTS FOR HEMOSTATIC DISORDERS

No single diagnostic test evaluates all hemostatic components. Consequently, several hemostatic tests are usually done to determine the nature of a hemostatic disorder.

Platelet Count

Stained blood smears should be examined each time platelet counts are done to verify that low platelet counts, determined manually or by machine, are valid. The presence of platelet clumps can result in erroneously low counts. Factors used to estimate platelet numbers vary depending on the microscope used, method of blood film preparation, and area of the film examined; however, the formula given below generally provides a reasonable platelet estimate.

$$\text{Platelets per } \mu\text{L} = \text{number of platelets per } 100 \times \text{oil field} \times 15,000.$$

Most electronic cell counters cannot accurately count cat platelets in whole blood, because cat platelets are larger than those of other domestic animals, making them difficult to separate from erythrocytes based on cell volume.

Mean Platelet Volume

The mean platelet volume (MPV) is the average volume of a single platelet in femtoliters. Impedance cell counters (such as the Coulter Counter S+4 and the Abbott Cell-Dyne 3500) can count platelets and determine the MPV in whole blood from dogs and horses, but not in whole blood from cats. Cat platelets are larger and more prone to aggregation during sample collection than those of the other species; consequently, it is not possible for impedance counters to accurately separate cat platelets from RBCs based on size.

Before the platelet count and MPV from a blood sample are considered valid, cell counters determine whether the size distribution of the platelets approximates the histogram normally expected for platelets. If the histogram is abnormal in shape or if insufficient numbers of platelets are present for accurate histogram construction (very low platelet counts), the values may not be reported. Consequently, whole blood platelet counts and MPV cannot be determined on every sample. Unfortunately, MPV values are often not reported in thrombocytopenic animals, where they might provide useful information.

Within the normal ranges of platelet counts and MPVs, there is an inverse correlation between platelet count and MPV in some species. Studies on the effects of anticoagulants and storage conditions on MPV are inconclusive. MPV values may be slightly higher when collected using EDTA *versus* citrate as an anticoagulant, and increases in MPV may be more likely when stored at 5° C *versus* room temperature. A high MPV value suggests that enhanced thrombopoiesis is present, but it can also be high in animals with myelodysplastic disorders and in otterhounds with a hereditary platelet function defect. A normal MPV does not rule out enhanced thrombopoiesis. The presence of small platelet aggregations in blood samples can result in an artificially increased MPV value. Decreased MPV (presence of microthrombocytes) has been associated with immune-mediated thrombocytopenia in dogs and humans, due to platelet fragmentation. Following appropriate therapy, MPV may increase above normal in these individuals with immune-mediated thrombocytopenia. MPVs have been reported to be slightly higher in hyperthyroid cats and slightly lower in hypothyroid dogs than in euthyroid animals. Healthy King Charles spaniel dogs may have higher MPV values because of the occurrence of a population of macroplatelets. Dogs with phosphofructokinase deficiency of RBCs and skeletal muscle have high MPVs with normal platelet counts.

Bleeding Time

The bleeding time is a simple but crude hemostatic test. It is prolonged in animals with platelet abnormalities. Since this test is expected to be prolonged in animals with low platelet counts, it provides no additional information in animals already known to have severe thrombocytopenia. The oral mucous membrane bleeding time is done to evaluate platelet function in animals with normal or near-normal platelet counts. Following penetration with a lancet, the site should bleed freely undisturbed. Bleeding will usually stop in less than 5 minutes.

Bleeding times determined by toenail clip in anesthetized dogs and cats evaluate not only platelet function, but may also detect severe coagulation defects, because the vessel injury caused by this technique is more substantial than that produced in the oral mucous membrane bleeding time.

Activated Clotting Time

The activated clotting time (ACT) evaluates the intrinsic and common coagulation pathways (Fig. 5–11). It must be done in close proximity to the animal being evaluated. The ACT requires a special collection tube containing siliceous earth (Vacutainer No. 3865; Becton, Dickinson and Company) and a method to maintain collection tubes at 37° C. Blood is collected into prewarmed tubes and maintained at 37° C until clotting has occurred. The ACT is usually less than 3 minutes 20 seconds in horses, 125 seconds in dogs, and 65 seconds in cats.

Activated Partial Thromboplastin Time

The activated partial thromboplastin time (APTT) test is also used to evaluate the intrinsic and common pathways. It is measured using plasma prepared from blood collected with 3.8% sodium citrate as the anticoagulant in a 9:1 mixture. Samples should be kept cool and assays should be done within 30 minutes of collection. A healthy control animal should be measured at the same time. The APTT is likely prolonged if the patient's time is more than 4 seconds longer than the control's time. The reference range will depend on the method used. The APTT is artifactually prolonged if the plasma to anticoagulant ratio is inappropriately low as occurs if insufficient blood is collected into a vacuum tube containing premeasured citrate solution or if erythrocytosis is present (e.g., if severe dehydration is present).

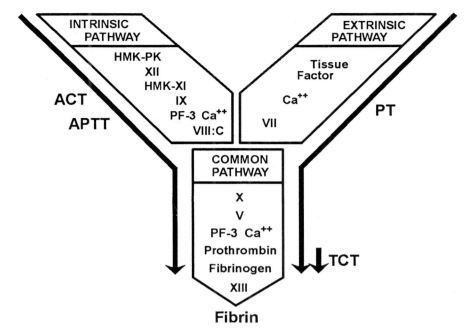

FIGURE 5–11. Parts of the coagulation cascade evaluated using activated clotting time (ACT), activated partial thromboplastin time (APTT), prothrombin time (PT), and thrombin clotting time (TCT) tests. HMK, high-molecular-weight kininogen; PK, pre-kallikrein; PF-3, platelet factor 3; Ca^{++}, calcium ions; VIII:C, the coagulant component of the factor VIII complex. Roman numerals refer to coagulation factors with these numbers and an associated "a" indicates the factor is activated.

Prothrombin Time

The prothrombin time (PT) test is used to evaluate the extrinsic and common pathways (Fig. 5–11). It also requires plasma prepared from blood collected with citrate as the anticoagulant. Samples should be kept cool and assays should be done within 30 minutes of collection. A healthy control animal should be measured at the same time. The PT is likely prolonged if the patient's time is more than 4 seconds longer than the control's time. The reference range will depend on the method used.

Thrombin Clotting Time

The thrombin clotting time (TCT) test is an indicator of quantitative and/or qualitative fibrinogen disorders. The TCT utilizes citrated plasma. Samples should be kept cool and assays should be done within 30 minutes of collection. A healthy control animal should be measured at the same time. The reference range will depend on the method used.

Fibrinogen

The heat precipitation test is a practical test for the estimation of fibrinogen, but it is not sensitive enough to differentiate low-normal from low fibrinogen values when it is determined by subtraction of total protein values using a refractometer. More accurate values can be obtained by ocular micrometry, but somewhat more time is required and a microscope with a calibrated ocular micrometer is needed.

Fibrin Degradation Products

The fibrin degradation products (FDP) test provides evidence of fibrinolysis *in vivo*. FDP produced by fibrinolysis have antihemostatic properties, thereby promoting hemorrhage which occurs as a sequela to disseminated intravascular coagulation (DIC). The serum FDP test is a latex bead agglutination test. It requires special collection tubes that promote complete coagulation and inhibit *in vitro* fibrinolysis. Some commercial collection tubes contain snake venom which can hemolyze animal RBCs. The presence of agglutination following the addition of serum is viewed as a positive test. Positive FDP tests occur in animals with fibrinolysis (secondary to DIC) and animals with fibrinogenolysis (*e.g.*, Eastern diamondback rattlesnake envenomation). Slightly increased values have been associated with exercise, anxiety, and stress in people. False positive results can result from the use of improper collection tubes or the collection of samples from heparinized patients.

SPECIALIZED TESTS FOR HEMOSTATIC DISORDERS

von Willebrand Factor (Factor VIII–Related Antigen)

vWF is a multimeric glycoprotein required for normal platelet adhesion. This factor is assayed when a platelet function defect is suspected. Inherited vWF deficiency (von Willebrand's disease) is especially common in certain breeds (up to 70% of Doberman pinschers) of dogs. Consequently, this factor may be measured prior to surgery or breeding of dogs from breeds in which the disease is prevalent. Some investigators have indicated that hypothyroidism may result in decreased vWF concentrations in plasma in dogs, but recent studies have been unable to confirm this relationship. vWF may increase in plasma as an acute phase reaction during inflammation. Increased concentrations have been reported in dogs with liver disease, during parturition, during endotoxemia, and following epinephrine infusion. vWF is generally quantified using rocket electroimmunodiffusion or enzyme-linked immunosorbent assay (ELISA). There is substantial temporal variation in individual dogs, making identification of carrier animals difficult. Consequently, multiple tests may be necessary to obtain a reliable estimate of vWF concentration.

Antithrombin III

Plasma antithrombin III can be measured using chromogen assays. It may be decreased in hypercoagulable states (*e.g.*, equine colic), DIC, protein-losing nephropathies, protein-losing enteropathies, and sepsis. Antithrombin III is increased in cats with various disease conditions, suggesting that it behaves as an acute phase protein in this species.

Platelet Function

Specialized platelet function tests are not done in most clinical pathology laboratories, but are typically done in hemostasis research laboratories. Platelet aggregation is evaluated in a platelet aggregometer following the addition of various agonists (e.g., ADP, thrombin, and collagen). Platelet adhesion can be measured by the retention of platelets in a glass bead column or a filter of standard size.

Antiplatelet Antibody

Increased platelet-bound immunoglobulins have been detected by flow cytometry and ELISA techniques in animals, but these tests are not readily available. Direct assays (patient's platelets) are preferred to indirect assays (patient's serum and normal canine platelets) because direct assays are more sensitive. Unfortunately, they must be done within a few hours after blood sample collection. Platelets naturally have some immunoglobulin absorbed to their surfaces and the amount of platelet-bound immunoglobulin can increase with time after sample collection; consequently, false positive tests are a significant problem in these assays. Positive test results may occur when immune complexes are absorbed to platelets as well as when antiplatelet antibodies are present.

Specific Coagulation Factors

Assays for specific coagulation factors are done in a few hemostasis research laboratories. Plasma from individuals with known coagulation factor deficiencies is utilized in these tests.

CLINICAL SIGNS OF HEMOSTATIC DISORDERS

If bleeding is excessive or unexplained, a defect in one or more of the components of hemostasis may be present. The type of hemorrhage observed may give some clue about the nature of the defect(s) present. Diffuse cutaneous or mucosal discoloration, resulting from hemorrhage and edema, suggests the presence of a vascular defect. Petechial and ecchymotic cutaneous and/or mucosal hemorrhages and epistaxis are suggestive of thrombocytopenia. The presence of inherited platelet defects is suspected in young dogs with epistaxis, mucosal bleeding, gingival bleeding, and excessive bleeding when shedding of teeth occurs. Spontaneous hematomas and hemarthrosis are more likely to result from coagulation defects than from vascular or platelet abnormalities.

PLATELET DISORDERS

Abnormal Platelet Morphology

The diameters of platelets vary depending on the species, with cats having larger platelets than other domestic animals. The presence of large platelets

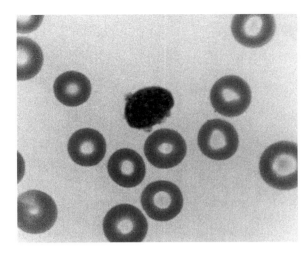

FIGURE 5–12. A macro-platelet in blood from a thrombocytopenic dog with enhanced thrombopoiesis.

(macroplatelets or megaplatelets) in a thrombocytopenic animal suggests that enhanced thrombopoiesis is present (Fig. 5–12), but macroplatelets may also be present in thrombocytopenic animals with myelodysplastic or myeloproliferative disorders. A population of macroplatelets may be seen in healthy nonthrombocytopenic King Charles spaniel dogs and in otterhound dogs with a hereditary platelet function defect.

When platelets are activated, their granules are crushed together by a surrounding web of microtubules and microfilaments. This central aggregate of platelet granules may be mistaken for a nucleus. Hypogranular platelets may result from platelet activation and secretion, but they have also been seen in animals with myeloproliferative disorders. Platelet aggregates form following platelet activation *in vitro*. If degranulation occurs, aggregates may be difficult to recognize, appearing as light blue material on stained blood films. The presence of platelet aggregates should be recorded because the platelet count may be erroneously decreased.

Ehrlichia platys is a rickettsial parasite that specifically infects dog platelets. Morulae appear as tightly packed basophilic clusters of organisms within the cytoplasm of platelets (Color Plate 4).

Thrombocytopenia

Thrombocytopenia denotes decreased blood platelets. Primary causes of thrombocytopenia include decreased production, increased platelet utilization in thrombus formation, and increased destruction. The distinction between the last two causes is not always clear and both processes may occur in some disorders. Less likely causes of thrombocytopenia include sequestration and acute massive external hemorrhage. Bone marrow examination is often indicated in the differential diagnosis of thrombocytopenia, especially in the absence of accompanying coagulation abnormalities.

Decreased Platelet Production. Aplastic anemia, myelophthisis, myeloproliferative disorders, and myelodysplastic syndromes (see Chapter 3) usually have associated thrombocytopenias. Late stages of infections with *Ehrlichia canis* and possibly other rickettsial diseases can have decreased platelet counts secondary to hypoplastic bone marrow. Most immune-mediated thrombocytopenias result from increased platelet destruction, but an immune-mediated destruction of megakaryocytes can result in decreased platelet production. Amegakaryocytic thrombocytopenia is rare in dogs and has been described only once in a cat. Mild cyclic thrombocytopenia occurs because of intermittently decreased platelet production in gray collie dogs with inherited cyclic hematopoiesis.

Increased Platelet Utilization. Increased platelet utilization occurs in disorders that induce DIC as will be discussed later. Increased platelet utilization also occurs in association with hemangiosarcoma in dogs, vasculitis, and other disorders that result in vascular injury.

Increased Platelet Destruction. The presence of increased immunoglobulin on the surface of platelets can result in increased phagocytosis of platelets and subsequent thrombocytopenia. Immune-mediated thrombocytopenia can be either primary or secondary. Autoantibodies are directed against platelet-specific epitopes in primary immune-mediated thrombocytopenia. Autoimmune thrombocytopenia (also called idiopathic thrombocytopenia purpura [ITP]) is a common cause of thrombocytopenia in dogs. Secondary immune-mediated thrombocytopenia results from external antigens (e.g., drugs) or antigen–antibody complexes being absorbed to the platelet surface.

Intravenous heparin frequently induces mild thrombocytopenia in some horses. The mechanism has not been determined, but heparin-induced thrombocytopenia appears to be immune mediated in people. Heparin binds to a platelet component (PF-4), and antibodies made against the heparin–PF-4 complex result in platelet activation and removal.

Thrombocytopenia can occur with a wide variety of bacterial, viral, rickettsial, and protozoal diseases. The most common infectious cause of thrombocytopenia in dogs appears to be *Ehrlichia canis*. This agent appears to cause immune-mediated platelet destruction in the acute phase of ehrlichiosis and decreased platelet production in the severe chronic phase of ehrlichiosis. The cause(s) of thrombocytopenias associated with other infectious agents is not always clear. Vascular injury and/or absorption of immune complexes to platelet surfaces may be involved. The administration of granulocyte-macrophage colony-stimulating factor (GM-CSF) to dogs results in shortened platelet life span and thrombocytopenia, apparently by activating the monocyte/macrophage system. This activation may be a mechanism of increased platelet destruction observed in a variety of diseases in which endogenous cytokine concentrations are increased. *Ehrlichia platys* is a rickettsial parasite that specifically infects dog platelets and causes a cyclic thrombocytopenia.

Sequestration of Platelets. Sequestration of platelets in the body may result in thrombocytopenia. Examples include splenomegaly and hypothermia in various species. Causes of splenomegaly include hereditary hemolytic anemias, immune-mediated diseases, infections, inflammation, splenic congestion, and infiltrative diseases. Increased platelet utilization or destruction also contribute to the development of thrombocytopenia in some of these disorders. When splenomegaly results in increased removal of platelets and/or other blood cells by the spleen, the term hypersplenism may be used.

Massive External Hemorrhage. Because of platelet storage in the spleen, acute hemorrhage usually causes minimal decreases in blood platelet counts. A thrombocytopenia may occur if massive external hemorrhage occurs, especially if the animal is subsequently given a large transfusion using packed RBCs or stored blood. Platelet counts seldom decrease below 100,000/μL from acute hemorrhage alone. Platelet counts are often increased in animals with chronic hemorrhage due to increased platelet production.

Pseudothrombocytopenia

It is essential that a blood smear estimation of platelet numbers be done as a quality control measure for each automated platelet count. The presence of platelet aggregates can result in erroneously low platelet counts. Platelet aggregates usually form when platelets are activated during blood sample collection and handling. EDTA-dependent pseudothrombocytopenia, secondary to platelet aggregation, has been reported in horses. Pseudothrombocytopenias may be reported in cats if whole blood platelet counts are performed using electronic cell counters, because cat platelets are large and difficult to separate from erythrocytes based on cell volumes. Healthy King Charles spaniel dogs exhibit a population of macroplatelets that may not be counted as platelets by electronic cell counters, resulting in frequent pseudothrombocytopenias in this breed.

Platelet Function Abnormalities

Acquired Platelet Function Defects. In addition to causing thrombocytopenia, antiplatelet antibodies may affect platelet function. This may be explained by the finding that the GPIIb/IIIa fibrinogen receptor is apparently the most frequent target antigen in immune-mediated thrombocytopenia in humans. Disorders such as multiple myeloma with high antibody concentrations can coat platelets and inhibit normal platelet function. Platelet defects may occur in association with uremia and following the administration of nonsteroidal antiinflammatory drugs such as aspirin and phenylbutazone, which inhibit TxA$_2$ synthesis. In addition, antihistamines, local analgesics, halothane, bile acids, and certain antibiotics may interact with platelets and interfere with normal platelet aggregation.

Inherited Platelet Function Defects. Several inherited platelet defects (thrombopathy, thrombopathia) have been reported in animals that result in excessive bleeding. Animals with these disorders usually have normal platelet counts and normal platelet morphology, but giant bizarre platelets are present in the thrombopathy reported in otterhound dogs. Deficiencies in the GPIIb/IIIa receptor account for platelet function defects in otterhounds and Great Pyrenees dogs. Platelet δ (dense) granule deficiency (platelet δ storage pool disease) has been reported in pigs and American cocker spaniel dogs. Platelet δ granule deficiency also occurs in Persian cats, Hereford cattle, and Aleutian mink as part of the inherited Chediak-Higashi syndrome. Animals with Chediak-Higashi syndrome have partial albinism with defects in granules of several tissues including skin, leukocytes, and platelets. The pathogeneses of the hereditary thrombopathies in foxhound, Scottish terrier, basset hound, and spitz dogs are unclear, but the mechanisms in the latter two breeds may involve signal transduction defects. Platelets from gray collie dogs with cyclic hematopoiesis appear to have signal transduction defects, but bleeding is not of clinical significance in this disorder.

von Willebrand's Disease.   vWD is a heterogeneous inherited bleeding disorder resulting from quantitative and/or qualitative defects of vWF. It is by far the most common bleeding disorder in dogs, having been recognized in more than 50 breeds. Decreased vWF concentrations are very common in corgi, Doberman pinscher, German shepherd, golden retriever, poodle, and Shetland sheepdog breeds. vWD also occurs in pigs, and has been reported in a Himalayan cat, a quarter horse, and a Simmental calf. Most cases of vWD result from decreased production of vWF by endothelial cells, but defects in the formation of intermediate and large vWF multimers have been described in German shorthair pointers, German wirehaired pointers, a quarter horse and a Simmental calf. Animals with vWD have prolonged bleeding times because vWF is needed for normal platelet adhesion to the subendothelium. Decreased vWF concentration may result in decreased factor VIII:C activity because the binding of VIII:C to vWF prolongs the half-life of VIII:C in the circulation, but the decrease in VIII:C is usually not sufficient to result in a significant prolongation of the APTT.

Thrombocytosis

Thrombocytosis refers to the presence in platelet counts above the normal reference range. It generally occurs secondary to increased production of thrombopoietin or other factors such as IL-1, IL-3, IL-6, and IL-11. Secondary thrombocytosis may occur following, or in association with, hemorrhage. This is especially common when ongoing hemorrhage results in iron deficiency anemia. It may also occur with some hemolytic anemias, with various chronic inflammatory diseases, and as a rebound response to thrombocytopenia. Transient thrombocytosis occurs with exercise and epinephrine secretion because splenic contraction moves the splenic platelet storage pool into the circulation. Thrombocytosis occurs within 1 week following splenectomy because the same number of platelets are produced, but the splenic pool has been removed. The platelet count may return to normal after several months following splenectomy. Primary thrombocytosis occurs independent of thrombopoietin or other growth factors. It may be present in some myeloproliferative disorders. The term "thrombocythemia" is usually used to describe a myeloproliferative disorder that is characterized primarily by persistent, markedly elevated platelet counts. It may be viewed as the platelet counterpart of polycythemia vera. The diagnosis of thrombocythemia is made by ruling out other causes of high platelet counts.

COAGULATION DISORDERS

Acquired Coagulation Disorders

Thrombosis.   The pathogenesis of thrombosis may involve endothelial injury, altered blood flow (turbulence or stasis), or hypercoagulable conditions. Thrombosis has been reported in dogs with heart disease, protein-losing nephropathy, hyperadrenocorticism, glucocorticoid therapy, local endothelial injury, and immune-mediated hemolytic anemia. Aortic thromboembolism often occurs in cats with cardiomyopathy. It does not appear to be the result of a hypercoagulable state in this disorder.

Hypercoagulable State. The increased tendency for coagulation to occur without clinical signs of thrombosis or laboratory evidence of fibrin deposition is termed the hypercoagulable state. Potential causes include initial reactions that ultimately result in DIC (see discussion below), antithrombin III deficiency (*e.g.*, nephrotic syndrome in dogs), and protein C deficiency (a hereditary disorder in horses). Horses with severe colic may develop a hypercoagulable condition as evidenced by decreased antithrombin III and protein C levels and increased thrombin–antithrombin (TAT) complexes in plasma. The presence of an antiphospholipid antibody may result in hypercoagulability and subsequent thrombosis. This antibody has been called a lupus "anticoagulant" when present in individuals with systemic lupus erythematosus (see Chapter 6), because it can cause prolongation of phospholipid-dependent coagulation tests such as the APTT.

Disseminated Intravascular Coagulation. The term "disseminated intravascular coagulation" (DIC) is used to describe a syndrome where diffuse thrombosis and secondary fibrinolysis occur in small vessels. DIC is not a primary disorder. It always occurs in association with other clinical conditions. The formation of thrombi in vessels can result in tissue hypoxia and organ damage (Fig. 5–13). The consumption of coagulation factors and platelets in the formation of these thrombi creates a tendency for hemorrhage. This propensity to bleed is increased by subsequent fibrinolysis, which not only breaks down the thrombi but produces FDP that interfere with normal platelet aggregation and fibrin polymerization. DIC often occurs as a life-threatening event with organ failure and/or hemorrhage, but may occur in a chronic form without severe clinical signs. DIC can result in shock, and shock can potentiate DIC, resulting in a vicious cycle of events. Extensive local intravascular coagulation may occur in some dogs with hemangiosarcoma. Laboratory findings in these cases are similar to those seen in DIC, making differentiation of DIC from local intravascular coagulation difficult.

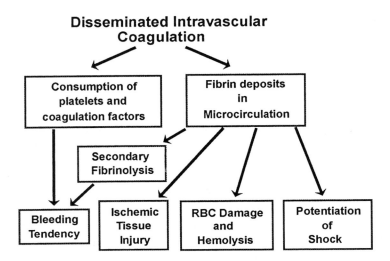

FIGURE 5–13. Pathophysiology of disseminated intravascular coagulation.

TABLE 5–1. Conditions Which May Result in Disseminated Intravascular Coagulation

Septicemia (various gram negative and gram-positive bacteria)

Viremia (infectious canine hepatitis, canine herpes, canine distemper, feline parvovirus, feline infectious peritonitis, African swine fever, blue tongue, and hog cholera)

Protozoal parasites (babesiosis, trypanosomiasis, sarcocystosis, leishmaniasis, and cytauxzoonosis)

Metazoal parasites (heartworms and lungworms)

Marked tissue injury (heatstroke, trauma, and surgical procedures)

Intravascular hemolysis

Obstetrical complications

Malignancy (hemangiosarcoma and disseminated carcinomas)

Traumatic shock

Liver disease

Pancreatitis

Gastric dilatation-volvulus

Toxins (snake and insect venoms, aflatoxin and insecticides)

DIC may occur in disorders where tissue factor is released into the circulation, in disorders where widespread vascular injury is present, in disorders resulting in widespread platelet activation, in disorders resulting in reduced blood flow, and in disorders with impaired removal of activated coagulation factors by the liver. Conditions that may induce DIC are shown in Table 5–1. Undoubtably other disorders will be added to this list over time.

Liver Disease. The liver is the primary site for the synthesis of coagulation factors. Consequently, generalized liver disease may result in an increased bleeding tendency due to decreased circulating coagulation factors. Because of these synthetic functions and the vascular nature of the liver, coagulation screening tests are generally done prior to performing liver biopsies. Liver disorders may also contribute to the development of DIC.

Vitamin K Deficiency. Vitamin K is essential in a carboxylation reaction that results in the formation of active coagulation factors II, VII, IX, and X. Vitamin K deficiency may occur in malabsorptive syndromes (*e.g.*, bile duct obstruction) or from sterilization of the gut by prolonged use of antibiotics. Dicumarol, a product of moldy sweet clover, inhibits the vitamin K–dependent carboxylation reaction. Consequently, dicumarol toxicity can result in hemorrhage in cattle and other species consuming moldy clover. This discovery led to the development of related compounds that are now used in rodenticides. Animals that consume these rodenticides develop life-threatening bleeding disorders. A PIVKA (proteins induced by vitamin K absence/antagonism) test is a simple, sensitive test for vitamin K deficiency that has been developed for human use. Preliminary studies indicate that it may also be useful in animals.

Snake Venoms. Snake venoms contain various proteolytic enzymes, some of which can activate coagulation or the fibrinolytic systems. The venom from the Eastern diamondback rattlesnake contains the enzyme crotalase, which degrades fibrinogen. The Western diamondback rattlesnake venom either directly or indirectly activates plasminogen to plasmin, which subsequently results in fibrinogen proteolysis. Envenomation from both species results in blood that does not clot after collection. Platelet counts may

be normal or decreased. Hemorrhage following rattlesnake bites is also potentiated by the presence of agents in venom that directly cause endothelial
injury. Hemostatic abnormalities are not clinically significant features of water moccasin, copperhead, or coral snake envenomations.

Hereditary Coagulation Disorders

An inherited coagulation factor deficiency is considered when unexplained
hemorrhage occurs or hemorrhage is protracted after surgery. Hereditary
coagulation defects appear to be much more common in dogs than in other
domestic animal species. The likelihood that a coagulation defect will result
in clinically significant hemorrhage varies with the nature of the defect.

Intrinsic Coagulation Pathway Defects. Animals with factor XII deficiency have prolonged APTT and ACT times, but they do not have a bleeding
disorder. Consequently, it is generally accepted that factor XII is not involved
in normal hemostasis. Like animals with factor XII deficiency, animals with
prekallikrein deficiency generally do not exhibit an increased bleeding tendency, although excessive hemorrhage has been reported after castration of
a Belgian horse with this deficiency. Factor XI deficiency has resulted in protracted bleeding after surgery in affected dogs and cattle.

Factor IX (hemophilia B) and factor VIII:C (classical hemophilia) deficiencies are transmitted as X chromosome–linked recessive traits; consequently,
these disorders are usually recognized in male animals. These deficiencies
generally result in severe bleeding disorders.

Extrinsic Coagulation Pathway Defect. Factor VII deficiency has been
reported in several breeds of dogs, occurring frequently in beagles. This
deficiency results in mild disease with no overt bleeding tendency, except for
increased bruising.

Common Coagulation Pathway Defects. Factor X deficiency results in
severe bleeding episodes in dogs. In American cocker spaniels, this deficiency
usually results in stillborn pups or fatal bleeding episodes in the neonatal
period. Prothrombin (factor II) deficiency has been reported in dogs with
mild bleeding tendencies. Fibrinogen (factor I) deficiency causes mild to severe bleeding episodes in affected dogs and goats.

Vitamin K-Dependent Coagulopathy. A vitamin K–dependent coagulopathy has been recognized in Devon rex cats. Affected cats are deficient in the
enzyme γ-glutamyl carboxylase, resulting in reductions in the activities of
factors II, VII, IX, and X. Some animals exhibit minimal bleeding tendencies,
but fatal hemorrhagic episodes have occurred in other affected cats.

INTERPRETATION OF HEMOSTATIC TEST PROFILES

The utilization of a number of hemostatic tests concomitantly helps differentiate causes of hemorrhage including simple thrombocytopenia; DIC; vWD;
vasculitis; rodenticide toxicity; liver disease; and inherited defects of the intrinsic, extrinsic, and common coagulation pathways. Examples of hemostatic test profiles and their interpretations are given below.

1. *Thrombocytopenia with normal APTT, PT, and FDP tests.* Thrombocytopenias without abnormalities in coagulation tests generally result from lack of production or enhanced platelet destruction. Bone marrow biopsies are needed to determine whether there is an abnormality in platelet production by megakaryocytes. Generalized marrow hypoplasia and aplasia are more common than pure amegakaryocytic thrombocytopenias, which are rare in animals. Myelophthisis resulting from marrow neoplasia can also result in thrombocytopenia. Enhanced platelet destruction is the most common cause of thrombocytopenia, often occurring as a result of an immune-mediated process.

2. *Thrombocytopenia with prolonged APTT and PT test results and a positive FDP test.* This profile suggests a consumption of both platelets and coagulation factors as occurs in DIC.

3. *Normal platelet count, prolonged APTT and PT test results, and a negative FDP test.* This profile suggests either multiple coagulation defects, as can occur in rodenticide toxicity and liver disease, or less likely an inherited defect in the common pathway. Platelet counts may sometimes be decreased in animals subsequent to marked blood loss associated with rodenticide toxicity. Collection of blood from a heparinized IV line should also be considered as a factitious cause of this hemostatic profile.

4. *Normal platelet count and PT, prolonged APTT, and a negative FDP test.* This profile suggests an inherited defect in the intrinsic pathway or hemoconcentration.

5. *Normal platelet count and APTT, prolonged PT, and a negative FDP test.* This profile suggests an inherited defect in the extrinsic pathway (*i.e.*, factor VII deficiency). It may also occur in early vitamin K deficiency because factor VII has the most rapid turnover of any coagulation factor.

6. *Normal platelet count, APTT, and PT, with a negative FDP test in the presence of a bleeding diathesis.* This profile suggests a platelet function defect or vascular injury. A concomitant prolonged bleeding time suggests a platelet function abnormality is present. Inherited platelet abnormalities or vWD could be present. vWD is diagnosed by measuring vWF in plasma in specialized laboratories. Some cases with severe vWF deficiency exhibit slightly prolonged APTT test results.

REFERENCES

Bauer KA, Rosenberg RD: Control of coagulation reactions. In Beutler E, Lichtman MA, Coller BS, Kipps TJ (eds): Williams Hematology, 5th edition. New York, McGraw-Hill, 1995, p 1239.

Benson RE, Catalfamo JL, Dodds WJ: A multispecies enzyme-linked immunosorbent assay for von Willebrand's factor. J Lab Clin Med 1992;119:420.

Boudreaux MK: Platelets and coagulation. An update. Vet Clin North Am Small Anim Pract 1996;26:1065.

Boudreaux MK, Kvam K, Dillon AR, et al: Type I Glanzmann's thrombasthenia in a Great Pyrenees dog. Vet Pathol 1996;33:503.

Brassard JA, Meyers KM: Evaluation of the buccal bleeding time and platelet glass bead retention as assays of hemostasis in the dog: The effects of acetylsalicylic acid, warfarin and von Willebrand factor deficiency. Thromb Haemost 1991;65:191.

Brooks M, Raymond S, Catalfamo J: Severe recessive von Willebrand's disease in German wirehaired pointers. J Am Vet Med Assoc 1996;209:926.

Brown SJ, Simpson KW, Baker S, et al: Macrothrombocytosis in cavalier King Charles spaniels. Vet Rec 1994;135:281.

Burton S, Miller L, Horney B, et al: Acute megakaryoblastic leukemia in a cat. Vet Clin Pathol 1996;25:6.

Callan MB, Bennett JS, Phillips DK, et al: Inherited platelet δ-storage pool disease in dogs causing severe bleeding: An animal model for a specific ADP deficiency. Thromb Haemost 1995;74:949.

Carr AP, Johnson GS: A review of hemostatic abnormalities in dogs and cats. J Am Anim Hosp Assoc 1994;30:475.

Chong BH: Heparin-induced thrombocytopenia. Br J Haematol 1995;89:431.

Cook AK, Werner LL, O'Neill SL, et al: Factor X deficiency in a Jack Russel terrier. Vet Clin Pathol 1993;22:68.

Dale GL, Wolf RF, Hynes LA, et al: Quantitation of platelet life span in splenectomized dogs. Exp Hematol 1996;24:518.

De Gopegui RR, Suliman HB, Feldman BF: Disseminated intravascular coagulation: Present and future perspective. Comp Haematol Int 1995;5:213.

Edens LM, Morris DD, Prasse KW, et al: Hypercoagulable state associated with a deficiency of protein C in a thoroughbred colt. J Vet Intern Med 1993;7:190.

Erslev AJ: Platelet morphology, biochemistry, and function. In Beutler E, Lichtman MA, Coller BS, Kipps TJ (eds): Williams Hematology, 5th edition. New York, McGraw-Hill, 1995, p 1161.

Estry DW, Mattson JC, Oesterle JR, et al: Basset hound hereditary thrombopathy: An inherited disorder with defective platelet aggregation despite normal fibrinogen binding and receptor mobility. Comp Haematol Int 1995;5:227.

Feldman BF: Diagnostic approaches to coagulation and fibrinolytic disorders. Semin Vet Med Surg Small Anim 1992;7:315.

Frances CW, Marder VJ: Mechanisms of fibrinolysis. In Beutler E, Lichtman MA, Coller BS, Kipps TJ (eds): Williams Hematology, 5th edition. New York, McGraw-Hill, 1995, p 1252.

Grindem CB, Breitschwerdt EB, Corbett WT, et al: Thrombocytopenia associated with neoplasia in dogs. J Vet Intern Med 1994;8:400.

Hammer AS, Couto CG, Swardson C, et al: Hemostatic abnormalities in dogs with hemangiosarcoma. J Vet Intern Med 1991;5:11.

Harvey JW: Ehrlichia platys infection (infectious cyclic thrombocytopenia of dogs). In Greene CE (ed): Infectious Diseases of the Dog and Cat, 2nd edition. Philadelphia, WB Saunders Co, 1997, in press.

Hinchcliff KW, Kociba GJ, Mitten LA: Diagnosis of EDTA-dependent pseudothrombocytopenia in a horse. J Am Vet Med Assoc 1993;203:1715.

Jesty J, Nemerson Y: The pathways of blood coagulation. In Beutler E, Lichtman MA, Coller BS, Kipps TJ (eds): Williams Hematology, 5th edition. New York, McGraw-Hill, 1995, p 1227.

Kitchens CS: Hemostatic aspects of envenomation by North American snakes. Hematol Oncol Clin North Am 1992;6:1189.

Lassen ED, Swardson CJ: Hematology and hemostasis in the horse: Normal functions and common abnormalities. Vet Clin North Am Equine Pract 1995;11:351.

Lewis DC, Meyers KM: Effect of anticoagulant and blood storage time on platelet-bound antibody concentrations in clinically normal dogs. Am J Vet Res 1994;55:602.

Lewis DC, Meyers KM, Callan MB, et al: Detection of platelet-bound and serum platelet-bindable antibodies for diagnosis of idiopathic thrombocytopenic purpura in dogs. J Am Vet Med Assoc 1995;206:47.

Littlewood JD, Shaw SC, Coombes LM: Vitamin K-dependent coagulopathy in a British Devon rex cat. J Small Anim Pract 1995;36:115.

Meyers KM, Wardrop KJ, Meinkoth J: Canine von Willebrand's disease: Pathobiology, diagnosis, and short-term treatment. Comp Contin Educ Pract Vet 1992;14:13.

Monreal L, Villatoro AJ, Monreal M, et al: Comparison of the effects of low-molecular-weight and unfractioned heparin in horses. Am J Vet Res 1995;56:1281.

Moser J, Meyers KM, Meinkoth JH, et al: Temporal variation and factors affecting measurement of canine von Willebrand factor. Am J Vet Res 1996;57:1288.

Nash RA, Burstein SA, Storb R, et al: Thrombocytopenia in dogs induced by granulocyte-macrophage colony-stimulating factor: Increased destruction of circulating platelets. Blood 1995;86:1765.

Northern J Jr, Tvedten HW: Diagnosis of microthrombocytosis and immune-mediated thrombocytopenia in dogs with thrombocytopenia: 68 Cases (1987–1989). J Am Vet Med Assoc 1992;200:368.

O'Brien SR, Sellers TS, Meyer DJ: Artifactual prolongation of the activated partial thromboplastin time associated with hemoconcentration in dogs. J Vet Intern Med 1995;9:169.

Panciera DL, Johnson GS: Plasma von Willebrand factor antigen concentration in dogs with hypothyroidism. J Am Vet Med Assoc 1994;205:1550.

Peng J, Friese P, George JN, et al: Alterations of platelet function in dogs mediated by interleukin-6. Blood 1994;83:398.

Pucheu-Haston CM, Camus A, Taboada J, et al: Megakaryoblastic leukemia in a dog. J Am Vet Med Assoc 1995;207:194.

Ramsey CC, Burney DP, Macintire DK, et al: Use of streptokinase in four dogs with thrombosis. J Am Vet Med Assoc 1996;780.

Rishniw M, Lewis DC: Localized consumptive coagulopathy associated with cutaneous hemangiosarcoma in a dog. J Am Anim Hosp Assoc 1994;30:261.

Sellon DC, Levine J, Millikin E, et al: Thrombocytopenia in horses: 35 cases (1989–1994). J Vet Intern Med 1996;10:127.

Sixma JJ, Van Zanten GH, Banga J-D, et al: Platelet adhesion. Semin Hematol 1995; 32:89.

Soute BAM, Ulrich MMW, Watson ADJ, et al: Congenital deficiency of all vitamin K-dependent blood coagulation factors due to a defective vitamin K-dependent carboxylase in Devon rex cats. Thromb Haemost 1992;68:521.

Stone MS, Johnstone IB, Brooks M, et al: Lupus-type "anticoagulant" in a dog with hemolysis and thrombosis. J Vet Intern Med 1994;8:57.

Sullivan P, Gompf R, Schmeitzel L, et al: Altered platelet indices in dogs with hypothyroidism and cats with hyperthyroidism. Am J Vet Res 1993;54:2004.

Sullivan PS, Grubbs ST, Olchowy TWJ, et al: Bleeding diathesis associated with variant von Willebrand factor in a Simmental calf. J Am Vet Med Assoc 1994;205:1763.

Sullivan PS, Manning KL, McDonald TP: Association of mean platelet volume and bone marrow megakaryocytopoiesis in thrombocytopenic dogs: 60 cases (1984–1993). J Am Vet Med Assoc 1995;206:332.

Thomas JS: von Willebrand's disease in the dog and cat. Vet Clin North Am Small Anim Pract 1996;26:1089.

Topper MJ, Prasse KW: Use of enzyme-linked immunosorbent assay to measure thrombin-antithrombin III complexes in horses with colic. Am J Vet Res 1996;57:456.

Van Winkle TJ, Bruce E: Thrombosis of the portal vein in eleven dogs. Vet Pathol 1993;30:28.

Wardrop KJ, Baszler TV, Reilich E, et al: A morphometric study of bone marrow megakaryocytes in foals infected with equine infectious anemia virus. Vet Pathol 1996;33:222.

Welles EG: Antithrombotic and fibrinolytic factors. Vet Clin North Am Small Anim Pract 1996;26:1111.

Welles EG, Boudreaux MK, Crager CS, et al: Platelet function and antithrombin, plasminogen, and fibrinolytic activities in cats with heart disease. Am J Vet Res 1994; 55:619.

6

Immunologic Disorders and Dysproteinemias

IMMUNE SYSTEM

The immune system is an integrated network composed of various cell types, numerous cytokines, and certain plasma proteins which work in synergy to eliminate infectious agents, parasites, and noxious antigens; consequently, defects in the immune response result in increased susceptibility to these foreign invaders. Inappropriate or exaggerated immune responses result in immune-mediated tissue injury. A thorough review of immunology is beyond the scope of this text; consequently, the reader is referred to current immunology textbooks for more detailed information.

Specific Immunity

Lymphocytes are the immunocompetent cells that respond to specific antigens. The production and function of lymphocyte types are discussed in Chapters 2 and 4, respectively. B-lymphocytes are primarily responsible for immunoglobulin (antibody) production; however, immunoglobulin production also requires the participation of T-lymphocytes and macrophages. In contrast to B-lymphocytes, which produce immunoglobulins that are carried in the blood (humoral immunity) to the site of a foreign antigen, T-lymphocytes can migrate to the site of a foreign antigen (cellular immunity). T-lymphocytes are involved in immune regulation, cytotoxicity, delayed-type hypersensitivity, and graft-*versus*-host reactions. T-helper (CD4+, CD8−) lymphocytes promote lymphocyte responses and T-suppressor/cytotoxic (CD4−, CD8+) lymphocytes down-regulate immunoglobulin production and play pivotal roles in cytotoxicity directed at fungi, protozoan organisms, and neoplastic cells.

Nonspecific Immunity

Nonspecific immunity involves neutrophils, macrophages, mast cells, eosinophils, basophils, and natural killer (NK) cells along with the complement system. In addition to their roles in phagocytosis and the production of various inflammatory cytokines, macrophages play a pivotal role in the processing and presentation of antigens to T-lymphocytes. The production and function of these various cell types are discussed in Chapters 2 and 4, respectively. The mucosal surfaces along with their secretions are another component of the nonspecific defense network.

TESTS FOR IMMUNE-MEDIATED DISORDERS

Examination for Red Blood Cell Agglutination. When red blood cells (RBCs) appear to clump in blood samples, it is important to differentiate autoagglutination (aggregation of RBCs together in clusters) from rouleaux (adherence of RBCs together like a stack of coins). Rouleaux formation is eliminated by washing RBCs in physiologic saline, but agglutination is not. This differentiation requires centrifugation of blood, removal of plasma, and resuspension of RBCs in saline. A rapid way to differentiate rouleaux from autoagglutination is to mix a drop of physiologic saline with a drop of blood on a glass slide and examine as a wet mount using a microscope. This dilution reduces rouleaux, but agglutination is not affected. The presence of autoagglutination indicates that the RBCs have increased surface-bound immunoglobulins. These immunoglobulins are usually of the IgM type because of the presence of 10 antigen-binding sites per molecule (Fig. 6–1). A direct antiglobulin test is not needed if autoagglutination is present in saline-washed samples.

Tests for Anti-RBC Antibodies

Tests for anti-RBC antibodies are done when autoagglutination is absent, but immune-mediated hemolytic anemia is still suspected.

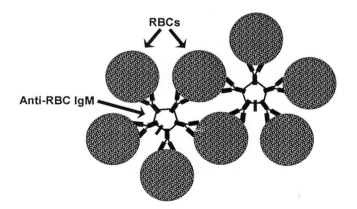

FIGURE 6–1. Anti-RBC IgM antibodies causing RBC agglutination.

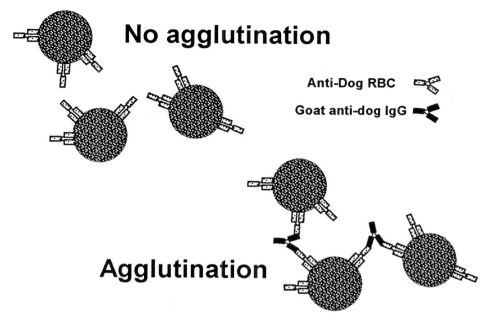

FIGURE 6–2. Direct antiglobulin test (Coombs' test). The addition of anti-dog IgG results in the agglutination of RBCs coated with IgG.

Direct Antiglobulin Test (DAT) or Coombs' Test. The DAT utilizes washed RBCs from the patient and species-specific antisera against IgG, IgM, and the third component of complement (C_3) to detect the presence of one or more of these factors on the surface of RBCs (Fig. 6–2). Unless clinical evidence of cold-agglutinin disease is present, this test is usually only conducted at 37°C, because a substantial number of normal animals exhibit positive test results when the test is run at cold temperatures. In addition to autoimmune hemolytic anemia, neonatal isoerythrolysis, and blood transfusion reactions, the DAT may be positive in association with various infectious, parasitic, neoplastic, inflammatory, and other secondary immune-mediated diseases. If a drug-induced immune-mediated disorder is suspected, the offending drug should be included in the assay system.

A negative DAT does not rule out an immune-mediated hemolytic anemia. A false negative test may occur if there are insufficient quantities of antibody or complement on RBCs, if the ratio of antiglobulin in the reagent to antibody or complement on RBCs is not appropriate, if the test is performed with an incorrect species-specific reagent or performed at an improper temperature, if the animal has been treated with glucocorticoid for a week or more, or if the drug was not added to the test for an animal with a drug-induced immune-mediated hemolytic anemia.

Direct Enzyme-Linked Antiglobulin Test (DELAT). DELAT is an enzyme-linked immunosorbent assay (ELISA) test that has been developed and evaluated for use in dogs. Regardless of the cause of the anemia, a majority of anemic dogs have increased RBC-bound immunoglobulin and/or complement when the DELAT is used. This test has high sensitivity but low specificity for the diagnosis of autoimmune hemolytic anemia.

Blood Typing

Large numbers of protein and complex carbohydrate antigens occur on the external surface of RBCs. Some antigens are present on RBCs from all members of a species and others (including blood group isoantigens) segregate genetically, appearing in some but not all members of a species. Blood group isoantigens are detected serologically on the surface of RBCs using agglutination and/or hemolysis tests. With detailed genetic studies, these isoantigens can be placed into blood groups (RBC isoantigen systems). Blood groups have individual chromosomal loci and each locus has from two to many allelic genes. Most blood groups derive their antigenicity from the carbohydrate composition of membrane-associated glycolipids and glycoproteins, with the amino acid sequence of membrane proteins accounting for the antigenic determinants in other blood groups.

Blood groups in domestic animals have been most extensively characterized in horses and cattle, where blood typing is routinely used for animal identification and parentage testing. Cattle have at least 11 blood groups with multiple alleles per group. Based on all the different combinations of factors that can occur, greater than 2 trillion distinctly different blood type profiles are possible in cattle.

Isoantigens vary markedly in their potential to cause hemolytic anemia. Many isoantigens are weak (do not induce antibodies of high titer) or induce antibodies that do not act at normal body temperature. Fortunately, only a few isoantigens appear to be important in producing life-threatening hemolytic disease in animals. Isoantigens of clinical significance include DEA-1.1 (and possibly DEA-1.2) in dogs, AB in cats, Aa and Qa in horses, and A and E in pigs.

Ideally, blood typing of donor and recipient animals for clinically significant isoantigens should be performed prior to all blood transfusions, as occurs in human medicine. This is generally not feasible in veterinary medicine, due to unavailability of in-house tests and/or cost considerations. A practical alternative is to send out blood samples from potential donors for blood typing and select blood donors that are negative for clinically significant isoantigens. The use of blood from these donors coupled with cross-matching of donor and recipient samples will minimize the likelihood of severe transfusion reactions.

Blood typing of animals may be done prior to mating to select animals of like blood types and minimize the possibility of subsequent hemolytic reactions (neonatal isoerythrolysis) in newborn animals. This is most frequently done in mares that have previously given birth to foals that developed neonatal isoerythrolysis. It may also be considered in certain breeds of cats where B-type blood is common (Table 6–1).

Blood Cross-Match Tests

Blood cross-match tests are used to detect the presence of hemagglutinating and hemolyzing antibodies in the serum of donor and recipient animals. Suspensions of washed RBCs are incubated with serum samples, centrifuged, and examined for the presence of hemolysis and gross and microscopic agglutination. The major cross-match tests for antibodies in the re-

TABLE 6–1. Frequency of Blood Type-B in Purebred Cats in the United States[a]

Type-B Frequency	Breeds
None	Siamese, and related breeds, Burmese, Tonkinese, Russian blue
1–10%	Main coon, Norwegian forest
11–20%	Abyssinian, Birman, Persian, Somali, sphinx, Scottish fold
20–45%	Exotic, and British shorthairs, Cornish, Devon rex

[a]Type-A frequency is determined by subtracting type-B frequency from 100% because type-AB is extremely rare. Data are from Giger U, Bucheler J, Patterson DF: Frequency, and inheritance of A, and B blood types in feline breeds of the United States. J Hered 1991;82:15.

cipient's serum that are directed against the donor's RBCs. The minor cross-match tests for antibodies in the donor's serum that are directed against the recipient's RBCs. Autoagglutination or severe hemolysis in the patients' blood sample precludes the accurate performance of cross-match tests.

The absence of agglutination or hemolysis in cross-match tests does not indicate that animals have similar blood types. It only indicates that preexisting antibodies were not detected and that an acute hemolytic transfusion reaction is highly unlikely. A delayed transfusion reaction can still occur if important isoantigen differences are present. The benefit of the transfusion is short-lived in delayed transfusion reactions because antibodies made against the donor's RBCs result in phagocytosis and removal of these RBCs within a few days.

Tests for Antinuclear Antibodies

The presence of circulating antinuclear antibodies (ANA) is associated with various autoimmune diseases in people and animals. ANA are most often measured in dogs suspected of having systemic lupus erythematosus (SLE). Studies indicate that ANA in dogs are primarily of the IgG type. They are directed against individual histones, but not against native DNA.

ANA Test. An indirect immunofluorescent antibody (IFA) technique is most widely used for ANA testing. Typically, dilutions of a patient's serum are placed on a glass slide with tissue cells fixed to the surface. After allowing time for ANA present to become bound to the nuclei, the slides are rinsed, and fluorescein-labeled antibodies to globulins of the same species as the patient are added. The slides are again rinsed and the presence or absence of nuclear fluorescence is determined using a fluorescent microscope. Frozen rodent liver sections have been used most frequently as the substrate in veterinary medicine (Fig. 6–3), but a human epithelial cell line (HEp-2) appears to be a superior ANA substrate because of its low reactivity with normal serum and the ease of discernment of the fluorescence pattern. Titers above 1/25 and 1/100 are considered positive in dogs when using HEp-2 and rat liver substrates, respectively.

Positive test results should be viewed with caution. Chronic bacterial infections (*e.g.*, bacterial endocarditis), parasitism (*e.g.*, heartworm disease),

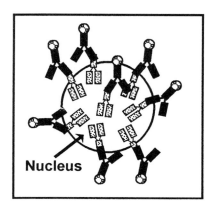

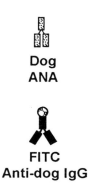

Dog
ANA

FITC
Anti-dog IgG

FIGURE 6–3. Antinuclear antibody (ANA) test. Sections of liver are incubated with test serum and following washing, the presence of antinuclear antibodies is demonstrated using fluorescein (FITC)-labeled antibodies against globulins of the same species as the patient.

rickettsial infections, viral infections (*e.g.*, feline leukemia virus [FeLV] and feline infectious peritonitis [FIP]) and neoplasia can give positive test results, although titers are usually low. The test must especially be interpreted with care in cats, because many normal cats are weakly ANA-positive.

LE Cell Test. A lupus erythematosus (LE) cell is a leukocyte (primarily a neutrophil) with a single large reddish purple amorphous inclusion that nearly fills the cytoplasm of the cell. This inclusion represents the nucleus of a damaged leukocyte that has been opsonized by antinuclear antibody and complement and phagocytized by an intact leukocyte. LE cells are occasionally seen in anticoagulated blood, bone marrow, and joint fluids that have been stored *in vitro.* The LE cell test is performed by rupturing leukocytes by forcing clotted blood through a sieve or mixing anticoagulated blood vigorously with glass beads, incubating the samples to allow time for LE cell formation, and then making buffy coat smears, staining, and examining for LE cell formation. Finding a single LE cell is considered a positive test result. With the ready availability of the ANA test, which is more sensitive and less labor intensive to perform than the LE cell test, the latter test is now seldom done in veterinary laboratories. The advantages of the LE cell test are that it does not require species-specific reagents and is more specific for SLE than is the ANA test.

Tests for Antiplatelet Antibodies

A number of tests have been developed to detect antiplatelet antibodies. These include the platelet factor 3 (PF-3) test for antibodies in serum, a direct immunofluorescent test of bone marrow megakaryocytes, and various ways of detecting immunoglobulin bound to platelet surfaces. In the PF-3 test, antiplatelet antibodies in test serum bind to platelets in the assay, resulting in the exposure of PF-3 and shortening of the coagulation time compared to control tests performed with normal serum added. This indirect test lacks sensitivity and is now seldom used. The microscopic detection of immunofluorescence of megakaryocytes is a subjective test that requires that a bone marrow aspirate be done to obtain megakaryocytes.

Increased platelet-bound immunoglobulins can be detected by microscopic platelet immunofluorescence, radioimmunoassay, flow cytometry, and ELISA techniques in animals, but these tests are not readily available. Direct assays (patient's platelets) are preferred to indirect assays (patient's serum and normal canine platelets) because direct assays are more sensitive. Unfortunately, direct assays must be done within a few hours after blood sample collection. Platelets naturally have some immunoglobulin absorbed to their surfaces and the amount of platelet-bound immunoglobulin can increase with time after sample collection; consequently, false positive tests are a significant problem in these assays. Positive test results may also occur when immune-complexes are absorbed to platelets. At this time, none of the tests for antiplatelet antibodies have been shown to be as readily available and cost-effective as the DAT for anti-RBC antibodies.

PRIMARY IMMUNE-MEDIATED DISORDERS

Some degree of immune-mediated cellular destruction occurs in many infectious, parasitic, neoplastic, inflammatory, and drug-induced diseases. Disorders presented in this section do not appear to be secondary to other diseases, but represent primary immune-mediated disorders.

Transfusion Reactions

Naturally occurring anti-RBC antibodies are defined as antibodies that occur in plasma in the absence of prior exposure to blood from another individual. In most animal blood groups, antibody formation results from prior exposure to different RBC isoantigens via transfusion, pregnancy, or vaccination with products containing blood group antigens. Fortunately, naturally occurring antibodies of clinical significance seldom occur in animals; consequently, severe hemolytic transfusion reactions to unmatched RBCs generally do not occur at the time of the first blood transfusion. However, exceptions may occur as in the case of the AB group in cats where B-positive cats have naturally occurring anti-A antibodies with high hemolytic titer. Less than 3% of domestic shorthair and longhair cats in the United States are type-B, but up to 45% of purebred cats in some breeds are type-B (Table 6–1). The transfusion of type-A blood into a type-B cat can result in a life-threatening intravascular hemolytic reaction the first time a transfusion is given. In contrast, cats with type-A blood have weak anti-B antibodies in their blood. Type-B blood transfusions given to type-A cats do not result in severe intravascular hemolysis, but the transfusion is not efficacious because the transfused RBCs are phagocytized and removed within a few days.

Although dogs have at least 12 blood groups, only the DEA-1.1 isoantigen regularly generates hemolysins in high enough titer to cause significant hemolytic transfusion reactions when dogs with antibodies to this blood group are again transfused with 1.1-positive blood. The DEA-1.2 blood type may not be responsible for life-threatening intravascular hemolytic reactions, but previously sensitized negative dogs exhibit phagocytosis and removal of transfused RBCs within 1 day after administration of 1.2-positive RBCs.

Neonatal Isoerythrolysis

Animals with neonatal isoerythrolysis (NI) are healthy at birth, but develop hemolytic anemia within a few hours to a few days after ingestion of colostrum. Aa and Qa isoantigens are responsible for most cases of NI in horses, where mares that are negative for these factors develop antibodies against them and transfer these antibodies to their newborn foals through colostrum. If the foals have acquired one or more of these RBC antigens from the sire, a hemolytic reaction can occur. The dams become sensitized to these foreign isoantigens from leakage of fetal RBCs through the placenta during pregnancy or from exposure to fetal RBCs of the same blood type during a previous parturition. Generally the first foal born is unaffected, but subsequent foals carrying the same foreign antigen(s) will likely develop hemolytic anemia. NI occurs more frequently in mule foals than in horse foals because of a RBC antigen not found in horses, but present in some donkeys and mules.

NI has been reported in some calves born to cows previously vaccinated for anaplasmosis or other bovine origin vaccines containing RBC membranes. The most important blood group isoantigens involved in this disorder in calves are uncertain. The mating of a DEA-1.1–negative bitch to a DEA-1.1–positive stud dog can result in neonatal hemolytic anemia in DEA-1.1–positive pups if the bitch has been sensitized to the DEA-1.1 isoantigen by past blood transfusion or prior pregnancy. NI can occur in type-A kittens born to primiparous type-B queens, because all adult type-B cats naturally have high anti-A antibody titers.

Blood typing of prospective breeding animals can be done to minimize the possibility of NI developing in offspring. The possibility of offspring developing NI can be evaluated by testing the sire's RBC against the dams serum during pregnancy. If the potential for NI is known to exist prior to parturition, colostrum can be withheld from the offspring until a cross-match can be done between the RBCs of the offspring and the serum of the mother. If an incompatibility is present, the neonatal animal can be foster fed for 2 days, before allowing it to nurse from the mother.

Autoimmune Hemolytic Anemia

Immune-mediated hemolytic anemias may be primary (autoimmune) or they may occur secondarily to rickettsial, bacterial, or protozoal infections; neoplasia (especially lymphomas); systemic lupus erythematous; and toxin or drug exposure. Vaccination with combination vaccines has been incriminated as a trigger of immune-mediated hemolytic anemia in dogs. In an autoimmune response, antibodies are directed against self-antigens on RBCs. In secondary immune-mediated disorders, the immune response is directed against foreign antigens or altered self-antigens, with inadvertent RBC injury. A diagnosis of immune-mediated hemolytic anemia is made if autoagglutination (persisting after saline washing of RBCs), a positive DAT, and/or spherocytosis are present. Spherocytes are accurately recognized only in dogs because the degree of central pallor is naturally less in other domestic animals. A diagnosis of autoimmune hemolytic anemia (AIHA), also called idiopathic immune-mediated hemolytic anemia, is reached by ruling out other disorders known to have concomitant immune-mediated hemolytic anemias.

AIHA is common in dogs, but not in other domestic animal species. Retrospective studies have indicated an increased incidence of AIHA in various breeds, with cocker spaniels consistently being recognized as a breed with an increased incidence. About two thirds of the cases of canine AIHA have spherocytosis and about two thirds have absolute reticulocytosis. A regenerative response to this hemolytic anemia may be lacking if the onset of anemia is acute or if antibodies and/or complement are directed against reticulocytes or bone marrow precursor cells. Bilirubinemia and marked bilirubinuria are usually present. Autoagglutination and/or hemoglobinemia with hemoglobinuria occurs in no more than 10% of cases. Most cases of AIHA in dogs are mediated by IgG antibodies. IgM antibodies and/or complement are most likely involved if autoagglutination or intravascular hemolysis is present.

A neutrophilia (often with a prominent left shift) is typically present in dogs with AIHA. A thrombocytopenia also occurs in more than half of the dogs with this disorder. In some instances the concurrent thrombocytopenia also appears to be autoimmune in origin (Evan's syndrome). In other instances the thrombocytopenia appears to result from increased platelet utilization as occurs in disseminated intravascular coagulation or multiorgan venous thrombosis, with pulmonary thrombosis being most common.

Autoimmune Thrombocytopenia

Immune-mediated thrombocytopenia (IMT) occurs when immunoglobulin (primarily IgG) is bound to the surface of platelets, resulting in the premature removal of platelets by macrophages. The presence of IMT is detected by measuring immunoglobulin bound to the patient's platelets (direct assays) or by measuring immunoglobulin in the serum of a patient that is capable of binding to platelets collected from a normal animal of the same species (indirect assay). Direct assays are generally more sensitive than indirect assays for detecting IMT (see the previous section on tests for platelet-bound immunoglobulins).

IMT may be primary (autoimmune) or it may occur secondarily to rickettsial, bacterial, viral, or parasitic infections; neoplasia; systemic lupus erythematous; rheumatoid arthritis; and drug administration. A diagnosis of autoimmune thrombocytopenia, also called idiopathic thrombocytopenic purpura (ITP), is made after ruling out other potential causes of IMT. A presumptive diagnosis of autoimmune thrombocytopenia is often confirmed by a positive response to glucocorticoid therapy, alone or in combination with vincristine, azathioprine, cyclophosphamide, danazol, or splenectomy.

Autoimmune thrombocytopenia is common in dogs, where it occurs twice as often in females compared to males. It tends to occur in middle-aged dogs, with an increased incidence consistently reported in cocker spaniels. Some dogs present with lethargy and weakness attributable to anemia, but many animals present with bleeding problems in the absence of other signs of illness. Megakaryocyte numbers are usually increased in the bone marrow in response to the thrombocytopenia, but rare cases of amegakaryocytic thrombocytopenia have been reported in dogs and a single case has been reported in a cat.

Systemic Lupus Erythematosus

SLE is a chronic autoimmune disease characterized by the production of a variety of autoantibodies (including antinuclear antibodies) that result in immune-mediated injury of multiple organs. SLE is fairly common in dogs, but is rare in cats and horses. Dogs with SLE have reduced suppressor/cytotoxic (CD8+) T-lymphocyte numbers in blood, suggesting that deficient suppressor activity may be responsible for the uncontrolled production of autoantibodies by B-lymphocytes. Possible manifestations of SLE are non-erosive polyarthritis, glomerulonephritis, persistent or recurring fever, anemia (often DAT positive), thrombocytopenia, lymphadenopathy, facial or mucocutaneous dermatitis, polymyositis, thyroiditis, and myocarditis. A diagnosis of SLE should be considered when several of these inflammatory processes are recognized in a patient. The presence of a positive ANA test or LE cell test helps confirm the diagnosis (see sections on tests for antinuclear antibodies).

TESTS FOR IMMUNE DEFICIENCY DISORDERS

Neutrophil Function Tests

Numerous steps are required for neutrophil chemotaxis, phagocytosis, and killing of bacteria; consequently, a variety of tests are needed to assess neutrophil function. These tests are not available in most commercial laboratories but are done in a limited number of research laboratories. Chemotaxis assays measure the ability of neutrophils to migrate in direction of various chemoattractants. The ability to phagocytize microbes can be determined microscopically and microbial phagocytosis and killing can be assayed by bacterial culture following incubation of bacteria, serum, and neutrophils together. The nitroblue tetrazolium (NBT) reduction test and the chemiluminescence test detect the presence of the oxidant burst needed for normal bacterial killing. The above tests are screening tests. More specialized tests are required to demonstrate the specific nature of an inherited defect.

Lymphocyte Assays

A majority of circulating lymphocytes are T-lymphocytes. Consequently, the presence of a normal absolute blood lymphocyte count tends to rule out a generalized defect in T-lymphocyte production. Lymphocyte blastogenic assays are used to determine the responsiveness of lymphocytes to various mitogens. Different mitogens tend to stimulate different types of lymphocytes. T-lymphocyte function may also be assessed *in vitro* using leukocyte migration inhibition assays, cytokine release assays, and cytotoxicity assays. Subpopulations of lymphocytes can be quantified using fluorescence labeling of surface molecules and flow cytometry. For example, cats with feline immunodeficiency virus (FIV) infections have been shown to have reduced populations of CD4+ lymphocytes using flow cytometry.

Serum Immunoglobulin Assays

A variety of methods may be used to determine if immunoglobulin deficiencies are present. Routine serum protein electrophoresis may be used as a screening test, because immunoglobulins account for all of the protein that migrates in the γ region and some of the protein that migrates in the β region of electrophoretic gels. Low γ-globulin concentration indicates an immunoglobulin (usually IgG) deficiency. Various immunoelectrophoresis techniques can be used to make qualitative and quantitative serum immunoglobulin measurements. Specific immunoglobulin classes may be quantified using various methods including single radial immunodiffusion, ELISA, rocket immunoelectrophoresis, and laser nephelometry. Several semiquantitative tests including zinc sulfate turbidity, glutaraldehyde coagulation, and sodium sulfite precipitation have been used to screen for the failure of the passive immunity via colostrum in neonatal animals. An ELISA screening test (CITE, IDEXX Laboratories) is available for serum IgG measurements in foals.

IMMUNE DEFICIENCY DISORDERS

Inherited Neutrophil Defects

A number of inherited defects of neutrophils have been described. These include the Chediak-Higashi syndrome in several animal species, β_2-integrin adhesion molecule deficiencies in dogs and cattle, bactericidal defects in dogs, and cyclic hematopoiesis in gray collie dogs. These disorders are discussed in Chapter 4.

Combined Immunodeficiency

The production of T- and B-lymphocytes is deficient in combined immunodeficiency (CID) syndromes. CID is transmitted as an autosomal recessive trait in Arabian foals. Affected foals have few or no circulating lymphocytes, hypoplasia of the primary and secondary lymphoid organs, and an inability to produce antibodies. Presuckle serum of foals normally contains some IgM, but not in CID foals. If affected foals suckle successfully shortly after birth, they acquire immunoglobulins from the mare and generally appear healthy. Once maternal immunoglobulins are catabolized, CID foals are susceptible to a variety of overwhelming infections by low-grade pathogens and die by 4 to 6 months of age. A similar syndrome has been described in an Angus calf.

An X-linked CID syndrome has been recognized in basset and cardigan Welsh corgi dogs. Affected male dogs fail to thrive, exhibit increased susceptibilities to bacterial and viral pathogens, lack palpable peripheral lymph nodes, and die by 4 months of age unless housed in a germ-free environment. These dogs are unable to make IgG or IgA, but the serum IgM concentration is normal. Blood lymphocyte counts are decreased or in the low normal range. B-lymphocyte percentages are normal and T-lymphocyte percentages vary from absent to near normal. Blood lymphocytes are unresponsive to T-lymphocyte mitogens. Two different mutations of the γ-chain of the interleukin-2 receptor have been shown to cause the X-linked CID syndrome in these dog breeds.

Serum Immunoglobulin Deficiencies

A defect in the synthesis of all immunoglobulin classes may be present as occurs in agammaglobulinemia in foals that have no identifiable B-lymphocytes. A number of selective immunoglobulin deficiencies have been described in domestic animals. These include IgM deficiency in horses and dogs, IgG deficiency in a foal, IgG_2 deficiency in cattle, and IgA deficiency in dogs. Animals with immunoglobulin deficiencies generally exhibit increased susceptibility to bacterial infections.

Complement Deficiency

An inherited deficiency of the third component of complement (C3) has been reported as an autosomal recessive trait in Brittany spaniel dogs. Homozygous affected animals suffer from recurrent sepsis, pneumonia, pyometra, and wound infections. Humoral immune response to both T-lymphocyte–dependent and T-lymphocyte–independent antigens is defective in affected dogs.

T-Lymphocyte Deficiencies

A T-lymphocyte deficiency has been reported in a family of Weimaraner dogs with immunodeficiency, and dwarfism. Affected dogs exhibited lethargy, emaciation, and recurrent infections in association with thymic atrophy. This syndrome is believed to result from a deficiency of growth hormone.

Cattle with hereditary parakeratosis (trait A-46) are deficient in T-lymphocytes, but exhibit normal antibody production. Affected animals exhibit severe skin infections, and die by 4 months of age unless treated with zinc. These animals probably have a reduced ability to absorb zinc, which is an essential component of the thymic hormone thymulin. A somewhat similar syndrome has been described in bull terrier dogs.

Viral Immune Deficiency Disorders

A number of viral immune deficiency disorders have been recognized in animals, a few of which are listed here. Feline acquired immunodeficiency syndrome (AIDS) is caused by the FIV. Infected cats may be asymptomatic for months to years before signs of severe chronic inflammatory diseases are observed. Increased susceptibility to infectious agents is associated with neutropenia and/or lymphopenia, and decreased numbers of CD4+ T-lymphocytes. A similar syndrome has been reported in primates with simian immunodeficiency virus (SIV) infections.

The FeLV is a potent immunosuppressive virus. Persistently infected cats often exhibit neutropenia and/or lymphopenia. Severe T-lymphocyte dysfunction is present, but B-lymphocyte function is generally only mildly impaired. FeLV-positive cats are predisposed to a variety of secondary infections. Other infectious diseases found to induce secondary immune deficiencies of T- and/or B-lymphocytes include canine distemper, fetal equine herpes virus I infection, and bovine viral diarrhea in calves.

Failure of Passive Transfer of Immunoglobulins

Failure of passive transfer of immunoglobulins is an acquired immunodeficiency disorder. Prior to suckling, newborn domestic animals have extremely low amounts of immunoglobulin in their plasma. Colostrum is rich in IgG and IgA, but also contains some IgM. Colostral immunoglobulins (especially IgG) can be absorbed intact through the small intestine of animals during the first day of life. If insufficient or poor-quality colostrum is produced, if the intake of colostrum is inadequate, or if there is a failure of intestinal absorption, the neonate may not obtain sufficient antibodies to provide the necessary protection against bacterial infections (especially septicemia). Refer to the section on serum immunoglobulin assays for tests used to detect the failure of passive transfer.

SERUM PROTEIN ELECTROPHORESIS

Basic Principles

Most serum proteins carry a negative charge when dissolved in alkaline buffers. When applied to cellulose acetate strips or agarose gels, serum proteins can be separated based on their charge densities, and resultant mobilities in an electric field. Albumin, a protein of low molecular weight and high negative charge, migrates with the greatest velocity toward the anode (positive pole). The negative charge density of the various globulins decreases from α- to β- to the practically uncharged γ-globulins which move little from the point of application. Following electrophoresis, the membrane or gel is stained with a protein stain and scanned in a densitometer. The width and density of each protein band are represented by the width and height of a peak on the densitometer tracing (Fig. 6–4). This tracing or graph is sometimes called an electrophoretogram. The area under each peak of the densitometer tracing is measured, the percentage of each protein fraction is determined, and absolute value for each protein fraction is calculated by multiplying the percentage of each fraction times the total serum protein concentration assayed chemically. With the exception of the albumin peak, each peak is composed of a variety of different proteins that can only be separated by more complicated immunoelectrophoretic techniques.

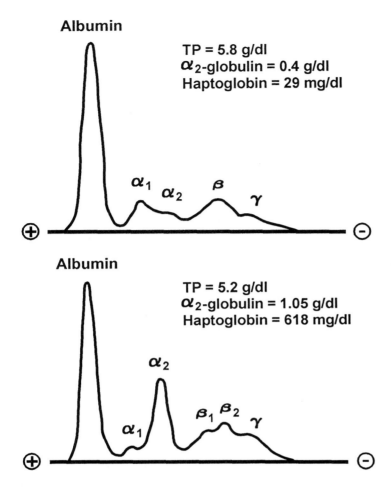

Albumin

TP = 5.8 g/dl
α_2-globulin = 0.4 g/dl
Haptoglobin = 29 mg/dl

α_1 α_2 β γ

⊕ ⊖

Albumin

TP = 5.2 g/dl
α_2-globulin = 1.05 g/dl
Haptoglobin = 618 mg/dl

α_2

α_1 β_1 β_2 γ

⊕ ⊖

FIGURE 6–4. Serum protein electrophoretograms from two dogs. The one at the top is from a dog with a normal serum protein electrophoretogram and low-normal haptoglobin concentration. The one at the bottom is from a dog with hepatic necrosis. The α_2-globulin and haptoglobin concentrations are increased.

Clinical Applications

Serum protein electrophoresis is usually performed when serum proteins are increased, but may be used as a screening test for immunoglobulin (primarily IgG) deficiency, because immunoglobulins account for all of the protein that migrates in the γ region, and some of the protein that migrates in the β region of electrophoretic membranes or gels. The absence and presence of IgG are demonstrated in serum electrophoretograms from a foal before and after absorption of colostrum (Fig. 6–5).

Serum protein electrophoresis can provide useful information in determining the cause of an increased total serum protein concentration. Except for animals with dehydration, increased total serum protein concentrations usually indicate increased concentrations of immunoglobulins. Substantial increases can occur in the concentrations of nonimmunoglobulin proteins migrating in the α and β regions, but these increases are usually not of sufficient magnitude by themselves to result in total protein concentrations above the reference range. An increase in the α_2-globulin is often observed in animals with inflammatory conditions. Studies in dogs have shown that most of this α_2-globulin increase can be attributed to an increase in the acute-

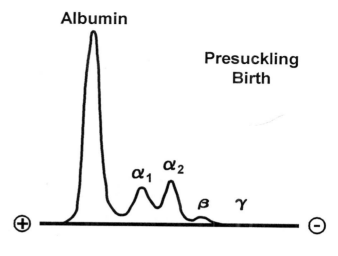

Albumin

Presuckling Birth

α_1 α_2 β γ

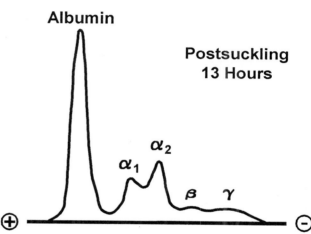

Albumin

Postsuckling 13 Hours

α_1 α_2 β γ

FIGURE 6–5. Serum protein electrophoretograms for a foal before and after suckling. The serum IgG concentration was less than 200 mg/dl before suckling and greater than 800 mg/dl after suckling.

phase reactant protein haptoglobin (Fig 6–4). The concentration of haptoglobin is also increased in dogs following glucocorticoid administration; consequently, increased α_2-globulin concentration does not necessarily indicate the presence of inflammation.

Increased serum immunoglobulin concentrations occur in either inflammatory or neoplastic conditions. When the increase appears as multiple peaks or a broad-based peak in the β and/or γ region of the electrophoretic tracing, the terms polyclonal hyperglobulinemia and polyclonal gammopathy are used to describe the increased immunoglobulin concentration (Fig. 6–6). Polyclonal hyperglobulinemia usually results from chronic inflammatory conditions. As discussed above, an increased α_2-globulin concentration may also be present.

When the increased immunoglobulin concentration results from a single protein that appears as a sharp, narrow-based peak (similar to that seen for albumin) in the electrophoretic tracing, the terms monoclonal hyperglobulinemia and monoclonal gammopathy are used (Fig. 6–6). Although a misnomer, the term monoclonal gammopathy is often used even when the abnormal protein migrates in the β region of the electrophoretic membrane

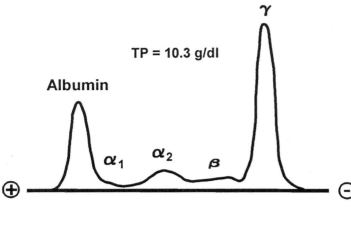

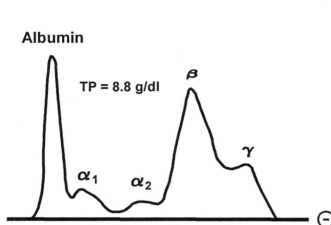

FIGURE 6–6. Serum protein electrophoretograms from a cat with multiple myeloma and a monoclonal gammopathy (top graph), and a dog with chronic pyoderma and a polyclonal gammopathy (bottom graph)

or gel. These abnormal proteins are sometimes referred to as M proteins or as paraproteins. Most monoclonal gammopathies are produced by clonal proliferations of neoplastic cells of the B-lymphocyte series (multiple myeloma, plasmacytoma, primary or Waldenström's macroglobulinemia, lymphoma, and chronic lymphocytic leukemia), but monoclonal gammopathies have also been reported rarely in animals with extensive nonneoplastic plasma cell proliferations (canine ehrlichiosis, plasmacytic gastroenterocolitis, and leishmaniasis), amyloidosis, and in the absence of an identifiable cause (idiopathic paraproteinemia or monoclonal gammopathy of undetermined significance). Biclonal gammopathies with two separate paraproteins have rarely been reported in animals with plasma cell tumors.

References

Barker RN, Elson CJ: Red cell-reactive non-specific immunoglobulins, and autoantibodies in the sera of normal, and anaemic dogs. Vet Immunol Immunopathol 1993; 39:339.

Barker RN, Gruffydd-Jones TJ, Elson CJ: Red cell-bound immunoglobulins, and complement measured by an enzyme-linked antiglobulin test in dogs with autoimmune haemolysis or other anaemias. Res Vet Sci 1993;54:170.

Barta O: Veterinary Clinical Immunology Laboratory, Blacksburg, BAR-LAB, Inc, 1993.

Baxter K: Haemolytic anaemia in an embryo transfer calf. Vet Rec 1996;138:339.

Bücheler J, Giger U: Alloantibodies against A, and B blood types in cats. Vet Immunol Immunopathol 1993;38:283.

Callan MB, Jones LT, Giger U: Hemolytic transfusion reactions in a dog with an alloantibody to a common antigen. J Vet Intern Med 1995;9:277.

Casal ML, Jezyk PF, Giger U: Transfer of colostral antibodies from queens to their kittens. Am J Vet Res 1996;57:1653.

Chabanne L, Fournel C, Caux C, et al: Abnormalities of lymphocyte subsets in canine systemic lupus erythematosus. Autoimmunity 1995;22:1.

Clough NEC, Roth JA: Methods for assessing cell-mediated immunity in infectious disease resistance, and in the development of vaccines. J Am Vet Med Assoc 1995;206:1208.

Cotter SM: Autoimmune hemolytic anemia in dogs. Comp Cont Educ Pract Vet 1992;14:53.

Day MJ, Penhale WJ: Immune-mediated disease in the old English sheepdog. Res Vet Sci 1992;53:87.

Diehl KJ, Lappin MR, Jones RL, et al: Monoclonal gammopathy in a dog with plasmacytic gastroenterocolitis. J Am Vet Med Assoc 1992;201:1233.

Drew ML, Fowler ME: Comparison of methods for measuring serum immunoglobulin concentrations in neonatal llamas. J Am Vet Med Assoc 1995;206:1374.

Duval D, Giger U: Vaccine-associated immune-mediated hemolytic anemia in the dog. J Vet Intern Med 1996;10:290.

Edwards DF, Parker JW, Wilkinson JE, et al: Plasma cell myeloma in the horse. J Vet Intern Med 1993;7:169.

Feldman BF: Demographics of canine immune-mediated haemolytic anaemia in the southeastern United States. Comp Haematol Int 1996;6:42.

Fenger CK, Hoffsis GF, Kociba GJ: Idiopathic immune-mediated hemolytic anemia in a calf. J Am Vet Med Assoc 1992;201:97.

Font A: Consider leishmaniasis in differential for monoclonal gammopathies in dogs. J Am Vet Med Assoc 1996;208:184.

Gaschen FP, Smith Meyer B, Harvey JW: Amegakaryocytic thrombocytopenia, and immune-mediated haemolytic anaemia in a cat. Comp Haematol Int 1992;2:175.

Giger U, Gelens CJ, Callan MB, et al: An acute hemolytic transfusion reaction caused by dog erythrocyte antigen 1.1 incompatibility in a previously sensitized dog. J Am Vet Med Assoc 1995;206:1358.

Ginel PJ, Margarito JM, Molleda JM, et al: Biotin-avidin amplified enzyme-linked immunosorbent assay (ELISA) for the measurement of canine serum IgA, IgG, and IgM. Res Vet Sci 1996;60:107.

Griot-Wenk M, Callan MB, Casal ML, et al: Blood type AB in the feline AB blood group system. Am J Vet Res 1996;57:1438.

Griot-Wenk M, Pahlsson P, Chisholm-Chait A, et al: Biochemical characterization of the feline AB blood group system. Anim Genet 1993;24:401.

Griot-Wenk ME, Giger U: Feline transfusion medicine—blood types, and their clinical importance. Vet Clin North Am Small Anim Pract 1995;25:1305.

Hale AS: Canine blood groups, and their importance in veterinary transfusion medicine. Vet Clin North Am Small Anim Pract 1995;25:1323.

Hansson H, Trowald-Wigh G, Karlsson-Parra A: Detection of antinuclear antibodies by indirect immunofluorescence in dog sera: comparison of rat liver tissue, and human epithelial-2 cells as antigenic substrate. J Vet Intern Med 1996;10:199.

Honeckman AL, Knapp DW, Reagan WJ: Diagnosis of canine immune-mediated hematologic disease. Comp Cont Educ Pract Vet 1996;18:113.

Hudgens KAR, Tyler JW, Besser TE, et al: Optimizing performance of a qualitative zinc sulfate turbidity test for passive transfer of immunoglobulin G in calves. Am J Vet Res 1996;57:1711.

Jones DRE, Gruffydd-Jones TJ, Stokes CR, et al: Use of a direct enzyme-linked antiglobulin test for laboratory diagnosis of immune-mediated hemolytic anemia in dogs. Am J Vet Res 1992;53:457.

Kato H, Momoi Y, Omori K, et al: Gammopathy with two M-components in a dog with IgA-type multiple myeloma. Vet Immunol Immunopathol 1995;49:161.

Klag AR, Giger U, Shofer FS: Idiopathic immune-mediated hemolytic anemia in dogs: 42 cases (1986–1990). J Am Vet Med Assoc 1993;202:783.

Kristensen AT, Weiss DJ, Klausner JS, et al: Comparison of microscopic, and flow cytometric detection of platelet antibody in dogs suspected of having immune-mediated thrombocytopenia. Am J Vet Res 1994;55:1111.

Larsen AE, Carpenter JL: Hepatic plasmacytoma, and biclonal gammopathy in a cat. J Am Vet Med Assoc 1994;205:708.

Lewis DC: Canine idiopathic thrombocytopenia purpura. J Vet Intern Med 1996;10:207.

Lewis DC, Meyers KM: Effect of anticoagulant, and blood storage time on platelet-bound antibody concentrations in clinically normal dogs. Am J Vet Res 1994;55:602.

Lewis DC, Meyers KM, Callan MB, et al: Detection of platelet-bound, and serum platelet-bindable antibodies for diagnosis of idiopathic thrombocytopenic purpura in dogs. J Am Vet Med Assoc 1995;206:47.

Mandel NS, Esplin DG: A retroperitoneal extramedullary plasmacytoma in a cat with a monoclonal gammopa. J Am Anim Hosp Assoc 1994;30:603.

McClure JJ, Koch C, Traub Dargatz J: Characterization of a red blood cell antigen in donkeys, and mules associated with neonatal isoerythrolysis. Anim Genet 1994;25:119.

McConnico RS, Roberts MC, Tompkins M: Penicillin-induced immune-mediated hemolytic anemia in a horse. J Am Vet Med Assoc 1992;201:1402.

Monestier M, Novick KE, Karam ET, et al: Autoantibodies to histone, DNA, and nucleosome antigens in canine systemic lupus erythematosus. Clin Exp Immunol 1995;99:37.

Peterson EP, Meininger AC: Immunoglobulin A, and immunoglobulin G biclonal gammopathy in a dog with multiple myeloma. J Am Anim Hosp Assoc 1997;33:45.

Somberg RL, Pullen RP, Casal ML, et al: A single nucleotide insertion in the canine interleukin-2 receptor gamma chain results in X-linked severe combined immunodeficiency disease. Vet Immunol Immunopathol 1995;47:203.

Tizard I: Veterinary Immunology. An Introduction, 4th ed. Philadelphia, WB Saunders Co, 1992.

7

Evaluation of Hepatobiliary System and Skeletal Muscle and Lipid Disorders

For the study of medical diseases of the liver, it is essential that the pathologist be apprised of the clinical findings and the results of laboratory tests and radiographic studies. The correct diagnosis is most likely to be reached by the pathologist and clinician working as a team.

—Kamal Ishak

PHYSIOFUNCTIONAL ANATOMY

Primary hepatic disease and the "reaction" of the liver to extrahepatic disease can cause both serum hepatic test and histomorphologic abnormalities. The secondary biochemical and morphologic response poses two diagnostic problems: (1) it mimics primary hepatic disease and (2) it diverts attention from the primary extrahepatic disease process. There are a variety of reasons why extrahepatic diseases secondarily involve the liver and complicate its diagnostic enzymology. These can be divided into anatomic and functional relationships. An insult or metabolic disturbance to one component of the liver will usually involve the others due to their complex functional interdependence.

The hepatocyte is the parenchymal cell that comprises approximately 60% of the liver. Each milligram of human liver contains approximately 170,000 hepatocytes. The remainder of the hepatic tissue is comprised of nonparenchymal cells, approximately 30,000 cells/mg. These consist of Kupffer cells, lipocytes (Ito cell), endothelial cells, and resident large granular lymphocytes (pit cells). The Kupffer cell accounts for approximately one third of this population. While we do not have clinical tests for this relatively large contribution to the structure of the liver, their involvement in the pathophysiology of disease can indirectly cause abnormal hepatic test values.

Hepatocytes have a remarkable capability to regenerate. Following partial hepatectomy, there is 80% regrowth within 5 days and it is complete within 3 weeks for the rat. For humans, it is approximately 8 months for complete regrowth. This regenerative process in the dog probably takes about 6 to 8 weeks, since the maximum regenerative response occurs 72 hours after hepatectomy for the dog and 24 hours for the rat. By inference, reparation following injury can be very rapid, days to weeks, depending on the severity of insult and the integrity of the delicate stromal scaffolding. This relatively unique ability of the liver to regenerate is one reason why repeat testing is a valuable strategy in assessing hepatic pathology and why both static tests and tests that evaluate function have complementary roles in the biochemical evaluation of the liver. Using the rat hepatectomy model as an example, the plasma total bile acid concentration, a hepatic function test discussed later, increases approximately eight-fold by 6 hours following surgery. The post-operative decrease in its serum concentration parallels the return of the normal hepatic mass: approximately four-fold increase on day 1, two-fold increase on day 5, and same as the control value on day 21.

One side of the hepatocyte faces the sinusoid/space of Disse, another the adjacent hepatocytes, and the third faces the canaliculus. The biliary system begins with the bile canaliculi, which are grooves on the surface of adjacent hepatocytes with special membrane functions that are actively involved in the process of bile secretion. The canalicular network drains into an enlarging epithelial-lined bile duct system which leads to the portal area and eventually drains into the duodenum via the common bile duct. These anatomic and functional relationships combine to form hepatic units; one termed the classic lobule and the other the liver acinus. The classic lobule is a six-sided parenchymal unit with a portal triad at each point and a vein (central) in the middle. It is more easily defined microscopically and often used for descriptive purposes when examining hepatic tissue histologically. The liver acinus is difficult to identify microscopically but is proposed to be more representative of a functional unit. Figuratively, it is similar to a grape-like cluster of hepatocytes surrounding a hepatic artery and portal vein that is approximately 2 mm in diameter and is comprised of approximately 100,000 hepatocytes (Fig. 7–1).

The liver has two blood supplies: the hepatic artery and the portal vein. The former provides nutrition and oxygen. The latter, which comprises approximately 80% of the total hepatic blood flow, delivers substances absorbed from the gastrointestinal tract and hormones from the pancreas. Hepatic integrity and function can be altered secondary to cardiovascular insufficiency, anemia, portosystemic shunts, and an increased exposure to intestinal bacteria or their products when the intestinal barrier is violated by disease. Blood enters the portal triad and flows sequentially through zones 1, 2, and 3 before draining via the terminal hepatic (central) vein (Fig. 7–1). Consequently, hepatocytes in zone 3 (centrilobular) are most susceptible to hypoxic conditions such as heart failure and shock. There is remarkable metabolic diversity of the hepatic zones in order to accommodate the numerous activities associated with protein, lipid, and carbohydrate metabolism. For example, albumin synthesis, gluconeogenesis for the synthesis of glucose and glycogen, cholesterol synthesis, amino acid metabolism, formation of urea, oxidative energy metabolism with β-oxidation, and removal of bile acids from the portal blood occur primarily in zone 1. Zone 3 supports

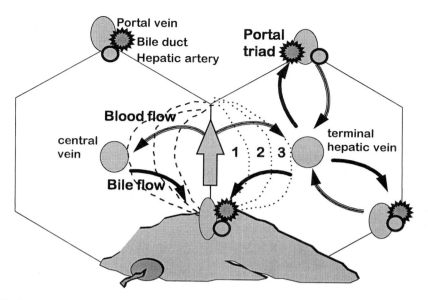

FIGURE 7–1. Microcirculatory hepatic unit illustrating the simple liver acinus. The confluence of blood from the terminal hepatic arteriole and terminal portal venule courses through the sinusoids comprising zones 1, 2, and 3 en route to the terminal hepatic venule. The canalicular bile enters the terminal interlobular ductules, which drain into an enlarging bile ductular system that carries bile in a direction opposite to that of blood flow. The ductules surround the terminal hepatic portal venules in a "spider web-like" way. The counterflow of this physioanatomic arrangement is an effective mechanism for effecting the exchange between the blood and bile constituents, notably the transfer of bile acids. The functional interrelationship is one reason that multiple hepatic test abnormalities are frequently associated with hepatic pathology of diverse causes.

liponeogenesis, formation of ketones, glycolysis, glycogen synthesis from glucose, glutamine formation, and xenobiotic metabolism. It is not surprising that the density of mitochondria and peroxisomes are highest in zones 1 and 3, respectively. Sometimes metabolic enzyme systems are in sequence as it is for ammonia metabolism. Hepatocytes in zone 1, rich in the urea cycle enzymes, predominate in the formation of urea nitrogen from ammonia when its concentration is less than 50 mmol. When the concentration is greater than 50 mmol, glutamine synthetase-rich hepatocytes in zone 3 are the predominate urea formers. Many of these functions are related to the intermediary role of hepatocyte metabolism between dietary sources of energy and extrahepatic tissue demands for energy. Therefore, metabolic diseases often involve the liver. Examples include hyperadrenocorticism, diabetes mellitus, hyperthyroidism, hypothyroidism, and lipid disorders.

The liver is also the predominant organ for the metabolism of xenobiotics, compounds that are foreign to the body. To support this function, hepatocytes, especially those located in zone 3, are rich in enzymes belonging to the cytochrome P-450 enzyme system (also termed monooxygenases or mixed function oxidase system). A xenobiotic can directly cause hepatic injury, or a metabolite produced during its elimination by the cytochrome P-450 enzyme system can be hepatotoxic.

Another cell type that plays a role in the extrahepatic manifestations of disease is the Kupffer cell, a member of the resident monocyte-macrophage system. It is involved interactively in the immune response by the liver and it "filters" bacteria and endotoxins in the portal circulation. When this role is amplified in response to extrahepatic disease, *e.g.*, bacterial translocation secondary to a diseased intestinal tract, the hepatocytes in the vicinity of the macrophage can be indirectly damaged causing biochemical and histopathologic findings consistent with focal hepatitis.

HEPATIC TESTS—SERUM ENZYME TESTS

> Dr. Watson: "This is indeed a mystery. What do you imagine it means?"
> Sherlock Holmes: "I have no data yet. It is a capital mistake to theorize before one has data. Insensible one begins to twist facts to suit theories, rather than theories to suit the facts."
> —A. Conan Doyle, *Scandal in Bohemia*

The serum hepatic enzyme tests are grouped into those that indicate hepatocellular injury/repair and those that reflect increased enzyme production stimulated by retained bile or drug induction. The magnitude and duration of increase in plasma enzyme activity is dependent on (1) its innate tissue activity; (2) its cellular location; (3) its rate of removal from the plasma; and (4) the type, severity, and duration of the injury/stimulus. The rate of removal seems to have molecule-specific and species-specific properties; neither is well characterized in veterinary medicine. Table 7–1 lists examples for the dog and cat. Species specificity applies to the other three factors as well. The magnitude of increase of the plasma enzyme activity does not prognosticate the irreversibility of liver disease at one point in time.

Leakage Enzymes

Alanine Aminotransferase (ALT)

There is a high activity of alanine aminotransferase (ALT) in hepatocellular cytoplasm of the dog, cat, and primate (Fig. 7–2); the equine, bovine, birds, and marmoset are notable exceptions (see Table 1–5). One can think of each hepatocyte like a little balloon filled with ALT. Altered permeability of the hepatocellular membrane caused by injury or a metabolic disturbance re-

TABLE 7–1. Approximate Plasma Half-Life of Hepatic Enzymes in the Dog and Cat

Enzyme	Dog	Cat
ALT	61 (or 40) hr[a]	3.5 hr
AST	12 hr	1.5 hr
GLDH	18 hr	—
ALP		
Hepatobiliary isoenzyme	66 hr	6 hr
Corticosteroid isoenzyme	74 hr	—
Intestinal isoenzyme	6 min	2 min

[a]References differ.
hr = hours; min = minutes.

FIGURE 7–2. The subcellular location of hepato-biliary enzymes. ALT, SD, and most of AST is located in the cytosol in high activity. GD and a component of AST are associated with the mitochondria. An alteration of the integrity of the hepatocellular membrane with subsequent "leakage" of these enzymes causes their initial increase in the plasma. ALT is not present in high enough activity to be diagnostically useful in the horse and ruminant. SD and GD are generally found in the liver of most species, although the magnitude does vary (see Table 1–5). ALP and GGT are associated with the cytomembranes of the canaliculi and biliary epithelium, respectively. They have a relatively low magnitude of tissue activity and their production must first be stimulated for their increase to be noted in the plasma.

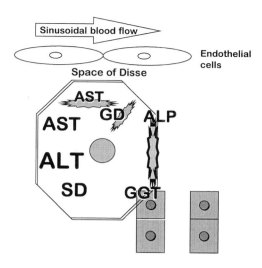

sults in a release of this soluble enzyme. Subsequent to an acute, diffuse injury, the magnitude of increase in the plasma crudely reflects the number of affected hepatocytes (Fig. 7–3).

Aspartate Aminotransferase (AST)

A variety of tissues, notably skeletal muscle and liver, contain high aspartate aminotransferase activity (AST) (see Table 1–5). The determination of the serum AST activity is used as a convenient screening test of hepatic injury in those species without high hepatic ALT activity when skeletal muscle injury is not present (Fig. 7–2). Skeletal muscle injury is best defined biochemically by the measurement of the serum creatine kinase (CK, CPK) activity, a specific skeletal muscle enzyme (see Table 1–5). By determining both enzymes in horses and ruminants, the serum AST activity is a more useful indicator of hepatic disease (Fig. 7–4). Hepatocellular injury can be further supported in these species by the measurement of other liver-specific enzymes such as

FIGURE 7–3. The relative magnitude and duration of increase of the plasma activities for SD, AST, GD, ALT, and ALP following an acute, severe, diffuse injury to the liver. An increase in the plasma ALT activity would not be detected in the horse or ruminant. The increase in the plasma ALP activity is most notable in the dog.

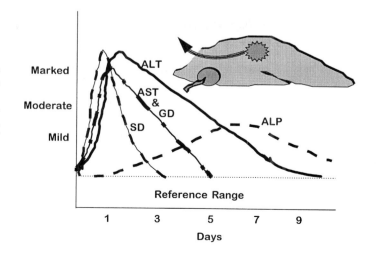

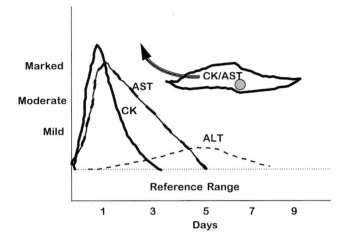

FIGURE 7–4. *A,* The relative magnitude and duration of increase of the plasma activities for CK, AST, and ALT following an acute severe diffuse injury to the skeletal muscle. *B,* Differentiation between hepatic and skeletal muscle injury based on the magnitude of increase of the plasma activities of CK, AST, and ALT.

Dog and cat:
ALT >>> AST ➡ hepatic injury
AST >>> ALT ➡ skeletal muscle injury
                        (CK will be increased)

Horse and ruminant:
↑AST & normal CK➡ hepatic injury
↑AST & CK ➡ skeletal muscle injury
   or both hepatic and skeletal muscle injury

sorbitol dehydrogenase (SD, SDH) or glutamate dehydrogenase (GD, GLDH) (see Figs. 7–2 and 7–3).

Our experience suggests that there is value in the interpretation of the serum activities of ALT and AST for liver disease in the dog and cat. Following an acute injury resulting in a moderate to marked increase in the serum ALT and AST activities, the serum AST activity will return to normal more rapidly (hours to days) than the serum ALT activity (days) due to their difference in plasma half-lives and cellular location. By determining these values every 2 to 5 days (note the species difference for plasma half-lives in Table 7–1) following an acute insult, a sequential "biochemical picture" indicative of resolution is obtained (Fig. 7–3). Persistent mild to moderate increases of the serum ALT and AST activities (documented multiple times over months) suggest a "smoldering" inflammatory process, chronic hepatitis. The persistent increase in the aminotransferase activities is probably a consequence of increased release subsequent to both cell injury and ongoing hepatocellular reparation (regeneration).

Novel Concept 1. Clinically, the decrease in the serum ALT and AST activities is often slower than their plasma half-lives would predict following a one-time release phenomenon subsequent to cellular injury. This is probably due in some cases to the temporary persistence of the insulting agent and the ensuing inflammatory reaction. An explanation that can be more generically applied to explain this discrepancy focuses on the relatively unique regenerative ability of the hepatocyte.

Studies in the rat indicate that 24 hours following carbon tetrachloride–induced hepatocellular injury, the expected increase in the plasma ALT and AST activities occurs. If the increase in the plasma was due solely to a one-time release from the damaged tissue, the corresponding hepatic tissue activity would be expected to be decreased. Recent studies demonstrate that the hepatic tissue activities for both aminotransferases are actually moderately increased at 24 hours. The finding suggests that the remaining viable hepatocellular tissue has increased its synthesis of the aminotransferases as a consequence of, and/or in support of, the reparative/regenerative process (Fig. 7–5). This concept is supported by repeating the carbon tetrachloride study and coadministering cyclohexamide, a nonspecific inhibitor of protein synthesis. Following the administration of this "cocktail" to rats, the rise in the plasma aminotransferase activities is blunted by approximately 60% compared to the group that received only carbon tetrachloride. Clinically, a precipitous decrease in the serum ALT and AST activities following their moderate increase may be suggestive of insufficient hepatic mass to support repair and a harbinger of fulminant hepatic failure (see Case 7–1).

Novel Concept 2. Hepatic AST appears to be released later and as a consequence of more severe injury than ALT. Perhaps this explains the finding in one study that an increase in the serum AST activity has high specificity (but low sensitivity) for hepatic disease in the dog. The subcellular location of AST activity is divided between a soluble cytosolic form (c-AST) and a

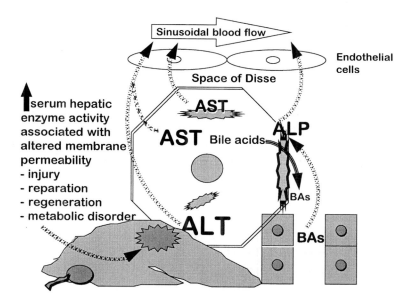

FIGURE 7–5. Following the initial release of ALT and AST to the plasma subsequent to an acute injury, it has been shown that the maintenance of their plasma activity is related to an increase in their tissue activity in association with the reparative process. A persistence of an increase in the plasma aminotransferase activity would suggest a chronic process of injury-repair. It is also possible that metabolic disorders could affect the processes responsible for maintaining the integrity of the cell membrane, resulting in enzyme "leakage." Impaired bile flow increases the duration of bile acid contact with the canalicular membrane. This initiates the liver's production of ALP, a sensitive plasma marker of cholestasis in the dog, less so in the cat, and of limited diagnostic value in the horse and ruminant.

mitochondrial form (m-AST) (Fig. 7–2). The c-AST is the predominant form. Experimental studies and clinical observations suggest that (1) the magnitude of increase is greater for serum ALT activity than for AST and (2) an increase in serum ALT activity precedes AST. Mitochondrial injury is necessary for m-AST to contribute to the serum AST activity. Since its release is consequent to necrobiosis, measurement by electrophoresis or immunochemistry is being investigated in human patients as an ''index'' of severity.

Reduced serum ALT and AST activities (less than the reference range) are noted with relative frequency in dogs and rats during preclinical studies of drugs under pharmaceutical development. In one study an approximate 40% decrease in both the plasma ALT and AST activities was shown to be associated with a concurrent reduction of similar magnitude of their activities in hepatic tissue. This finding further supports the close plasma/hepatic tissue relationship of these enzymes. Marketed drugs such as phenothiazines and cefazolin have been reported to cause decreased serum aminotransferase activities in humans and animals, potentially precluding their use as markers of hepatic injury in those patients.

The activity of ALT and AST are dependent on a cofactor, pyridoxal 5'-phosphate, the active metabolite of vitamin B_6. Pyridoxine appears to be activated in the liver by the zinc-containing metalloenzyme alkaline phosphatase. Consequently, another possible cause for decreased aminotransferase activity as well as alkaline phosphatase activity may be zinc or vitamin B_6 deficiency. A syndrome in bull terriers attributed to zinc deficiency was consistently associated with reduced serum ALT and ALP activities.

Sorbitol Dehydrogenase (SD, SDH), Glutamate Dehydrogenase (GD, GLDH)

Both SD and GD are located primarily in the liver in high activity for most species (see Table 1–5 and Fig. 7–2). They are particularly valuable diagnostically in those species that lack ALT (see Case 7–2). Following an acute insult to the liver, SD rises rapidly (12 to 24 hours) and returns to the reference range within 48 to 72 hours (Fig. 7–3). The enzyme kinetics of SD have both advantages (indicator of acute injury) and limitations (not useful for chronic hepatic injury). Either can be used as a liver-specific test to determine if an increased serum AST activity is of liver or skeletal muscle origin. Their routine use in veterinary medicine is limited by the unavailability of convenient methodology.

Lactate Dehydrogenase (LD, LDH)

Lactate dehydrogenase is an enzyme located in multiple tissues (see Table 1–5) for which there are five isoenzymes. The popularity of its diagnostic use has waned and no longer has value in veterinary medicine.

Markers of Cholestasis and Drug Induction

Alkaline Phosphatase (ALP) and γ-Glutamyltransferase (GGT)

Alkaline phosphatase and γ-glutamyltransferase (γ-glutamyltranspeptidase, GGTP) show minimal activity in normal hepatic tissue (see Table 1–5) but can become markedly increased in the plasma subsequent to increased enzyme production stimulated by either impaired bile flow or drugs. The increased synthesis begins within hours with subsequent appearance in the plasma by release mechanisms that are not clearly defined. These enzymes have a membrane location; ALP associated with the canalicular membrane and GGT associated with epithelial cells comprising the bile ductular system (Fig. 7–2).

Alkaline phosphatase is an enzyme located on the membrane of a variety of tissues (see Table 1–5) but only two are diagnostically important: hepatobiliary and bone. Each tissue has an ALP isoenzyme that can be separated by electrophoresis. With the exception of the growing animal or the patient with bone disease, an increased serum ALP activity is of hepatobiliary origin. There is considerable species variation for the diagnostic application of ALP. The reference range is wide for horses and ruminants, limiting its diagnostic sensitivity. The hepatobiliary tissue of the cat has a limited capacity for accelerated ALP production. The diagnostic sensitivity and magnitude of increase in the cat is further attenuated by a plasma half-life of 6 hours. In contrast, the dog liver has a robust ability to increase ALP production and a relatively long plasma half-life of 66 hours.

There is minimal increase in the plasma following an acute, severe insult (in contrast to ALT and AST) (see Case 7–1). Any initial rise is probably a reflection of enzyme activity on cell membrane fragments released to the plasma as a consequence of the damage. Disruption of the hepatobiliary architecture causes local impairment to bile flow, which stimulates increased ALP production within hours. During hepatic reparation following an injury, the serum aminotransferase activity slowly decreases while the serum ALP activity often increases until the "local" cholestasis has resolved. Consequently, the serum ALP activity is usually the last serum hepatic enzyme test to return to normal in the dog following resolution of an acute insult (Fig. 7–3).

A primary event that obstructs the flow of bile, whether intrahepatic or extrahepatic, is initially associated with an increase in the serum ALP activity (Fig. 7–6). The retention of bile acids is linked to initiation of alkaline phosphatase synthesis by an ill-defined mechanism (Fig. 7–5). If the insult is protracted and severe, increased serum total bile acid concentration, bilirubinuria (notably dog), and finally hyperbilirubinemia occur, resulting in jaundice (Fig. 7–6). The magnitude of increase in the serum ALP activity is not a reliable index for differentiating extrahepatic and intrahepatic cholestatic disorders. Lesser increases in the serum aminotransferase activities often develop either as a consequence of the primary pathologic event and/or the detergent effects of the retained hydrophobic bile acids altering membrane permeability.

An increase in the serum ALP activity is associated with the use of glucocorticoids and anticonvulsant medications. There is remarkable individual variation in the magnitude of these increases and there is no concomitant hyperbilirubinemia. In the dog, the increased serum ALP activity associated with corticosteroids has been attributed to an induction of the synthesis of a novel ALP (CIALP) isoenzyme that can be distinguished from the cholestatically induced liver ALP (LALP) isoenzyme by several procedures. The CIALP isoenzyme has been used diagnostically for hyperadrenocorticism. Unfortunately, an increase in this isoenzyme can be associated with hepatobiliary disease, diabetes mellitus, hypothyroidism, acute pancreatitis, and

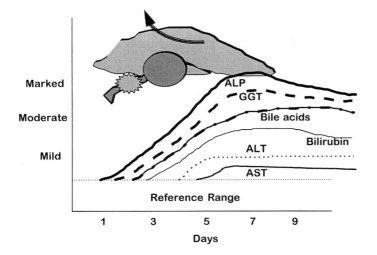

FIGURE 7–6. The relative magnitude and sequence of increases of the plasma ALP, GGT, ALT, and AST activities and concentrations of total bile acids and bilirubin following the ligation of the common bile duct. The increase of the plasma ALP activity is less dramatic in the horse and ruminant. Since the retained hydrophobic bile acids are potent detergents, their prolonged contact with the cell membrane will result in the "leakage" of the cytosolic enzymes.

phenobarbital treatment. Its judicial use in the context of the patient's history and other biochemical findings may have supportive differential diagnostic value for hyperadrenocorticism. A moderate to marked increase in serum ALP activity without concurrent hyperbilirubinemia and minimal increase in the aminotransferases is most compatible with a corticosteroid effect and warrants a review of the patient's history (topical or systemic corticosteroids) or evaluation of adrenal function. Occasionally this biochemical pattern mimics primary hepatic disease, especially early cholangiohepatitis, and a hepatic biopsy is required for the differentiation.

In cats with hyperthyroidism, the serum ALT, AST, ALP activities and bilirubin concentration can be increased; an abnormal ALP value is most common. A rise in the activity of isoenzymes from the liver, bone, and an unidentified source all contribute to the raised plasma ALP activity. While hyperthyroidism in humans has been associated with increased osteoblastic and osteoclastic activity, the mechanisms responsible for the increase in the other ALP isoenzymes or the rise in the other hepatic tests are not known.

Anticonvulsant medications (phenobarbital, phenytoin, and primidone) can increase the serum ALP activity in the dog. The aminotransferase activities may be increased to a lesser magnitude and there is no hyperbilirubinemia. This is important to realize because these medications can occasionally cause chronic hepatitis. A prominence of the serum ALT activity in these patients during treatment, especially if accompanied by an increased serum GGT activity, warrants further investigation, *e.g.*, measurement of the serum total bile acid concentration or biopsy.

The serum ALP activity has been shown to increase rapidly following a meal in humans and rats; the increase can be dramatic in the latter. The magnitude of increase is related to the lipid component of the meal. The mechanism for the increase appears to be related to the secretion of a particulate ALP onto the apical surface of the enterocyte with subsequent release into both the lymphatics and the intestinal lumen. If this does occur in the dog and cat, the effect would not be noted clinically in the fasted animal due to the short plasma half-life of intestinal ALP (6 minutes). A possible exception would be a delayed clearance of this isoenzyme resulting in an increased plasma ALP activity (see below).

Novel Concept. The variable, unique increase of ALP in dogs associated with corticosteroids may be related to a novel concept pertaining to the formation of the CIALP isoenzyme. Experimental findings in the dog clearly demonstrate that the hepatic ALP isoenzyme is the one that initially increases subsequent to the administration of corticosteroids. It is the predominant component of the total serum ALP activity for at least 30 days with a smaller contribution by the CIALP isoenzyme after about 1 week.

A fascinating study measured the rate of clearance for the intestinal ALP isoenzyme by the asialoglycoprotein receptor pathway both *in vivo* and *in vitro* using isolated hepatocytes from dogs treated with corticosteroids. The findings indicate that the structurally related intestinal and CIALP isoenzymes may be metabolically related through the asialoglycoprotein receptor endocytosis pathway. A portion of the intestinal ALP isoenzyme normally endocytosed through this pathway in corticosteroid-treated dogs may be recycled and hyperglycosylated to form the isoenzyme measured as the CIALP rather than being degraded by the hepatocyte (Fig. 7–7). This "abnormal" isoenzyme is not cleared as rapidly as the intestinal isoenzyme (plasma half-life of 74 hours and 6 minutes, respectively) and accumulates in the plasma. The electrophoretically isolated CIALP isoenzyme has been shown to be a

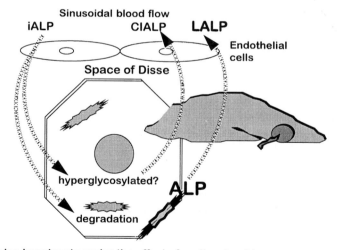

Canine hepatocyte under the effect of corticosteroids

FIGURE 7–7. Corticosteroids cause an increase in the plasma ALP activity in the dog. They have been shown to stimulate the production of the canine liver isoenzyme of ALP (LALP) and they are associated with the appearance in the plasma of a novel isoenzyme of ALP (CIALP). One proposed mechanism for the increased plasma CIALP activity is an induction of its hepatic synthesis as well. A second possibility is that the terminal carbohydrate moiety of the intestinal isoenzyme of ALP (IALP), with a plasma half-life of 6 minutes, is changed during its hepatic clearance by hepatocytes that are metabolically altered by corticosteroids, resulting in the formation of CIALP. The metabolic alteration of the "newly" formed isoenzyme gives it a different electrophoretic mobility and delays its plasma clearance (half-life of 74 hours).

product of the same gene as the intestinal ALP isoenzyme with only a slight difference in their carbohydrate moiety.

This concept is not new in medicine and has been documented in humans, both juvenile and adult, with viral infections, hepatic cirrhosis, diabetes mellitus, chronic renal failure, and undergoing hemodialysis. The increase of the serum activities of ALP (or GGT) in these conditions has been shown to be due to a decreased clearance. An alteration of the terminal carbohydrate moiety (increased sialic acid content) has been suggested to affect receptor recognition, which impairs its clearance. Following a viral infection, for example, the temporary increase of serum ALP activity may last weeks or months. Altered clearance has been shown to occur for the macroenzymes, resulting in increased plasma activity. It is possible that the relatively high serum ALP values in cats with hepatic lipidosis, an intrahepatic disorder, also may be due to delayed clearance. Certainly more studies are indicated. The added message is that increased plasma enzyme activity can be a consequence of predominantly increased release, predominantly increased formation and release (the traditional concepts), or predominantly decreased removal.

Benign familial hyperphosphatasemia refers to an inherited condition in human beings in which a markedly raised serum ALP activity is serendipitously identified in childhood and persists into adulthood. The cause of the increased enzyme activity is not known but it is not associated with underlying pathology, hence the term benign. It is a biochemical curiosity with no adverse effect other than potentially causing an unnecessary evaluation for bone or hepatic disease. A biochemically similar condition has been described in Siberian husky pups.

GGT is an enzyme that is located on the membrane of a variety of tissues (see Table 1–5). Increased serum GGT activity is associated with impaired bile flow and glucocorticoid administration in the dog. Anticonvulsant medications cause minimal to no increase in the serum GGT activity in the dog, which is in contrast to the response in humans. The serum GGT activity is a useful marker of biliary tract disease in the horse and ruminant (see Case 7–2). It may also be more diagnostically sensitive than ALP in the cat. Acute, severe hepatic injury can cause a mild increase in the serum GGT activity in the horse and ruminant because of the relatively high activity associated with the biliary tissue. This increased serum activity may be a consequence of these enzyme-rich membrane fragments from the damaged tissue reaching the peripheral circulation. The magnitude of this increase is much less than that associated with predominantly cholestatic disease in these species. Bone does not contain GGT; therefore, growth and bone disease are not associated with increased serum GGT activity. Colostrum and milk have high GGT activity and nursing animals develop increased serum GGT activity. Consequently, it can be used as a marker in a passive transfer monitoring program as an indirect indication of the plasma immunoglobulin concentration in the neonate. For neonatal dairy calves, it has been proposed that age-related serum GGT values should exceed 200, 100, 75, and 65 IU/L in 1, 4, 7, and 10 day old calves, respectively.

The renal tubular epithelial cells have a relatively high GGT tissue activity (see Table 1–5). Acute tubular injury results in a rapid increase in the activity of GGT in the urine (but not the serum). The measurement of urine GGT activity is a useful indicator of early nephrotoxicity secondary to the use of aminoglycoside antibiotics in all species (see Table 10–1).

Macroenzymes

In human patients, unexplained persistent increases in serum enzyme activity has been demonstrated with increasing frequency to be the result of macroenzymes. The enzymes reported include ALT, AST, ALP, GGT, CK, LD, lipase, and amylase. These high-molecular-mass enzyme forms can be immunoglobulin-bound or nonimmunoglobulin-bound. In either case the enzyme clearance is reduced. In dogs with proteinuria, an immunoglobulin-amylase complex (macroamylase) resulting in an increased serum amylase activity without clinical signs of pancreatitis has been reported. An increased serum enzyme activity without clinical and/or histomorphologic abnormalities should prompt the consideration of a macroenzyme.

HEPATIC TESTS: EVALUATION OF HEPATOBILIARY FUNCTION

Biochemical Analytes Produced by the Hepatocyte

Albumin

Albumin production is solely dependent on the liver and an adequate nutritional input. The dog, cat, horse, and ruminant have a tremendous reserve capacity for its production, limiting its use as an early indicator of hepatic dysfunction. A reduced serum concentration is associated with chronic hepatic insufficiency (see Case 7–3). Increased loss in the urine or gastrointestinal tract, malnutrition, and down-regulation of albumin production secondary to hyperglobulinemia are extrahepatic causes of hypoalbuminemia. A reduction of the serum globulin concentration accompanies the reduced serum albumin concentration in some diseases (Table 7–2) (see Case 7–1).

Glucose

Although the liver participates in maintaining a normal blood glucose concentration, it is an insensitive liver function test. Hypoglycemia may develop secondary to fulminate hepatic necrosis (see Case 7–1). A decreased or low

TABLE 7–2. Causes of Hypoalbuminemia

Decreased production
    Hyperglobulinemia-induced down-regulation of synthesis
    Chronic hepatic insufficiency
    Prolonged reduced protein diet
    Prolonged insufficient caloric intake
    Maldigestion (exocrine pancreatic insufficiency)
    Malabsorption
Increased loss
    Protein-losing nephropathy (see Case 10–1)
    Protein-losing enteropathy[a]
    Hemorrhage[a] (internal body cavity, tissue planes, or external-exterior
      gastrointestinal tract)
    "Third space" sequestration (subcutaneous, body cavity)
    Extensive skin lesion (burns)[a]

[a]Globulins decreased concurrently.

normal serum glucose concentration does occur in dogs and cats with congenital portosystemic shunts. It should be monitored during surgical procedures, especially in the cat.

Coagulation Factors

The liver synthesizes all the coagulation factors with the exception of the endothelium-produced factor VIII. It is not surprising that the prothrombin time and, more commonly, the activated partial thromboplastin time may be abnormal in liver disease (see Case 7–3). Factors II, VII, IX, and X are vitamin K-dependent, and insufficient bile (cholestasis) in the intestinal tract impairs the absorption of this fat-soluble vitamin, resulting in abnormal coagulation tests. While the prothrombin time is classically prolonged in humans with extrahepatic cholestasis, it appears to be less characteristic in the dog. The Thrombotest is a simple, sensitive test of vitamin K deficiency. It measures the plasma appearance of proteins induced by vitamin K absence/antagonism (PIVKA). These proteins represent the inactive vitamin K–dependent coagulation factors and indicate inadequate vitamin K activation required for their functional activity. The subcutaneous administration of vitamin K to the icteric patient at least 12 hours prior to invasive procedures is a prudent consideration (see Case 7–3). The bleeding time may be prolonged in jaundiced dogs due to abnormal platelet function; the increased serum bile acids may be causative of this functional disturbance.

Ammonia and Urea Nitrogen

The urea cycle is the major pathway for the conversion of intestinal-derived ammonia to urea nitrogen (Fig. 7–8). Hepatic insufficiency can result in a reduced serum urea nitrogen (BUN) concentration relative to the serum creatinine concentration and a raised plasma ammonia concentration (see Cases 7–1 and 7–4). Ammonia, along with other protein-derived metabolic

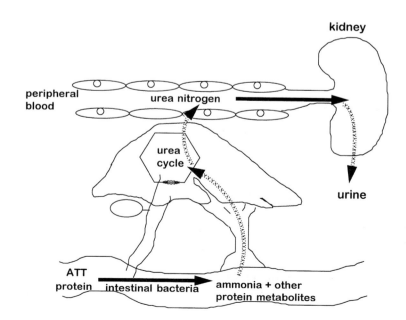

FIGURE 7–8. The ammonia derived from protein or given during the ammonia tolerance test (ATT) is rapidly converted to urea nitrogen by the hepatocellular urea cycle and excreted in the urine.

products that escape hepatic metabolism, can alter the function of the central nervous system, resulting in a syndrome referred to as hepatic encephalopathy (see Cases 7–1, 7–2, 7–3, 7–4, and 7–5). The determination of the plasma ammonia concentration can be used to support the presence of hepatic encephalopathy secondary to congenital portal vascular anomalies, cirrhosis, or an enzyme deficiency of the urea cycle (Fig. 7–9). The serum total bile acid concentration is increased concurrently in the former two disorders but is normal in the latter. In the ruminant, ammonia intoxication may occur secondary to the ingestion of large quantities of urea in the diet.

Uric acid is a degradation product of purine catabolism. In contrast to humans, most mammals oxidize most of it to allantoin in the liver by the activity of uricase. Dalmatians are a notable exception. Despite high hepatic uricase activity, the breed has a hepatic uptake defect for uric acid which results in the common finding of urate crystals in the urine. In other breeds and cats, urate crystalluria is an indication of hepatic insufficiency. The finding of ammonium (bi)urate crystals in the urine is most common in association with congenital portosystemic shunts because of the frequency and duration of hyperammonemia (Fig. 7–9) (see Case 7–4).

Since a fasting plasma ammonia concentration will be normal in some cases, we adapted an ammonia tolerance test (ATT) from the medical literature to challenge this hepatic metabolic function (Fig. 7–9). Ammonium chloride at a dose of 100 mg/kg (3 g maximum), dissolved in 20 to 30 mL of water, is given orally or rectally. A second blood sample is taken approxi-

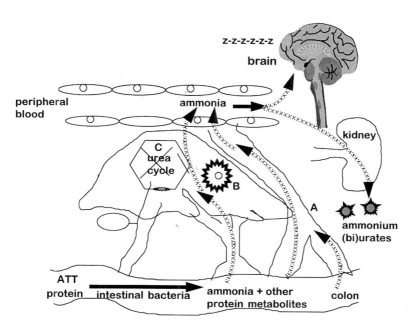

FIGURE 7–9. Hyperammonemia, resulting in encephalopathy, can be caused by three disorders: (*A*) congenital portosystemic shunts, (*B*) loss of parenchymal mass secondary to chronic hepatitis (with or without acquired portosystemic shunts), and (*C*) a congenital deficiency of one of the five enzymes comprising the urea cycle. Ammonium urate crystalluria can be associated with the first two disorders. In the ruminant, the ingestion of large quantities of urea in the diet can result in hyperammonemia.

mately 30 minutes following its administration. There is usually less than a two-fold increase compared to the fasting value. An increase greater than three-fold or a value above the reference range is indicative of hepatic insufficiency. The ATT should not be performed in patients with signs of hepatic encephalopathy prior to the determination of the fasting ammonia concentration. The dry chemistry-based reagent system conveniently supports the in-house use of the ATT. Since ammonia is volatile, the heparinized sample should be kept on crushed ice and assayed within 1 hour.

Cholesterol

Altered lipid metabolism (dyslipoproteinemia) often accompanies hepatic disease but their evaluation is not a sensitive clinical marker of hepatic dysfunction. The association of poikilocytes with chronic hepatic insufficiency may be an indirect indication of abnormal lipid metabolism. Cholesterol enrichment of the erythrocyte membrane reduces bulk lipid fluidity and decreases its resiliency subsequent to deformation resulting in abnormal shapes (irregularly spiculated erythrocytes) (see Case 7–4). Because cholesterol is eliminated from the body through both the formation of bile acids and its dissolution in bile, hypercholesterolemia develops in cholestatic disease. Hypocholesterolemia may be found in association with congenital portosystemic shunts; the reason is not known. Table 7–3 lists the more common causes of abnormal cholesterol concentrations in the plasma. The dyslipoproteinemia of hepatic disease does not usually cause visually observable lipemia. Other diseases that cause hyperlipemia are listed in Table 7–4.

Biochemical Components Dependent on Hepatocellular Uptake, Metabolic Processing, and Excretion

Bilirubin

Bilirubin is a pigmented compound produced largely from the degradation of the heme by the macrophage system from aged erythrocytes (Fig. 7–10). A smaller proportion is derived from hepatic cytochromes and ineffective erythropoiesis. The iron and globin from hemoglobin are recycled and the water-insoluble, unconjugated (indirect-reacting) bilirubin circulates to the

TABLE 7–3. Causes of Rises or Reductions of the Serum Cholesterol Concentration

Hypercholesterolemia
Hypothyroidism
Nephrotic syndrome (see Case 10–1)
Cholestasis
Pheochromocytoma
Hypocholesterolemia
Exocrine pancreatic insufficiency
Congenital portosystemic shunts
Malabsorption

TABLE 7–4.   Causes of Hyperlipidemia Due to Either Hypercholesterolemia or Hypertriglyceridemia

Postprandial[a]
Primary
    Familial: miniature schnauzer
    Familial: lipoprotein lipase deficiency of cats
    Hyperchylomicronemia of cats
    Equine hyperlipidemia syndrome (usually ponies)
Secondary
    Acute pancreatitis
    Diabetes mellitus
    Hypothyroidism[b]
    Hyperadrenocorticism[b]
    Nephrotic syndrome[b]
    Cholestatic hepatic disease
    Equine hyperlipidemia syndrome associated with systemic disease

[a]The triglyceride-rich chylomicron particles in plasma will float to the top of a refrigerated specimen within 8 hours. It is a good indication of the cause of the lipemia, and the "cleared" plasma can be harvested for biochemical analysis.

[b]Lipemia is usually not observed. If a primary hyperlipidemia is suspected after eliminating the more common secondary causes, lipoprotein lipase activity can be measured following the administration of heparin, and a lipoprotein electrophoresis of fresh plasma (refrigerated but not frozen) can be pursued.

liver bound to albumin. A carrier-mediated process dissociates it from albumin at the hepatocyte membrane and it is subsequently bound with cytosolic ligandin. The uptake site for bilirubin is also shared by other organic anions such as sulfobromophthalein (BSP) and indocyanine green (ICG) but not bile acids (Fig. 7–11).

Conjugation with glucuronic acid, catalyzed by uridine diphosphate glucuronosyltransferase (UDPGT, bilirubin UGT), results in the formation of conjugated bilirubin (direct-reacting), a water-soluble compound. Conjugation is necessary for its efficient excretion by the canalicular membrane. Excretion of bilirubin into the canalicular lumen is against a high concentration gradient and is the rate-limiting step in its elimination. The canalicular transport is a carrier-mediated process competitively shared by, once again, BSP and ICG, and cholecystographic dyes but not bile acids.

Comparative Interest.   In most nonmammalian vertebrates (birds, reptiles, amphibians), heme degradation terminates at the heme oxygenase step with the resulting water-soluble, green-blue biliverdin easily eliminated from the body. The reason is not understood why certain vertebrates convert the biologically innocuous biliverdin to bilirubin, which requires additional metabolic processing.

Bile acids are largely responsible for driving the flow of bile (bile acid–dependent flow), carrying along with it constituents such as bilirubin, through the biliary system within the liver to the common bile duct. Within the intestinal tract, colonic bacteria initially hydrolyze the conjugated bilirubin to unconjugated bilirubin and finally to a group of colorless compounds termed urobilinogens. Spontaneous oxidation of these compounds to orange-colored urobilins contributes to the fecal color. A small amount of urobilinogen is reabsorbed by the colon and reexcreted by the liver (enterohepatic circulation) (see Fig. 7–15); a physiologic reason for the recycling is not known. A

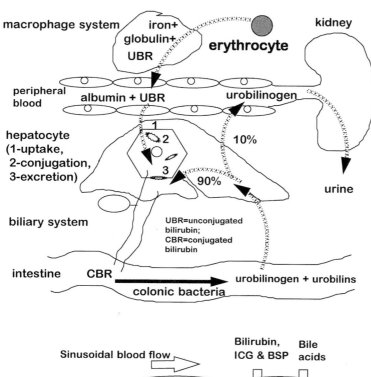

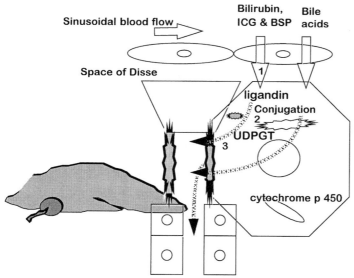

FIGURES 7–10 AND 7–11. Bilirubin (unconjugated) is formed predominantly from the degradation of aged erythrocytes, taken up by the hepatocytes, "captured" intracellularly by ligandin (glutathione-S-transferase B), conjugated with a carbohydrate moiety that is catalyzed by uridine diphosphate glucuronyltransferase (UDPGT), and excreted in the bile. Its hepatocellular uptake is shared by other organic anions such as indocyanine green (ICG) and sulfobromophthalein (BSP); both are dyes that are used as tests of hepatobiliary function. The site of bile acid uptake is distinct from the bilirubin pathway. The recycling of urobilinogen is an example of an "enterohepatic circulation." Its measurement in the urine with the reagent test strip was once used for the differential diagnosis of extrahepatic biliary obstruction.

small fraction of the reabsorbed urobilinogen may escape into the systemic circulation, where it is promptly eliminated in the urine. The measurement of urobilinogen in urine with reagent strips used to be used as a test in the differential diagnosis of jaundice. Its determination is no longer considered clinically reliable because factors such as orally administered antibiotics and intestinal transit time affect its formation and recirculation.

A rise in the plasma total bilirubin concentration imparts a yellow color to the plasma at greater than 1 mg/dL (17 μmol/L) and to other tissue at greater than 2 to 3 mg/dL (34 to 51 μmol/L). The yellow discoloration of tissue is referred to as jaundice or icterus. The slight variability in the expression of this clinical sign is due to the variable avidity of tissues for bilirubin and the predominant plasma fraction; conjugated being water soluble and unconjugated having a high affinity for lipid. Generally, one of three pathophysiologic events affecting the kinetics of bilirubin metabolism is responsible for an increase in the serum bilirubin concentration. Jaundice occurs when there is an accelerated destruction of erythrocytes, relatively severe primary intrahepatic disease, or impairment to bile flow in the common bile duct (extrahepatic) (Fig. 7–12). The use of the ratio of the unconjugated and conjugated bilirubin values comprising the total serum bilirubin concentration was used historically in the differential diagnosis of jaundice. The concept, largely extrapolated from the medical literature, appears like an attractive approach based on the kinetics of bilirubin metabolism. More recent studies in veterinary medicine indicate that species variation in the metabolism of bilirubin precludes the reliable diagnostic use of the ratio, predominant component of the total bilirubin concentration, or the magnitude of increase of the total serum bilirubin concentration in the differentiation of the cause of jaundice. Conjugated hyperbilirubinemia generally occurs in the dog and cat even in association with hemolytic disorders. Unconjugated hyperbilirubinema occurs predominantly in horses and ruminants even in association with obstruction of the extrahepatic bile duct.

Linking the clinical sign of jaundice to the evaluation of the patient's hematology, serum hepatic enzymes, and adjunct procedures is a valuable approach. Accelerated destruction of erythrocytes is associated with a moderate to marked reduction in the packed cell volume (PCV). Examination of the blood film may provide additional information; autoagglutination, Heinz bodies, or erythrocytic parasites. Biochemically, a marked increase in the serum ALT (dog, cat) and AST activities with a mild increase in the serum ALP activity indicates acute, severe hepatocellular damage (see Case 7–1). Mild to moderate, variable increases in the serum ALT, AST, and ALP activ-

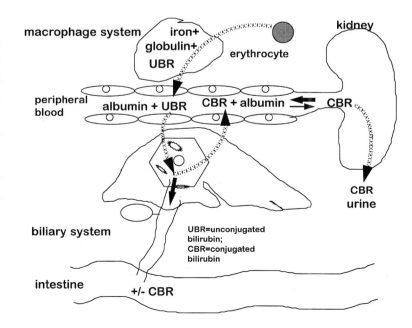

FIGURE 7–12. Three events most commonly result in hyperbilirubinemia: (1) an increased destruction of erythrocytes; (2) impaired hepatocellular uptake, conjugation, or canalicular excretion; and (3) extrahepatic obstruction to bile flow. Refer to the text for a discussion of the renal threshold concept for bilirubin. In the horse, fasting commonly causes an unconjugated hyperbilirubinemia. Free fatty acids or other metabolites that accumulate during the fast may interfere with the uptake bilirubin or its binding to ligandin.

macrophage system

iron+
globulin+
UBR

erythrocyte

kidney

peripheral
blood

albumin + UBR

CBR + albumin

CBR

CBR

biliary system

UBR=unconjugated
bilirubin;
CBR=conjugated
bilirubin

CBR
urine

intestine

+/- CBR

ities in association with hyperbilirubinemia suggest intrahepatic disease and the need for additional diagnostics. Ultrasonography is a valuable tool for assessing the extrahepatic biliary system.

A physiologic phenomenon involving bilirubin metabolism occurs in the horse. Fasting (anorexia) for more than 24 hours often results in jaundice. The cause is not known but appears to be related, in part, to competition or interference with uptake by free fatty acids or other metabolic constituents that accumulate during fasting. The differential diagnosis of jaundice in the "sick" horse therefore can be even more problematic than in the other species. The determination of the serum total bile acid concentration can be helpful (see Cases 7–2 and 7–5). As noted earlier, bile acid uptake utilizes a site that is distinct from the one used by bilirubin (Fig. 7–11). Studies have shown that the factors that affect bilirubin uptake do not impair the uptake of bile acids. Although fasting does decrease the portal blood flow, resulting in a reduced clearance of bile acids, their high hepatic extraction efficiency results in only a small increase in the plasma concentration. Therefore, a serum total bile acid concentration greater than 20 μmol/L is suggestive of hepatobiliary disease.

Novel Concept.   The existence of an additional bilirubin moiety in patients with cholestasis was discovered recently by the use of more sensitive methods of measurements. Biliprotein (originally referred to as delta bilirubin because of its location after separation of the total serum bilirubin with high-performance liquid chromatography) is a fraction of conjugated bilirubin that is irreversibly bound to albumin by covalent binding. Its formation as a consequence of cholestasis is not completely understood and the amount formed is variable. In jaundiced dogs and cats, it can range from virtually none to more than 90% of the total serum bilirubin concentration. Because of its irreversible binding to albumin, its degradation parallels that of albumin, approximately 14 days. Consequently, if it is the predominant component of the total bilirubin, the decrease in the serum total bilirubin concentration following resolution of the disease process will be protracted. For example, in cats with surgical ligation of the common bile duct for 3 weeks followed by reestablishment of bile flow, we demonstrated that the reversibly bound conjugated bilirubin decreased within 3 days, while the biliprotein slowly decreased over 10 to 14 days. The decrease in the total serum bilirubin concentration paralleled these changes dependent on the predominant conjugated bilirubin fraction. Because some of the dry-chemistry reagent systems can directly measure biliprotein, its determination along with the total bilirubin concentration should be evaluated in jaundiced patients.

Bilirubin can appear in the urine in cholestatic disease. Its occurrence is associated with an increase in the plasma concentration of the one fraction of conjugated bilirubin that has a relatively loose bond to albumin. As the concentration of this fraction of conjugated bilirubin increases, a small amount dissociates from albumin (Fig. 7–12). When the concentration of this "free" conjugated bilirubin is high enough, it is detected in the urine by the reagent strip test. The plasma concentration of the "free" conjugated bilirubin at which it enters the glomerular filtrate is referred to as the "renal threshold." In the dog, a small amount of bilirubinuria in a concentrated urine is acceptable. However, a moderate bilirubinuria will occur early in the time course of the cholestatic process in the dog (see Case 7–1). The serum ALP activity and total bile acid concentration should be concurrently increased. In the cat, bilirubinuria occurs about the same time that jaundice becomes apparent and is therefore a less valuable screening test. If a patient is jaundiced with only a small amount of bilirubin (or none) detected in the urine, it suggests that most of systemic bilirubin is in the form of biliprotein since albumin cannot enter the glomerular filtrate.

Bilirubinuria can occur in association with hemolytic disease. Since unconjugated bilirubin is not water soluble and remains bound to albumin, its increase cannot explain the finding. Two possible explanations are proposed. The large amount of unconjugated bilirubin presented to the liver for conjugation and elimination saturates canalicular excretion. Some of the conjugated bilirubin may be "regurgitated" into the systemic circulation and appear in the urine. Secondly, the canine kidney (especially in male dogs) can metabolize free hemoglobin into bilirubin. In intravascular hemolysis, the high plasma hemoglobin concentration exceeds haptoglobin binding and results in hemoglobinuria. This hemoglobin can be directly metabolized to bilirubin. Therefore, both hemoglobinuria and bilirubinuria should be present in this disease condition.

Reminder. Lipemia often causes an artifactually high serum bilirubin value when measured by "wet" chemistry systems (see Chapter 1). The possibility should be considered when the patient is not jaundiced or there is an absence of bilirubinuria.

Bile Acids

Bile acids of mammals and birds are amphipathic steroids (hydroxy cholanoic acids) containing monoanionic side chain and hydroxyl groups in various numbers and positions resulting in a variety of individual bile acids in different species. They are planar molecules with hydrophilic groups on one side and the hydrophobic steroidal part of the molecule projecting on the opposite. This arrangement facilitates micellar formation and permits them to act as biologic detergents for the solubilization of lipids in bile and aid in the digestion and absorption of fats in the intestine—physiologically good news. These same physiochemical properties also enable bile acids to solubilize biologic membranes when left in prolonged contact resulting in cytotoxicity—pathologically bad news.

The primary bile acids are synthesized from cholesterol in hepatocytes by its hydroxylation mediated by 7 α-hydroxylase. This enzymatic step is rate limiting and receives negative feedback from bile acids (predominantly chenodeoxycholic acid) in the portal blood. Glucocorticoids and thyroxine also can have an influence on this enzymatic step. Cholic acid (CA) is the predominant bile acid formed in the dog, cat, and bovine, while chenodeoxycholic acid (CDCA) is the major bile acid in the horse and human. Following their synthesis from cholesterol, these primary bile acids are conjugated with glycine and/or taurine before secretion into bile. The liver of the cat uses taurine exclusively for conjugation, the dog and horse livers use taurine predominantly for conjugation, and the bovine and human liver use glycine predominantly for conjugation. The conjugated primary bile acids are secreted by the canalicular membrane into the canaliculus (Fig. 7–13). This energy-dependent event provides the major driving force for bile flow (bile acid–dependent flow). Canalicular transport of bile acids is the rate-limiting step in their excretion.

Most of the bile acids are usually stored in the gallbladder (except the horse of course) prior to secretion into the duodenum. Approximately 50 to 70% of the newly formed bile (100% for the horse) is continuously secreted into the duodenum in support of bile acid recycling during the fasting period. This component contributes to the fasting serum total bile acid (FBA) concentration. Within the intestinal lumen, the primary bile acids, CA and CDCA, are dehydroxylated by bacteria to deoxycholic acid (DCA) and lithocholic acid (LCA), respectively. DCA and LCA are referred to as secondary bile acids. Intestinal bacterial enzymes also deconjugate a small percentage of the primary and secondary conjugated bile acids. The bile acids are efficiently reabsorbed by the terminal ileum mediated by a sodium-potassium ATPase active transport system (Fig. 7–13). Only 5 to 10% of bile acids are lost in the feces during any one enterohepatic cycle; the minimal loss being replenished by hepatic synthesis of primary bile acids.

After their reabsorption into the portal circulation, they are carried to the liver and efficiently extracted from the sinusoidal blood by the hepatocytes located in zone 1 and reexcreted into the biliary system. The physioanatomic counterflow relationship of the portal blood and bile in this region of the liver facilitates this process (Fig. 7–1). The relatively bile acid–rich portal blood flows through zone 1 in one direction while the relatively bile acid–poor bile flows in the opposite. As the bile acids are actively transported against a gradient into bile, its counter flow aids in whisking them out of the liver.

The hepatic-intestinal "recycling" of bile acids is termed "enterohepatic circulation." The high extraction efficiency (75 to 90%) for bile acids limits the quantity that "escapes" into the peripheral circulation. The concentration of all the bile acids measured in the peripheral blood following a meal is referred to as the postprandial serum total bile acid concentration (PPBA). In the horse only one random sample is necessary for the determination of the serum total bile acid concentration.

The FBA and PPBA concentrations are a reflection of the efficiency and integrity of the enterohepatic circulation. Their measurement aids in the (1) detection of congenital portosystemic shunts, (2) identification of chronic hepatitis/cirrhosis prior to the development of jaundice, and (3) monitoring of the progression or resolution of hepatic disease with therapy (Figs. 7–14

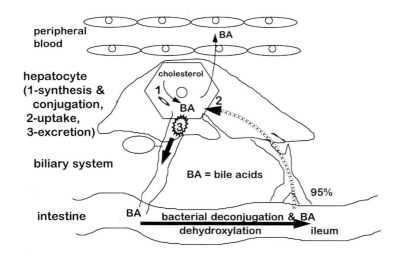

FIGURE 7–13. The enterohepatic circulation of bile acids (BA). The primary BA are synthesized from cholesterol, conjugated, and excreted into bile. The bacterial dehydroxylation of the primary BA results in the secondary BA. Bacterial deconjugation is minimal in health. BA are efficiently absorbed by the ileum and efficiently removed from the portal blood for reexcretion. It is this functional integrity of BA recycling that is primarily responsible for maintaining the enterohepatic BA "pool."

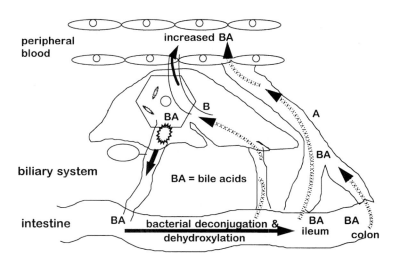

FIGURE 7–14. Congenital abnormalities of the portal circulation result in an increase in the plasma total bile acid concentration. *A,* Single or multiple macroscopic portosystemic shunts are more common than (*B*) abnormalities of the microcirculation ("microscopic" portosystemic shunts or hepatoportal microvascular dysplasia).

and 7–15). In the horse, the measurement of the serum total bile acid concentration additionally assists in the differential diagnosis of fasting hyperbilirubinemia. The measurement of the serum total bile acid concentration in the ruminant is problematic due to the wide range of reported normal values, hourly fluctuations up to 60 μmol/L during hay feeding, and the occasional moderately increased value measured in an apparently healthy animal. However, they appear to have value when applied to the evaluation of a herd situation, especially if the animals are off feed. The following generalizations are suggested as serum total bile acid concentrations indicative of hepatic dysfunction: greater than 100 μmol/L in sheep and most nonlactating and lactating cows except those in peak lactation where the range is too wide, and greater than 125 μmol/L in beef cattle.

The most common indications for the determination of the serum total bile acid concentration include: (1) increased serum ALT and/or AST in a patient with clinical signs suggestive of hepatobiliary disease (see Cases 7–2 and 7–3), (2) persistently increased serum ALT (±AST) activity in the dog

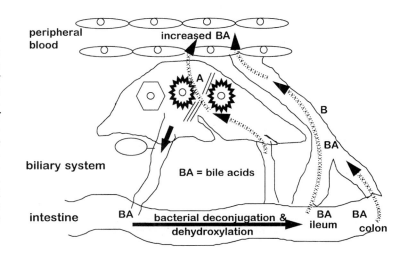

FIGURE 7–15. *A,* An impairment to hepatocellular uptake and/or excretion of bile acids secondary to hepatic pathology results in an increase in the plasma total bile acid concentration (conceptually, a form of acquired "intrahepatic shunting"). *B,* Acquired extrahepatic portosystemic shunting develops in response to an increased resistance to the hepatic portal blood flow (portal hypertension) caused by the progression of chronic hepatic disease.

and cat or serum AST activity in the horse (Fig. 7–16), (3) juvenile animals with clinical signs of hepatic insufficiency (hepatic encephalopathy, poor growth, nonspecific neurologic or behavioral signs) consistent with congenital portosystemic shunts (Fig. 7–16; see Cases 7–4 and 7–5), and (4) monitoring patients with known hepatic disease.

The FBA sample is obtained after an overnight fast (8 to 12 hours) and the PPBA sample taken approximately 2 hours after feeding 1/2 to 1 can (depending on size of dog) or 3 tablespoons of a Prescription Diet—P/D (dogs), C/D (cats), respectively. Using the same food consistently provides the same fat stimulus for gallbladder contraction. Larger quantities of food are not necessary for this purpose and may result in lipemia, which can interfere with the assay (see Chapter 1). In sick patients that resist food intake or are showing signs suggestive of hepatic encephalopathy, the FBA concentration alone usually provides the needed information. FBA and PPBA values of less than 5 and 15 μmol/L, respectively, for the dog, and less than 2 and 15 μmol/L, respectively, for the cat, and a single value of less than 15 μmol/L for the horse and less than 22 μmol/L for the llama are generally within the reference range for these species. These are guidelines and individual variation occurs. For example in the healthy dog, the PPBA can approach 30 μmol/L within the 95% confidence interval. This in turn relates to the value placed on the sensitivity and specificity of a test. Raising the cutoff of the upper end of the reference range enhances the specificity of a test at the expense of sensitivity. A relatively good positive predictive value of histopathologic changes is achieved with values of greater than 25 μmol/L for the dog and greater than 20 μmol/L for the cat and horse. These cutoffs suggest that

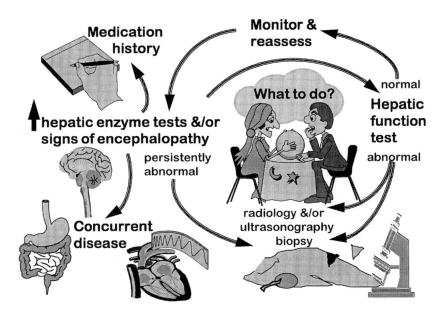

FIGURE 7–16. A simplified algorithm for the investigation of abnormal hepatic tests in an animal without severe anemia. An assessment of all medications given is an important first step, especially for the dog. Concurrent extrahepatic diseases such as lymphocytic-plasmacytic enteritis, pancreatitis, heart failure, and endocrinopathies can cause hepatic tests to be abnormal.

FIGURE 7–17. Chronic hepatic injury with its attendant reparation/regeneration processes results in persistently raised plasma aminotransferase activity. The plasma total bile acid concentration increases when there is sufficient histopathology to distort the intrahepatic architecture and disrupt the efficiency of their enterohepatic circulation.

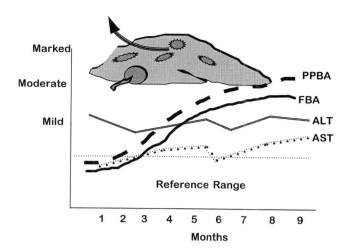

there is sufficient alteration of the enterohepatic circulation secondary to chronic disease to be detected histologically especially when linked with the evaluation of the serum aminotransferase activity (Fig. 7–17). This does not imply that a histologic diagnosis of a disease entity will be achieved; only that there will be descriptive histopathologic findings.

Occasionally the FBA value is greater than the PPBA value in the dog. The reason for this disparity is probably multifactorial: (1) fasted dogs only store approximately 30 to 50% of the newly formed bile in the gallbladder, a variability that may impact the FBA concentration; (2) meal-stimulated gallbladder bile release varies between 5 and 65%, a variability that may affect the PPBA concentration; and (3) postprandial lipemia can predispose the sample to hemolysis, which artifactually lowers the measured total bile acid value. A fourth possibility is linked to the fact that lipoproteins can bind bile acids. Their removal by ultracentrifugation or chemical precipitation to "clear" a lipemic postprandial serum specimen would probably remove the bound bile acids as well. At relatively low serum concentrations, the erroneous value could result potentially in a PPBA value less than the FBA. A final noteworthy possibility is based on the fact that intestinal bacterial overgrowth greatly enhances the formation of unconjugated bile acids. These can passively diffuse into the portal circulation anywhere along the intestinal tract during the fasted period. They are less efficiently removed from the sinusoidal blood during first pass through the liver and enter the peripheral circulation where they contribute to the measurement of the FBA concentration. Following the meal stimulation of bile flow, the conjugated bile acids are efficiently removed from the portal blood and the physiologic postprandial increase in total hepatic blood flow facilitates the removal of the unconjugated bile acids from the peripheral circulation. The overall effect could result in a lesser PPBA concentration compared to the FBA value.

BIOCHEMICAL PATTERNS OF HEPATIC DISEASE AND THEIR APPLICATION

Many of the hepatic tests discussed are routinely available on a biochemical profile. Because of the functional interdependence of the anatomic components of the hepatobiliary system (Fig. 7–1), multiple test abnormalities are frequently measured. However, abnormal serum hepatic test values do not imply primary hepatic disease. Frequently, extrahepatic disease indirectly causes the liver to "react" to gut-derived endotoxins, hormone excesses or deficiencies associated with endocrinopathies, and the perturbation of cytokines generated in response to inflammation (Fig. 7–18). Mild histopathologic changes can accompany the raised serum hepatic test values. Through

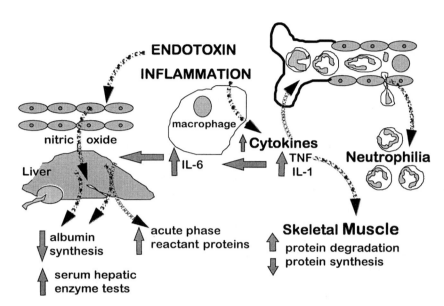

FIGURE 7–18. Cytokines are a group of hormone-like molecules, consisting of interferons, interleukins, and hematopoietic growth factors, that form a complex network of interactive signals. An increase in their systemic activity as a consequence of tissue injury and inflammation can have multiple and varied effects on organs. The more common clinically recognizable effects are those associated with tumor necrosis factor (TNF, "cachectin"), interleukin-1 (IL-1), and interleukin-6 (IL-6). The latter also plays a prominent role in regulation of hepatic-specific genes resulting in the accelerated production of multiple proteins referred to as "acute-phase reactants." Most of these migrate to the α_1 or α_2 position of the protein electrophoresis. The acute-phase response is well preserved throughout phylogeny and probably plays an important role in the host defense against tissue damage and infection. Fibrinogen is involved in blood clotting and wound healing. Nonspecific, potent inhibitors of protease include α_2-macroglobulin, α_1-antichymotrypsin, and α_1-antitrypsin. α_1-Acid glycoprotein may be a useful marker of inflammation in multiple species and of malignant neoplasia. C-reactive protein can opsonize bacteria, immune complexes, and parasites and enhance their removal by the macrophage system. Activation of the Kupffer cells for this process can cause focal hepatic histologic changes (often give a morphologic diagnosis of hepatitis) with a mild increase in the serum hepatic enzyme tests. This probably happens with relative frequency in association with severe enteritis and the translocation of bacteria and endotoxins from the intestinal tract into the portal circulation. Through poorly understood mechanisms, the stimulation of the hepatic "acute-phase response" is often associated with a concurrent reduction in albumin synthesis. Nitric oxide (NO) can also decrease albumin synthesis and alter hepatocellular function. Endotoxin can stimulate nitric oxide synthetase of blood vessels to increase the production of endothelium-derived nitric oxide and it can induce nitric oxide formation in both Kupffer cells and hepatocytes. This can have a direct effect on Kupffer cells, but the induction of hepatocellular nitric oxide synthetase appears to require multiple cytokines including IL-1 and TNF.

the judicious use of the enzyme markers and function tests, the biochemical "patterns" can provide a clue to the underlying hepatic disease process. Approaches to the evaluation of a patient with raised serum hepatic enzymes or signs of encephalopathy are outlined in Figure 7–16 and Algorithms 7, 8, and 9.

OTHER QUANTITATIVE TESTS OF HEPATIC FUNCTION

The liver is responsible for more than 600 anabolic, catabolic, and storage processes. In *Diseases of the Liver and Biliary System*, Dr. Sheila Sherlock summarized the goal to develop a succinct testing strategy to evaluate hepatic function with the following statement: ". . . the multiple functions of the liver are exceeded in number only by the biochemical methods designed to test them." The following tests have been characterized in experimental and clinical studies of the dog and in naturally occurring hepatic disease in humans. They are accepted as having clinical value as sensitive indicators of hepatic function but are generally restricted to facilities with investigative capabilities. Indocyanine green and lidocaine (see below) are examples of "flow-limited" substrates, *i.e.*, they reflect the rate at which they are presented to the hepatocyte. "Capacity-limited" substrates evaluate the intrinsic drug-metabolizing capacity of the liver by determining their clearance. Antipyrine and caffeine are examples; both are metabolized by components of the hepatic P-450 cytochrome oxidase system. The recent availability of an enzyme-multiplied immunoassay technique (EMIT) for the measurement of caffeine may provide access to a practical, sensitive test for the assessment of the liver's metabolic capacity.

Other function tests that may have investigative application include the measurement of specific bile acids (*e.g.*, cholic acid or the cholic acid to chenodoxycholic acid ratio), serum hyaluronate concentration (function of the sinusoidal endothelial cell and marker of fibrosis), erythromycin breath test (selectively measures P450lllA activity, a major xenobiotic metabolizing enzyme), MEGX test (following an intravenous bolus of lidocaine, it is converted to monoethylglicinexylidide [MEGX] through hepatic cytochrome P-450), and scintigraphic evaluation of functional liver cell mass using ^{99m}Tc-galactosylneoglycoalbumin.

SKELETAL MUSCLE TESTS

Skeletal muscle contains high activities of creatine kinase (CK, creatine phosphokinase, CPK), AST, and lactate dehydrogenase (LD). Cell injury with subsequent leakage of the enzymes is the most common cause of their increased plasma activities (see Cases 7–2 and 7–6). CK catalyzes the reversible reaction of creatine phosphate in the presence of ADP to form creatine and ATP (Fig. 7–18); an energy store to support muscle metabolism. Creatinine is irreversibly formed from creatine by its nonenzymatic dehydration. It rapidly diffuses into the plasma at a relatively constant rate proportionate to muscle mass. It freely enters the glomerular filtrate and is excreted in the urine (Fig. 7–19).

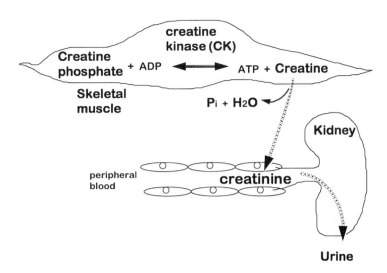

FIGURE 7–19. Skeletal muscle contains a high activity of CK, which catalyzes the reversible reaction with creatine and creatine phosphate as an energy source of muscle metabolism. Both CK and creatine are released to the plasma following skeletal muscle injury; CK is the one routinely measured. Creatinine is formed within the muscle from creatine by its nonenzymatic dehydration, rapidly diffuses into the plasma at a relatively constant rate, and is freely filtered by the glomeruli. The measurement of creatinine in the plasma and urine is commonly used as an index of the glomerular filtration rate. Pi = inorganic phosphorus.

CK is tissue specific (not present in the liver) and is useful diagnostically for identifying skeletal muscle disease. There are three isoenzymes that comprise CK: CK3 or CK-MM in the skeletal muscle, CK2 or CK-MB in the myocardium, and CK1 or CK-BB in the brain. The measurement of CK-BB in the cerebrospinal fluid has been used as a marker of central nervous system (CNS) disease. Because of the paucity of myocardial disease in veterinary medicine, most increases in the plasma CK activity are associated with skeletal muscle injury. The type and magnitude of injury and the species variation in tissue mass affect the magnitude of the plasma CK activity. As noted in Table 1–5, the cat has relatively less CK than the other species. This, in combination with the relatively sparse muscle mass, means that even a small increase in the serum CK activity is meaningful diagnostically in the cat. Anorectic cats can have mild to marked rises in the serum CK activity which begins to decrease within 2 to 3 days of appropriate supportive alimentation. It may be a clinically useful biochemical marker for monitoring the nutritional status in cats.

Metabolic diseases such as phosphofructoskinase deficiency, hypothyroidism, hyperadrenocorticism, and malignant hyperthermia in the dog and muscular dystrophy in the dog and cat are associated with increased plasma CK activity. AST is generally increased in parallel to the CK but to a much lesser magnitude and decreases relatively slower (Fig. 7–4) (see Case 7–6). ALT is present in skeletal muscle in very low activity quantitatively. Sufficient skeletal muscle injury can cause a slight increase in the plasma ALT activity in the dog. However it should be noted that, in contrast to hepatic injury in the dog, the serum AST activity will be higher than the serum ALT activity and will be accompanied by a moderate to marked increase in the plasma CK activity (Fig. 7–4).

Additional Reading

Ballmer PE, Ballmer-Hofer K, Repond F, et al: Acute suppression of albumin synthesis in systemic inflammatory disease: An individually graded response. J Histochem Cytochem 1992;40:201–206.

Baumgartner U, Sellinger M, Ruf G, et al: Change of zone bile acid processing after partial hepatectomy in the rat. J Hepatol 1995;22:474–480.

Billiar TR, Curran RD, Stuehr DJ, et al: An L-arginine-dependent mechanism mediates Kupffer cell inhibition of hepatocyte protein synthesis in vitro. J Exp Med 1989; 169:1467–1472.

Butcher NR: Experimental aspect of hepatic regeneration. N Engl J Med 1967;277: 686–696.

Chamuleau RA, Bosman DK: Liver regeneration. Hepatogastroenterology 1988;35: 309–312.

Craig AM, Pearson EG, Rowe K: Serum bile acid concentrations in clinically normal cattle: Comparison of type, age, and stage of lactation. Am J Vet Res 1992;53: 1784–1786.

Counsell LJ, Lumsden JH: Serum bile acids: Reference values in healthy dogs and comparison of two kit methods. Vet Clin Pathol 1988;17:71–74.

Day AP, Feher MD, Chopra R, et al: Triglyceride fatty acid chain length influences the post prandial rise in serum intestinal alkaline phosphatase activity. Ann Clin Biochem 1992;29:287–291.

De Broe ME, Van Hoof VO: Multiple forms of alkaline phosphatase in plasma of hemodialysis patients. Clin Chem 1991;37:783–784.

De Bruijne JJ, Rothuizen J: The value of serum bile acid and GLDH in the screening for canine liver function disorders. In Blackmore DJ, Evans GO, Sommer H, et al (eds): Animal Clinical Biochemistry. Cambridge, Cambridge University Press, 1988, pp 175–180.

Elialim R, Mahmood A, Alpers DH: Rat intestinal alkaline phosphatase secretion into lumen and serum is coordinately regulated. Biochim Biophys Acta 1991;1091:1–8.

Francavilla A, Porter KA, Benichow J, et al: Liver regeneration in the dog: Morphologic and chemical changes. J Surg Res 1978;25:409–419.

Garry FB, Fettman MJ, Curtis CR, et al: Serum bile acid concentrations in dairy cattle with hepatic lipidosis. J Vet Intern Med 1994;8:432–438.

Gilson SD, Withrow SJ, Wheeler SL, et al: Pheochromocytoma in 50 dogs. J Vet Intern Med 1994;8:228–232.

Golden DL, Spano JS, Wilson RC, et al: Application of an enzyme-multiplied immunoassay technique for determination of caffeine elimination kinetics as a test of liver function in clinically normal dogs. Am J Vet Res 1994;55:790–794.

Haukey CM, Hart MG: Fibrinogen levels in mammals suffering from bacterial infections. Vet Rec 1987;121:519–521.

Hoffmann WE, Everds N, Pignatello M, et al: Automated and semiautomated analysis of rat alkaline phosphatase isoenzymes. Toxicol Pathol 1994;22:633–638.

Horney BS, Farmer AJ, Honor DJ, et al: Agarose gel electrophoresis of alkaline phosphatase isoenzymes in the serum of hyperthyroid cats. Vet Clin Pathol 1994;23:98–102.

Ishak K: Hepatic histopathology. In Schiff L, Schiff E (eds): Diseases of the Liver, 7th edition. Philadelphia, JB Lippincott Co, 1993, p 145.

Jalan R, Hayes PC: Review article: Quantitative tests of liver function. Aliment Pharmacol Ther 1995;9:263–270.

Kuhlenschmidt M, Hoffmann W, Rippy M: Glucocorticoid hepatopathy: Effect on receptor-mediated endocytosis of asialoglycoproteins. Biochem Med Metab Biol 1991;46:152–168.

Kuwana T, Rosalki SB: Intestinal variant alkaline phosphatase in plasma in disease. Clin Chem 1990;36:1918–1921.

Lautt WW, GreenWay CV: Conceptual review of the hepatic vascular bed. Hepatology 1987;7:952–963.

Lawler DF, Keltner DG, Hoffman WE, et al: Benign familial hyperphosphatasemia in Siberian huskies. Am J Vet Res 1996;57:612–617.

Morimoto T, Tsujinaka T, Yano M, et al: Regulation of albumin synthesis after hepatectomy and in the acute inflammation phase of rat liver. J Nutr Biochem 1995; 6:522–527.

Muller F, Tyler JW, Parish SM, et al: Stability of γ-glutamyltransferase activity in calf sera after refrigerated or frozen storage. Am J Vet Res 1997;58:354–355.

Ogilvie GK, Walters LM, Greeley SH, et al: Concentration of alpha 1-acid glycoprotein in dogs with malignant neoplasia. J Am Vet Med Assoc 1993;203:1144–1146.

Panteghini M: Benign inherited hyperphosphatasemia of intestinal origin: Report of two cases and a brief review of the literature. Clin Chem 1991;37:1449–1452.

Pappas NJ Jr: Source of increased serum aspartate and alanine aminotransferase: Cycloheximide effect on carbon tetrachloride hepatotoxicity. Clin Chim Acta 1986;154:181–190.

Pearson EG, Craig AM, Rowe K: Variability of serum bile acid concentrations over time in dairy cattle, and effect of feed deprivation on the variability. Am J Vet Res 1992;53:1780–1783.

Rothuizen J, de Vries-Chalmers Hoynck van Papendrecht R, van den Brom WE: Post prandial and cholecystokinin-induced emptying of the gall bladder in dogs. Vet Rec 1990;126:505–507.

Rothuizen J, van den Brom WE, Fevery J: The origins and kinetics of bilirubin in healthy dogs in comparison with man. J Hepatol 1992;15:25–34.

Rothuizen J, van den Ingh T: Covalently protein-bound bilirubin conjugates in cholestatic disease in dogs. Am J Vet Res 1988;49:702–704.

Saini PK, Webert DW: Application of acute phase reactants during antemortem and postmortem meat inspection. J Am Vet Med Assoc 1991;198:1898–1901.

Sanecki RK, Hoffmann WE, Gelberg HB, et al: Subcellular location of corticosteroid-induced alkaline phosphastase in canine hepatocytes. Vet Pathol 1987;24:296–301.

Shepper J de, Stock J van der: Influence of sex on the urinary bilirubin excretion at increased free plasma haemoglobin levels in whole dogs and in isolated normothermic perfused dog kidneys. Experientia 1971;27:1264–1265.

Shuichi S, Ochi M, Horiuchi T, et al: Intestinal type alkaline phosphatase hyperphosphatasemia associated with liver cirrhosis. Clin Chim Acta 1992;210:63–73.

Siraganian PA, Mulvihill JJ, Mulivor RA, et al: Benign familial hyperphosphatasemia. JAMA 1989;261:1310–1312.

Solter PF, Hoffmann WE, Chambers MD, et al: Hepatic total 3 alpha-hydroxy bile acids concentration and enzyme activities in prednisolone-treated dogs. Am J Vet Res 1994;55:1086–1092.

Stark ME, Szurszewski JH: Role of nitric oxide in gastrointestinal and hepatic function and disease. Gastroenterology 1992;103:1928–1949.

Sutherland RJ, Deol HS, Hood PJ: Changes in plasma bile acids, plasma amino acids, and hepatic enzyme pools as indices of functional impairment in liver-damaged sheep. Vet Clin Pathol 1992;21:51–56.

Washizu T, Tomoda I, Kaneko JJ: Serum bile acid composition of the dog, cow, horse, and human. J Vet Med Sci 1991;53:81–86.

Yamamoto S, Shida T, Okimura T, et al: Determination of C-reactive protein in serum and plasma from healthy dogs and dogs with pneumonia by ELISA and slide reversed passive latex agglutination test. Vet Q 1994;16:74–77.

Zoli M, Marchesini H, Melli A: Evaluation of liver volume and liver function following hepatic resection in man. Liver 1986;6:286–291.

Skeletal Muscle

Aktas M, Auguste D, Lefebvre HP, et al: Creatine kinase in the dog: A review. Vet Res Commun 1993;17:353–369.

Fascetti AJ, Mauldin GE, Mauldin GN: Correlation between serum creatinine kinase activities and anorexia in cats. J Vet Intern Med 1997;11:9–13.

Finco DR, Brown SA, Vaden SL, et al: Relationship between plasma creatinine concentration and glomerular filtration in dogs. J Vet Pharmacol Ther 1995;18:418–421.

Valentine BA, Blue JT, Shelley SM, et al: Increased serum alanine aminotransferase activity associated with muscle necrosis in the dog. J Vet Intern Med 1990;4:140–143.

8

Evaluation of Pancreatic and Intestinal Tract Disorders

Endocrine and Exocrine Deficiencies; Intestinal Tests*

> *One must attend in medical practice not primarily to plausible theories, but to experience combined with reason.*
>
> —Hippocrates

The pancreas has two types of functions: hormonal (endocrine) and digestive (exocrine).

THE ENDOCRINE PANCREAS

Carbohydrate Metabolism

Insulin

The release of insulin by the pancreatic β-cells is regulated primarily by the feedback effect of glucose on the pancreas. When the plasma glucose concentration is increased insulin secretion increases, and when the plasma glucose concentration decreases so does insulin release. Studies suggest that the serum insulin concentration is near zero when the blood glucose approaches 30 mg/dL (1.65 mmol/L). This is the rationale for including the value of 30 mg/dL in the formula for the amended insulin to glucose ratio (AIGR) that is used to aid in the diagnosis of hyperinsulinism.

---

*See Algorithms 13, 14, and 15.

Fatty acids, selected amino acids, and ketones also have a stimulatory effect on insulin secretion. Glucagon, in small amounts, will stimulate insulin secretion. Growth hormone, glucocorticoids, estrogen, and progesterone increase peripheral resistance to the action of insulin amplifying its pancreatic secretion.

Glucagon

Glucagon is produced by pancreatic α-cells and cells in the wall of the duodenum and stomach.

Glucagon is also regulated by plasma glucose concentrations. A rise in glucose causes decreased secretion, whereas fasting causes increased secretion. Glucagon increases the glucose concentration primarily through hepatic glycogenolysis and gluconeogenesis (Fig. 8–1).

Diabetes Mellitus; Hyperglycemia

Glucose, in the absence of insulin, is utilized inefficiently by muscle, adipose tissue, and the liver. Insulin deficiency along with the continued activity of glucagon results in hyperglycemia and glycosuria (Fig. 8–2). Diabetic animals may also develop weight loss and polyphagia because, in spite of large quantities of blood glucose, body tissues are starved, resulting in the catabolism of fat and muscle. The longer hypoinsulinism exists, the more likely ketoacidosis will develop. Diabetes mellitus may also occur in patients with hypersomatotropism.

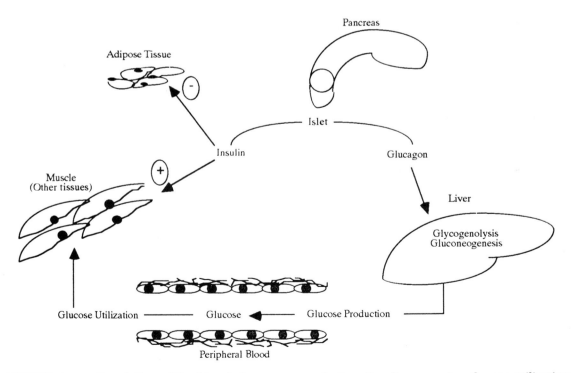

FIGURE 8–1. Regulation of the blood glucose concentration. Insulin promotes glucose utilization and inhibits lipolysis. Glucagon facilitates glucose production.

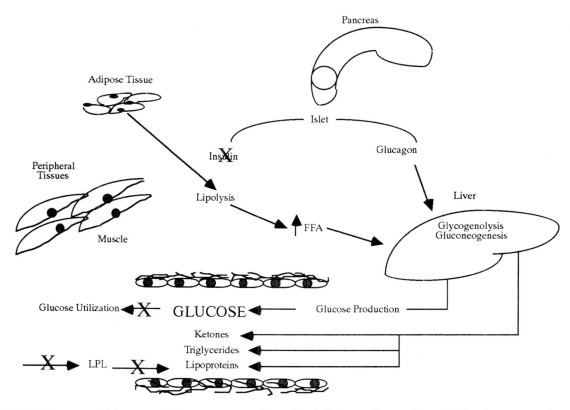

FIGURE 8–2. Diabetes mellitus. Because of insulin deficiency, hyperglycemia develops secondary to decreased utilization. Insulin deficiency permits lipolysis to generate free fatty acids (FFA) that are transported to the liver, where some are stored as triglycerides (fatty liver) and some are converted to lipoproteins (resulting in lipemia). Lipoprotein lipase (LPL) activity declines with insulin deficiency, contributing to the hyperlipoproteinemia. The altered glucagon to insulin ratio also activates fatty acid oxidation, resulting in ketone production.

Laboratory findings, in addition to hyperglycemia and glycosuria, include hypercholesterolemia (plasma is frequently lipemic), increased serum alkaline phosphatase and alanine aminotransferase activities as a consequence of hepatic lipidosis, and ketonemia and ketonuria.

Non-insulin-dependent diabetes mellitus (Type II) is a common form in the cat. Finding a fasting serum insulin concentration of greater than the mean of the reference range 117 pmol/L (16 μU/mL) concurrent with hyperglycemia is supportive of the diagnosis. Unfortunately, a lesser value can be measured in some cats with non-insulin-dependent diabetes mellitus limiting its use as a reliable marker. What is the reason for this apparent dichotomy? Chronic hyperglycemia appears to impair the ability of functional beta cells to respond appropriately to secretagogues in some patients. The effect is reversed subsequent to dietary management or oral sulfonylurea drugs. Chronic hypersecretion of growth hormone secondary to pituitary neoplasia (acidophil adenoma) causes acromegaly and hyperglycemia in cats. The condition is characterized by an insulin-resistant diabetes mellitus, organomegaly, cardiomyopathy, arthropathy, and central nervous system signs.

Other causes of hyperglycemia are summarized in Table 8–1.

TABLE 8–1. Causes of Hyperglycemia

Postprandial (monogastric animals)
Exertional epinephrine (very common in cats)
Increased glucocorticoids (stress hyperadrenocorticism, administration of corticoids or ACTH)
Diabetes mellitus
Growth hormone excess (acromegaly)
Acute pancreatitis
Drug induced (thiazide diuretics, morphine, intravenous fluids with glucose, Ovaban in some cats, ethylene glycol)
Glucagon-secreting pancreatic tumor (no ketonuria)

Uremic animals often have a diabetic-like glucose tolerance curve. The fasting glucose may not be increased, but hyperglycemia may develop after parenteral or oral administration of glucose. This is thought to occur because of peripheral resistance to insulin. Since insulin is catabolized by the kidney, it is ironic that glucose intolerance develops despite plasma insulin concentrations in the high normal range.

The increase in plasma glucose concentration associated with excess glucocorticoid activity is usually not marked. However, stressed cats frequently have a marked transient increase in plasma glucose as well as glycosuria, and this must be differentiated from diabetes. Measurement of the serum fructosamine concentration can make the distinction in problematic cases (Case 8–1).

Hyperglycemia occurs frequently in animals poisoned with ethylene glycol. The mechanism is not well understood, but it is thought that there may be (1) an inhibition of glycolysis and the Krebs cycle by aldehydes; (2) increases in glucocorticoid and epinephrine activity; and (3) inhibition of insulin release because of hypocalcemia.

Glucose tolerance tests may be used in patients that are mildly hyperglycemic (125 to 180 mg/dL) (6.875 to 9.9 mmol/L) to determine if they are latent diabetics. Intravenous glucose tolerance is the most common test performed. There are several protocols for the glucose tolerance test and the clinician should contact the laboratory being used. Prediabetic animals have a prolonged hyperglycemia after glucose administration. A recent report indicates that occasional wide inter- and intraindividual variability of the intravenous glucose tolerance test occurs in cats necessitating caution in its interpretation, especially in stressed cats.

Monitoring the plasma glucose concentration during the treatment of diabetes mellitus can be problematic for some patients, notably cats. The measurement of the serum fructosamine concentration can facilitate the management of diabetes mellitus. Fructosamine represents glycated serum proteins that form as a result of the nonenzymatic reaction between glucose and the amino group on the lysine residues of the proteins. The reaction is irreversible. Consequently, its measurement reflects the average plasma glucose concentration over 1 to 3 weeks. It is unaffected by acute changes in glucose metabolism associated with food intake and stress, and is stable for at least several days at 4° C and a month at −20° C. The measurement of the serum fructosamine concentration has been shown to be a useful indicator in the management of canine and feline diabetes mellitus. The upper limit of the reference range is approximately 3.5 mmol/L for the dog and the cat. Cats with hyperthyroidism appear to have serum fructosamine concentrations below the reference range.

Hyperinsulinism, Hypoglycemia

Hyperinsulinism is associated with pancreatic β-cell neoplasia (insulinoma).

Excessive production of insulin results in fasting hypoglycemia. Affected animals have a history of intermittent periods of episodic weakness and collapse.

A tentative diagnosis of hyperinsulinism can be made by demonstrating fasting hypoglycemia or marginally normal blood glucose associated with an inappropriate insulin concentration in a patient with a typical history. Since hyperinsulinemia is not consistently present at the time of sampling in dogs with insulinoma, multiple measurements have been suggested for diagnostic enhancement. The patient is hospitalized and fasted for approximately 8 hours while being carefully observed for signs of hypoglycemia. A blood sample is collected following the fast and three more are collected approximately one hour apart. Each sample is immediately assayed for the glucose concentration and an aliquot from each of the four samples is sent to the laboratory for the measurement of insulin. The sampling strategy increases the probability of finding an incongruent glucose-insulin relationship. Other causes of hypoglycemia are summarized in Table 8–2.

AIGR. The amended insulin to glucose ratio has been used to assist in the diagnosis of hyperinsulinism using the following formula:

$$\frac{\text{Serum insulin } (\mu U/mL) \times 100}{\text{Serum glucose (mg/dL)} - 30} = \text{AIGR.}$$

AIGR values greater than 30 support the diagnosis of an insulin-producing neoplasm; however, the formula is not unique to insulinomas.

TABLE 8–2.   Causes of Hypoglycemia

Delayed separation of serum from erythrocytes
Hepatic disease (severe)
Congenital portosystemic shunts
Hyperinsulinism (islet cell neoplasm or insulin therapy)
Extrapancreatic tumors (smooth muscle tumors)
Idiopathic in toy breed, puppies, hunting dogs
Septicemia/endotoxemia
Endocrine hypofunction (hypopituitarism, hypoadrenocorticism, hypothyroidism)
Canine renal glycosuria (severe cases)
Drug induced (salicylates, sulfonyurea, exogenous insulin, ethanol)
Hepatic glycogen storage disease
Starvation

THE EXOCRINE PANCREAS

The function of the exocrine pancreas is to produce and secrete digestive enzymes. Most of these enzymes are stored in the pancreas as inactive precursors (zymogens). Amylase and lipase are notable exceptions. The secretions respond to both neural and hormonal stimuli (Fig. 8–3).

Exocrine pancreatic disorders can be classified as inflammatory (pancreatitis, acute or chronic) or insufficiency (reduced production and secretion of digestive enzymes).

Inflammatory Disease

Amylase and *lipase* are the two enzymes that are measured most frequently as markers of acute pancreatitis. Although the majority of normal plasma activity of amylase and lipase is not of pancreatic origin, marked increases of both occur subsequent to experimental pancreatitis in the dog. In naturally occurring disease, the association is less consistent for unknown reasons. Additionally, controversy continues to surround which enzyme is the better marker of acute pancreatitis. It appears prudent to determine both, with a greater than two-fold increase in serum activity considered supportive of acute pancreatitis. Recurrence of the disease (chronic pancreatitis) results in a scarred organ with limited capacity for the production of digestive enzymes. Neither amylase nor lipase would be expected to increase (or decrease) in the plasma at this stage of the disease process. Electrophoresis of serum amylase results in several isoamylases. Although abnormal isoamylase patterns develop subsequent to acute pancreatitis, an overlap with other diseases occurs. Perhaps with improved methodology for separation and clinical utility the procedure will find future application.

There are numerous causes of acute pancreatitis, but in most cases the underlying etiology is not known (idiopathic). Some associated causes include

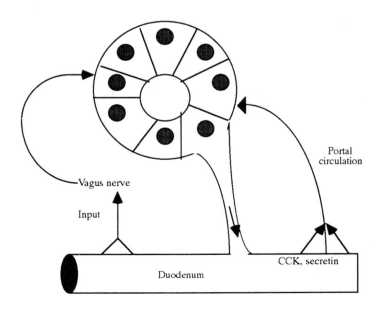

FIGURE 8–3. The exocrine pancreas is responsive to both neural and hormonal stimuli. Gastric acid and long-chain fatty acids cause secretin release into the portal circulation, which causes pancreatic water and bicarbonate secretion. Cholecystokinin (CCK) is released secondary to fat and protein digestion and stimulates the secretion of pancreatic enzymes (and relaxation of the sphincter of Oddi and contraction of the gallbladder).

diets rich in fat, drugs (glucocorticoids, azathioprine, sulfa antibacterials, organophosphates), trauma, and ischemia. The underlying pathophysiologic events appear to occur within the pancreatic acinar cells and involve impaired secretion of the inactive digestion enzymes. Eventually, intracellular lysosomal hydrolases, normally shielded from the zymogens, activate the enzymes, which initiates autodigestion of the organ (Fig. 8–4). It remains unclear how extrapancreatic events (inflammation, spasm, or obstruction of the pancreatic duct) are related to the intracellular activation of the digestive enzymes.

The kinetics of both amylase and lipase is affected by kidney function. *Chronic renal insufficiency* can cause an increase in one or both enzymes. In some dogs with kidney disease and proteinuria, the formation of macroamylasemia (amylase bound to immune complexes) has been shown to contribute to the hyperamylasemia. The hepatic removal of this enzyme-protein complex is probably impaired, resulting in the raised plasma amylase activity independent of pancreatic disease. Since acute pancreatitis can be associated with acute renal decompensation and the clinical signs can appear similar, values for amylase greater than three- to four-fold are supportive of acute pancreatitis when there is concurrent renal insufficiency.

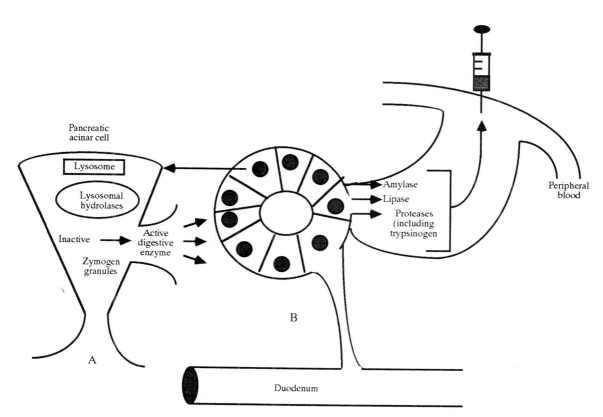

FIGURE 8–4. *A,* Impaired cellular secretion of zymogen granules results in the fusion of the zymogen granules and lysosome. Subsequent activation of the digestive enzymes by the lysosomal hydrolases causes autodigestion, allowing release of the enzymes into the peripheral circulation. *B,* The degree of tissue pathology may limit the exposure of the enzymes to the peripheral blood affecting the magnitude of their increase.

**TABLE 8–3. Causes of Increased Serum
Amylase or Lipase**

Pancreatic inflammation, necrosis, and neoplasia
Obstruction of pancreatic ducts
Chronic renal insufficiency
Macroamylasemia
Slight increase with glucocorticoids (lipase only)
Intestinal perforations

Although pancreatitis occurs in the cat, very little is known regarding the clinical disease process or its diagnosis. It should be noted that feline pancreatitis differs from that in the dog in that vomiting is not a prominent feature. Loss of appetite, lethargy, nondescript abdominal discomfort, and a painful mass in the anterior abdomen on palpation are the more common findings. Experimental pancreatitis in the cat was associated with a minimal increase (two-fold) in lipase and a decrease in amylase. Based on that study and on clinical experience, the biochemical diagnosis of pancreatitis differs from the dog. Most cats with acute pancreatitis have serum amylase and lipase activities within the reference range. Occasionally, the serum lipase activity is slightly raised in nonazotemic cats but is much less consistent than in the experimental model. The measurement of plasma trypsin-like immunoreactivity may be diagnostic in dogs and cats for acute pancreatitis when the assay becomes available for clinical use. Ultrasonographic evaluation of the pancreas is a value tool for the identification of acute pancreatitis in the cat. When localized fluid is identified and sampled, we have measured high lipase activity and found a nonseptic, suppurative exudate cytologically. The measurement of amylase in the abdominal fluid also has been suggested as a diagnostic test in horses. However, it is probable that it is also increased in the peritoneal fluid in association with obstructive disease involving the upper intestinal tract; a more common disorder.

The administration of glucocorticoids can cause a mild increase in plasma lipase activity and a decrease in plasma amylase activity without causing clinical or histologic evidence of pancreatitis in the dog. An exploratory laparotomy can also result in a mild increase in plasma lipase activity without evidence of pancreatitis. Other associations with hyperlipasemia and/or hyperamylasemia are listed in Table 8–3.

Hepatic Enzyme Tests

Abnormal hepatic enzyme tests and function reflected as hyperbilirubinemia can occur in association with acute pancreatitis. Although mechanical obstruction of the common bile duct may occur secondary to the closely associated inflamed peripancreatic/pancreatic tissue, direct release of proteases into the portal circulation with alteration of intrahepatic cellular structure and function probably occurs with greater frequency (Fig. 8–5). The observation of abnormal liver tests in a dog with acute, repetitive vomiting should prompt the determination of serum lipase and amylase activities. The abnormal liver tests will return toward normal within 7 to 10 days as the pancreatitis resolves. Persistence of hyperbilirubinemia beyond 10 days implies an extrahepatic obstructive process that should be pursued diagnos-

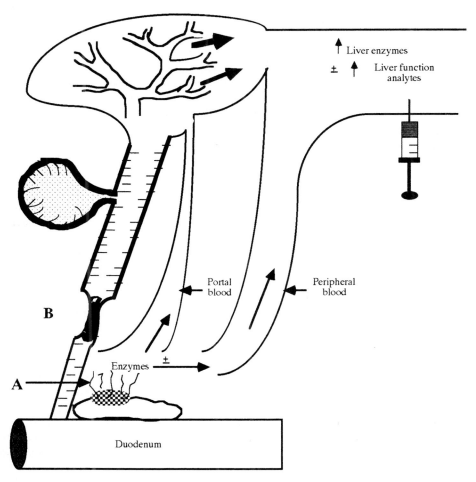

FIGURE 8–5. Acute pancreatitis may be associated with abnormal liver tests by *A*, release of active digestive enzymes into the portal circulation with subsequent intra-hepatic injury or *B*, obstruction (temporary or permanent) of the common bile duct due to the impingement of the inflamed pancreatic/peripancreatic tissue. (Modified from Meyer DJ, Burrows CB: The liver. Part 2: Biochemical diagnosis of the hepa-tobiliary disorders in the dog. Comp Contin Educ Small Anim Pract 1982;5:706, with permission.)

tically with ultrasonography and with surgery as a consideration. Icterus and raised serum hepatic enzyme tests were reported to be a relatively common finding in cats with acute pancreatitis with only anorexia, lethargy, and weight loss primarily demonstrated clinically. There is also a relatively high inci-dence of acute pancreatitis associated with the feline hepatic lipidosis syn-drome. These cats have a worse prognosis than those without concurrent acute pancreatitis.

Maldigestion and Malabsorption

The *exocrine pancreas* and *small intestine* are integral in facilitating digestion and absorption of ingested nutrients. Dysfunction of one or both organs results in chronic diarrhea and weight loss. Numerous serum and fecal tests have been developed for diagnostic use, indicative of the difficulty in evaluating the function of these organs. Because of the pragmatic limitations in adapting many of these tests for clinical use or because of unreliable results the following tests are not recommended: Sudan staining for fecal fat (before and after addition of acetic acid), iodine staining for fecal starch, assessment for fecal muscle fibers, fecal trypsin-gel tube or radiographic film digestion, plasma turbidity test, oral glucose tolerance test, and xylose absorption. The *most reliable* approach to the differential diagnosis of canine maldigestion/ malabsorption is by concurrently assessing the function of the exocrine pancreas and small intestine combined with endoscopic/surgical biopsy of the small intestine when indicated. Exocrine pancreatic insufficiency should always be ruled out in all cases of *chronic diarrhea* and/or *weight loss* so that the diagnostic focus can be shifted to the assessment of small intestinal function.

Trypsin-like Immunoreactivity

Trypsinogen (measured as trypsin-like immunoreactivity [TLI]) is organ specific for the pancreas. The reference range for the plasma TLI is solely dependent on a healthy, functioning pancreas. TLI is measured by use of a radioimmunoassay (RIA), which is species specific, *i.e.*, no cross-reaction with the assay developed for humans. The plasma TLI appears to increase rapidly subsequent to acute pancreatitis and rapidly decline within hours to days; clinical studies are required to confirm these findings from experimental studies. Chronic renal insufficiency causes a rise of the plasma TLI.

The serum TLI test was developed for the evaluation of pancreatic function (Fig. 8–6). It has become the biochemical "cornerstone" for the diagnosis of exocrine pancreatic insufficiency (EPI) due to its simplicity and high sensitivity and specificity. A decreased plasma TLI is diagnostic of EPI. No pancreatic enzyme supplements should be given at least 1 week prior to testing. A radial enzyme diffusion test to measure accurately the fecal proteolytic activity using an azocasein substrate has been shown to be useful for the diagnosis of EPI in the cat. Three fecal samples, not necessarily sequential, should be measured. Fresh or frozen samples stored at $-20°$ C can be used. Commercial availability is the primary limitation. The recent validation of a feline specific TLI assay will obviate the need for this distasteful testing strategy.

Folate and Cobalamin

Although the accurate biochemical diagnosis of EPI has been enhanced greatly, functional assessment of the small intestine is hampered by the tremendous surface area of the affected organ and by varying degrees of pathology. Folate is absorbed primarily in the proximal small intestine, and cobalamin (vitamin B_{12}) is absorbed predominantly by the ileum (Fig. 8–6). Pathology sufficient to result in chronic diarrhea can cause decreased serum values depending on the diseased site. Bacterial overgrowth, which appears to complicate both pancreatic and intestinal diseases secondarily, can cause increased serum folate values because of increased bacterial production. Oc-

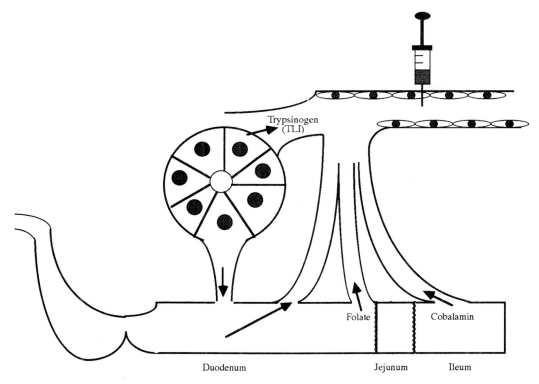

FIGURE 8–6. Exocrine pancreatic function is assessed with the measurement of serum TLI. The absorptive function of the proximal part of the small intestine can be assessed by measurement of serum folate concentration and distal small intestine function by the serum cobalamin concentration.

casionally bacterial consumption of cobalamin is sufficient to cause a concurrent decrease. Marked increases in both folate and cobalamin suggest B-vitamin supplementation. The concentration of folate and cobalamin in the diet can also alter their plasma concentrations.

Biochemical assessment of pancreatic and intestinal disorders in the equine remain problematic and restricted to institutions with research interests.

Additional Reading

Akol KG, Washabau RJ, Saunders HM, et al: Acute pancreatitis in cats with hepatic lipidosis. J Vet Inter Med 1993;7:205–209.

Baker RH: Acute necrotizing pancreatitis in a horse. J Am Vet Med Assoc 1978;172:268–270.

Bellah JR, Bell G: Serum amylase and lipase activities after exploratory laparotomy in dogs. Am J Vet Res 1989;50:1638–1640.

Cook AK, Breitschwerdt EB, Levine JF, et al: Risk factors associated with acute pancreatitis in dogs: 101 cases (1985–1990). J Am Vet Med Assoc 1993;203:673–679.

Corazza M, Tognetti R, Guidi G, et al: Urinary alpha-amylase and serum macroamylase activities in dogs with proteinuria. J Am Vet Med Assoc 1994;205:438–440.

Fittschen C, Bellamy JEC: Prednisone treatment alters the serum amylase and lipase activities in normal dogs without causing pancreatitis. Can J Comp Med 1984;48:136–140.

Hill RC, Van Winkle TJ: Acute necrotizing pancreatitis and acute suppurative pancreatitis in the cat. J Vet Intern Med 1993;7:25–33.

Jacobs RM: The origins of canine serum amylases and lipases. Vet Pathol 1989;26:525–527.

Jensen AL: Serum fructosamine as a screening test for diabetes mellitus in non-healthy middle-aged to older dogs. J Vet Med A 1994;41:480–484.

Karanjia ND, Widdison AL, Jehanli A, et al: Assay of trypsinogen activation in the cat experimental model of acute pancreatitis. Pancreas 1993;8:189–195.

Kitchell BE, Strombeck DR, Cullen J, et al: Clinical and pathologic changes in experimentally induced acute pancreatitis in cats. Am J Vet Res 1986;47:1170–1173.

Lutz TA, Rand JS, Watt P, et al: Pancreatic biopsy in the cat. Aust Vet J 1994;71:223–227.

Montgomery TM, Nelson RW, Feldman EC, et al: Basal and glucagon-stimulated plasma C-peptide concentrations in healthy dogs, dogs with diabetes mellitus, and dogs with hyperadrenocorticism. J Vet Intern Med 1996;10:116–122.

Parry BW, Crisman MV: Serum and peritoneal fluid amylase and lipase reference values in horses. Equine Vet J 1991;23:390–391.

Peterson ME, Taylor RS, Breco DS, et al: Acromegaly in 14 cats. J Vet Intern Med 1990;4:192–201.

Polzin DJ, Osborne CA, Stevens JB, et al: Serum amylase and lipase activities in dogs with chronic primary renal failure. Am J Vet Res 1983;44:404–407.

Reusch CE, Liehs MR, Hoyer M, et al: Fructosamine. J Vet Intern Med 1993;7:177–182.

Siliart B, Stambouli F: Laboratory diagnosis of insulinoma in the dog: A retrospective study and a new diagnostic procedure. J Small Anim Pract 1996;37:367–370.

Simpson KW, Shiroma JT, Biller DS, et al: Antemortem diagnosis of pancreatitis in four cats. J Small Anim Pract 1994;35:93–99.

Simpson KW, Simpson JW, Morton DB, et al: Effect of pancreatectomy on plasma activities of amylase, isoamylase, lipase, and trypsin-like immunoreactivity in dogs. Res Vet Sci 1991;51:78–82.

Sparkes AH, Adams DT, Cripps PJ, et al: Inter- and intraindividual variability of the response to intravenous glucose tolerance testing in cats. Am J Vet Res 1996;57:1294–1298.

Steiner JM, Medinger TL, Williams DA: Development and validation of a radioimmunoassay for feline trypsin-like immunoreactivity. Am J Vet Res 1996;57:1417–1420.

Sugimoto Y, Hayakawa T, Kondo T, et al: Peritoneal absorption of pancreatic enzymes in bile–induced acute pancreatitis in dogs. J Gastroenterol Hepatol 1990;5:493–498.

Thoresen SI, Bredal: Clinical usefulness of fructosamine measurements in diagnosing and monitoring feline diabetes mellitus. J Small Anim Prac 1996;37:64–68.

Traverso L, Longmire W, Tompkins R: A study of experimental canine pancreatitis. J Surg Res 1976;21:247–253.

Williams DA, Batt RM: Sensitivity and specificity of radioimmunoassay of serum trypsin-like immunoreactivity for the diagnosis of canine exocrine pancreatic insufficiency. J Am Vet Med Assoc 1988;192:195–201.

Williams DA, Reed SD, Perry L: Fecal proteolytic activity in clinically normal cats and in a cat with exocrine pancreatic insufficiency. J Am Vet Med Assoc 1990;197:210–212.

Williams DA: New tests of pancreatic and small intestinal function. Comp Contin Educ Pract Vet 1987;9:1167–1174.

9

Evaluation of Endocrine Function*

Dr. Watson: "What say Holmes?"
Sherlock Holmes: ". . . we are suffering from a plethora
of surmise, conjecture, and hypothesis. The difficulty is
to detach the framework of fact—absolute undeniable
fact—from the embellishments of theories and reporters.
Then having established ourselves upon this sound basis,
it is our duty to see what inferences may be drawn, and
which are the special points upon which the whole mys-
tery turns."
—A. Conan Doyle, *The Adventure of Silver Blaze*

PARATHYROID GLAND

Calcium And Phosphorus Homeostasis

The orchestration of calcium homeostasis is mediated through the integrated actions of parathyroid hormone (PTH), vitamin D, and calcitonin (Fig. 9–1). The former two are the most important mediators. The bone, the small intestine, and the kidney are the three principal target organs. Estrogens, glucocorticoids, somatotropin, glucagon, and thyroxine can influence calcium metabolism but their adverse effects are not a common clinical concern in veterinary medicine.

Plasma calcium exists in three forms: ionized or free (~50%), bound to albumin (~45%), and bound to anions (~5%). Ionized calcium is the physiologically active form. The pH of extracellular fluids and the plasma protein concentration can change its plasma concentration. Acidosis promotes an increase of the ionized form, whereas alkalosis has the opposite effect. An increase of the plasma protein concentration results in an increase in the total calcium concentration. A reduced plasma protein concentration has the converse effect. The protein-calcium binding is a freely reversible process that is related to a dissociation constant. As long as the protein-bound cal-

---

*See Algorithms 16, 17, 18, and 19.

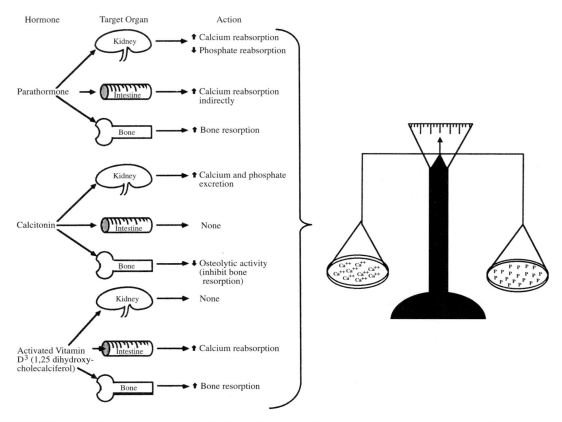

FIGURE 9–1. Endocrine control of mineral balance depends on the interaction of PTH from the parathyroid glands, calcitonin from the parafollicular cells of the thyroid gland, and vitamin D after activation to 1,25-dihydroxycholecalciferol by the kidney.

cium concentration to free protein concentration ratio remains constant, the ionized calcium concentration will remain constant. This relationship permits the use of nomograms for the estimation of ionized calcium using the total calcium and protein concentrations. Ion-selective electrode measurement of ionized calcium is the most accurate assessment.

The total serum calcium concentration can be "adjusted" for changes in the plasma albumin concentration using the following formula. The formula is only valid for the canine species.

1. Using the serum albumin (g/dL) and calcium (mg/dL) concentrations:

$$\text{Adjusted calcium} = \text{calcium} - \text{albumin} + 3.5.$$

2. SI conversion using serum albumin (g/L) and calcium (mmol/L):

$$\text{Adjusted calcium} = \left[\text{calcium} \times \left(4 - \frac{\text{albumin}}{10} \right) + 3.5 \right] \times 0.25.$$

3. Using serum total protein (mg/dL) and calcium (mg/dL):

$$\text{Adjusted calcium} = \text{calcium} - (0.4 \times \text{total protein}) + 3.3.$$

4. SI conversion using serum total protein (g/L) and calcium (mmol/L):

$$\text{Adjusted calcium} = \left[\text{calcium} \times 4 - \left(\frac{\text{total protein}}{10} \right) + 3.3 \right] \times 0.25.$$

PTH functions to raise the plasma ionized calcium concentration and reduce the plasma phosphorus concentration. The former event is mediated through osteoclast-activated bone resorption and the latter through an effect on the proximal renal tubule resulting in phosphaturia. Although the magnitude of the effect is poorly understood, there is a concurrent reduction of sodium, calcium, and bicarbonate reabsorption in the proximal tubule and an enhanced calcium reabsorption in the distal tubule. PTH stimulates the renal synthesis of 1,25-dihydroxycholecalciferol (the active vitamin D metabolite) resulting in enhanced calcium absorption from the small intestine. Hypercalcemia suppresses PTH secretion from the parathyroid gland by way of a finely tuned negative feedback loop.

The diet is the primary source of cholecalciferol (vitamin D_3), which is converted by the liver to 25-hydroxycholecalciferol and finally to 1,25-dihydroxycholecalciferol by the renal proximal tubules. Its production is controlled by a negative feedback loop; the hypocalcemic induction of PTH release stimulates its renal production. Hypercalcemia reduces its production through suppression of the PTH secretion. It primarily functions to enhance calcium absorption in the small intestine independent of PTH activity.

Calcitonin is produced and secreted in response to hypercalcemia by C-cells, a component of the amine precursor uptake and decarboxylation (APUD) system, represented as parafollicular in the thyroid gland. Although calcitonin is a pharmacologically potent calcium regulator causing a reduction of calcium and phosphorus, an essential physiologic role in calcium homeostasis is not well defined.

The bone, the kidney, and the small intestine are also the key organs involved in the homeostasis of phosphorus. About 85% of the phosphorus, measured as inorganic phosphorus, is present in bone as hydroxyapatite; the remainder is linked to organic substances such as phospholipids and biochemical energy storage compounds. Most of the inorganic phosphorus in extracellular fluid is present in two types of pH-dependent phosphate ions, HPO_4^- and $H_2PO_4^-$. Dietary intake is the main source of phosphorus. Ingestion of phosphate-rich food can increase the plasma phosphorus concentration. Absorption is enhanced by vitamin D and growth hormone, the latter probably responsible for the increased serum phosphorus concentration during growth. Most of the plasma phosphorus undergoes glomerular filtration with the majority reabsorbed by the tubules. PTH inhibits that reabsorptive process.

PTH is derived from ProPTH, an intermediate precursor polypeptide which is cleaved from a larger precursor molecule, PreProPTH. A mixture of these components circulates but only the PTH is biologically active with a half-life of minutes. The kidney clears the other components with half-lives of hours to days. Early assays for PTH directed at the C-terminal and mid-molecule sequences gave inaccurate measurements due to the interference of the inactive components. Newer assays referred to as two-site immunoradiometric or N-terminal radioimmunoassay are more consistently reliable for the determination of intact PTH in the serum of animals. The measurement should be used as an adjunct to the clinical presentation and correlated to the serum total calcium concentration, or, preferably, the serum ionized calcium value. A normal to increased serum PTH concentration in association with hypercalcemia is inappropriate and indicative of primary hyperparathyroidism. Conversely, a reduced PTH concentration in concert with hypocalcemia is compatible with primary hypoparathyroidism. The measurement of the serum PTH concentration in dogs with renal failure and hypercalcemia is problematic for discerning which is the primary disorder, renal or parathyroid gland. The serum PTH concentration is usually normal or reduced in association with malignancy-induced hypercalcemia. In this paraneoplastic disorder, there are PTH-like biochemical mimes that cause hypercalcemia. In addition to cytokines such as interleukin-1 and tumor necrosis factor, there is a factor referred to as PTH-related protein (PTHrP) that has been identified in humans with humoral hypercalcemia of malignancy and in dogs with lymphoma and apocrine gland adenocarcinomas of the anal sac.

Magnesium Metabolism

Magnesium is considered in the discussion of calcium and phosphorus homeostasis because the same conditions and hormones tend to control the excretion of all three ions, a consequence of their role as the major constituents of bone mineral. Severe hypomagnesemia impairs PTH secretion; magnesium supplementation being required to raise the plasma PTH concentration and, subsequently, the plasma calcium concentration. Magnesium is an abundant intracellular cation, second only to potassium, that is an activator of a wide variety of enzyme systems. Approximately one third is bound to albumin; the remainder exists as the free ion. Homeostasis appears to be maintained primarily by renal excretion/reabsorption. The determination of the plasma magnesium concentration correlates poorly with the total body status. Its accurate assessment necessitates cumbersome metabolic balance studies. A high incidence of hypomagnesemia appears to be associated with critical care patients; cardiac dysfunction may be one consequence. Since the total body magnesium is difficult to quantify, the concurrent change of another electrolyte may serve as a surrogate marker. Hypokalemia appears to be that clinically useful indicator based on preliminary work.

Hypercalcemia (Table 9–1)

Primary Hyperparathyroidism. This condition is caused by a functional neoplasm or idiopathic hyperplasia of the parathyroid gland. In the early stages there is a significant hypercalcemia accompanied by hypophosphatemia (Fig. 9–2). If renal calcinosis develops secondary to hypercalcemia, the serum phosphorus will increase as renal function deteriorates and is accompanied by azotemia and other laboratory changes associated with renal failure. If bone lesions develop the increased metabolic activity in the bone may result in an increase in serum alkaline phosphatase. The condition can be confirmed biochemically by demonstration of an increase in the serum PTH concentration.

Idiopathic parathyroid hyperplasia has been reported in German shepherd puppies.

TABLE 9–1. Disorders Causing Hypercalcemia

Hyperalbuminemia (dehydration)
Hypercalcemia of neoplasia (pseudohyperparathyroidism)
Primary hyperparathyroidism
Hypoadrenocorticism
Hypervitaminosis D
Renal disease (horse and cow, uncommonly in dog)
Osteolytic bone lesions (*e.g.*, septic osteomyelitis, myeloma)
Plant toxicity (jasmine in dogs and cats, *Cestrum* sp. and *Solanum* sp. [nightshade] in herbivores)
Calciferol-containing rodenticides
Certain granulomatous diseases (*e.g.*, canine blastomycosis)

Humoral Hypercalcemia of Malignancy (Pseudohyperparathyroidism). Laboratory findings associated with the paraneoplastic syndrome are similar to those seen in primary hyperparathyroidism with hypercalcemia and hypophosphatemia in the early stages followed by hyperphosphatemia and azotemia if renal calcinosis develops. In contrast, the serum PTH concentration is normal to decreased. Neoplasms that have been associated with hypercalcemia include malignant lymphoma, mammary gland adenocarcinoma, squamous cell carcinoma, pancreatic carcinoma, and nasal adenocarcinoma. Some of these neoplasms produce a PTH-related protein that affects calcium and phosphorus metabolism. The paraneoplastic syndrome is the most common cause of hypercalcemia.

Vitamin D Intoxication. Overzealous owners who supplement a diet with excess quantities of vitamin D may induce hypercalcemia accompanied by hyperphosphatemia. Hyperphosphatemia often occurs prior to renal damage from calcinosis.

Renal Disease. The horse is biochemically unusual with regard to renal disease as hypercalcemia commonly develops secondary to decreased urinary excretion. Serum phosphorus is low or low normal (Fig. 9–3). Hypercalcemia occurs in cattle and occasionally in the dog in the late stages of renal disease. The mechanism is not well established.

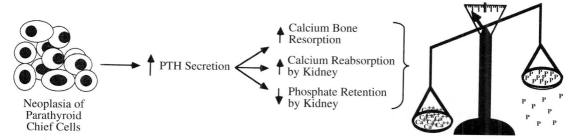

FIGURE 9–2. Effect of primary hyperparathyroidism on mineral balance. Increased production of PTH increases calcium from bone reabsorption and reabsorption by the kidney. It also causes increased phosphate loss (reduced retention). The net result is hypercalcemia and hypophosphatemia. *Note*: If the condition exists for some time renal calcinosis may develop, and when this occurs hyperphosphatemia may develop.

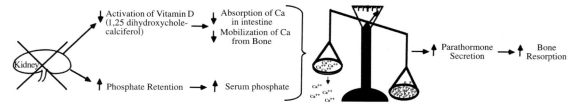

FIGURE 9–3. Effect of renal failure on the balance of calcium and phosphorous. Renal failure causes an increase in phosphate retention. This results in an increase in total mineral mass, and calcium excretion is increased. Vitamin D activation is also dependent upon renal function, and with renal failure vitamin D activation is reduced, causing decreased intestinal absorption of calcium and decreased bone mobilization. The cumulative effect is a decrease in serum calcium which in turn stimulates PTH secretion by the parathyroid gland and an increase in the mobilization of calcium from the bone.

Hypoadrenocorticism in the Dog. An increase in serum calcium occurs in some dogs with adrenal insufficiency. Increased renal tubular resorption of calcium is thought to be involved.

Osteolytic Bone Lesions. Hypercalcemia may occur after marked bone resorption. Neoplasia of the bone in which hypercalcemia has been reported include carcinoma, osteosarcoma, myeloma, and lymphosarcoma. Hypercalcemia may occur with severe osteomyelitis, particularly blastomycosis. It has been suggested that humans infected with blastomycosis have a hyperreactivity to vitamin D.

Plant Intoxication. The ingestion of jasmine (*Cestrum* sp.) by dogs and cats and *Solanum* and *Cestrum* sp. by herbivores will produce hypercalcemia and soft tissue mineralization. As the disease progresses the serum calcium will fall. The mechanism for this alteration is not known.

Cholecalciferol-Containing Rodenticides. Some rodenticides contain cholecalciferol (vitamin D_3) and will cause hypercalcemia. Such occurrences have been reported in both cats and dogs. One should consider the possible ingestion of either rodenticide or poisoned rodent in a dog and cat with unexplained hypercalcemia. The development of clinical signs is dose dependent and can be divided into neurologic, gastrointestinal, cardiovascular, and renal signs. The PTH concentration will be low normal to low.

Hypocalcemia (Table 9–2)

Hypoalbuminemia and Alkalosis. When the serum albumin concentration is reduced or an animal is alkalotic (especially ruminants) the serum calcium will be below the reference range. In an animal with metabolic alkalosis (increased total CO_2 or bicarbonate) there will be a reduction in the ionized calcium concentration and if sufficient may produce neuromuscular signs. These factors should be considered prior to attempting differentiation of the cause of the hypocalcemia.

Hypoparathyroidism. This condition is characterized by hypocalcemia and a normal or slightly increased serum phosphorus; serum PTH concentration is low. Hypoparathyroidism may appear after parathyroidectomy for removal of parathyroid neoplasms, in association with lymphocytic parathyroiditis, or secondary to infection with canine distemper virus.

TABLE 9–2. Disorders Causing Hypocalcemia

Hypoalbuminemia
Alkalosis (especially in ruminants)
Hypoparathyroidism
Secondary renal hyperparathyroidism
Ethylene glycol toxicity (dogs and cats)
Necrotizing pancreatitis
Dietary imbalance (hypovitaminosis D, excess phosphorus)
Eclampsia (bitch, mare, ewe) or parturient paresis (cow)
Hypomagnesemic tetany in ruminants (three fourths of cases)
Intestinal malabsorption (dog)
Blister beetle poisoning in horses
Hypercalcitonism
Transport tetany (sheep)
Factitious (EDTA used for sample collection)
Iatrogenic, after thyroidectomy (bilateral)
Bicarbonate treatment for salicylate toxicity

Renal Disease.   Hypocalcemia may occur in renal failure even though there is increased parathyroid activity. This occurs because there is a decreased conversion of vitamin D to its active form (1,25-dihydroxycholecalciferol), the reduction in calcium in response to hyperphosphatemia and decreased responsiveness to PTH.

These mineral changes are seen in both acute and chronic renal failure, and with postrenal urinary obstruction in the cat. If there is systemic acidosis clinical signs associated with the hypocalcemia may be masked as there is an increase in ionized calcium. However, rapid correcting of the altered acid-base state may cause a reduction of ionized calcium and precipitate clinical signs of tetany.

Dietary Imbalances.   Hypocalcemia as a result of excess dietary phosphorus, lack of vitamin D, or a dietary calcium deficiency is rare. Secondary hyperparathyroidism will occur with any of those conditions. If there is a dietary lack of calcium, serum phosphorus is normal or decreased. It is increased or normal if there is excess dietary phosphorus.

Parturient Paresis and Hypomagnesemic Tetany (Cattle) and Eclampsia (Horse, Dog, Sheep).   Hypocalcemia is a consistent finding in parturient paresis and hypomagnesemic tetany (cattle) and eclampsia (horse, dog, sheep) and is secondary to lactation and the subsequent depletion of calcium. It most commonly occurs in cattle that have been fed a prepartum diet of high calcium, which has a tendency to depress PTH secretion. Prolonged suppression prevents rapid mobilization of bone calcium which is needed when a negative calcium balance occurs with the beginning of lactation.

In hypomagnesemic tetany the majority of affected cows also have hypocalcemia. Hypomagnesemic tetany can be differentiated from parturient paresis by measuring urine magnesium. Magnesium is markedly decreased in urine of cattle with hypomagnesemic tetany (normal = about 50 mg/dL [25 mmol/L] urine).

Acute Pancreatitis.   In dogs this condition occasionally may be accompanied by hypocalcemia. The mechanism is probably multifactorial. If fat necrosis accompanies pancreatitis, calcium is bound to free fatty acids in the area. It has also been suggested that increased glucagon release associated with pancreatitis produces a decrease in ionized calcium via an increase in calcitonin.

Ethylene Glycol Toxicity (Dogs and Cats). This toxicity may be accompanied by hypocalcemia as calcium oxalate crystals are formed in excess.

Other Causes of Hypocalcemia. Hypocalcemia may also be caused by blister beetle poisoning in horses, intestinal malabsorption in dogs, hypercalcitonism secondary to neoplasia of thyroid parafollicular (C) cells in cattle, transport tetany in sheep, and idiopathic acute hypocalcemic tetany in horses. Hypocalcemia produced by these mechanisms is poorly understood.

Hyperphosphatemia (Table 9–3)

Young Animals. Serum phosphorus concentrations are above adult normals in growing animals.

Renal Disease. Hyperphosphatemia associated with renal disease in the dog and cat is a result of a reduction in glomerular filtration and is preceded by azotemia. Hyperphosphatemia (as well as azotemia) is not consistent in herbivorous animals with renal failure since phosphorus can also be eliminated via the digestive tract.

Exogenous Phosphorus. Administration of phosphorus-containing fluids and phosphorus (Fleet) enemas will result in hyperphosphatemia if given in excessive volume.

Other Causes of Hyperphosphatemia. Hypervitaminosis D (preceding renal calcinosis), osteolytic bone disease, jasmine (*Cestrum* sp.) toxicity (dog and cat), excess dietary intake of phosphorus, and hypoparathyroidism are accompanied by hyperphosphatemia in addition to the serum calcium changes described earlier. The high phosphate content of older antifreeze mixtures causes an abrupt rise in the serum phosphorus concentration following its ingestion. Its rise can precede the functional markers of renal failure associated with ethylene glycol toxicity. Serum held too long on RBCs will often have a high serum phosphorus concentration. This is because of

TABLE 9–3. Disorders Causing Hyperphosphatemia

Reduced glomerular filtration rate (renal, prerenal, or postrenal azotemia from any cause)
Factitious; sample held too long before analysis (phosphorus released from erythrocytes)
Growing animals
Dietary phosphorus excess
Phosphorus enema or administration of phosphorus-containing fluids
Hypervitaminosis D
Osteolytic bone disease (neoplasia)
Jasmine toxicity
Massive cell lysis (chemotherapy, rhabdomyolysis)
Hypoparathyroidism with normal glomerular filtration
Hypercalcemia of malignancy with normal glomerular filtration
Hyperthyroidism in casts without renal insufficiency
Slight increases occasionally from drug treatment (anabolic steroids, furosemide, minocycline, hydrochlorothiazide
Ethylene glycol toxicity (abrupt rise)
Hypersomatotropism

its release from erythrocytes. Excessive hemolysis will also produce a falsely increased serum phosphorus.

Based on the mass law of interactions between the calcium and phosphate ions, hyperphosphatemia leads to a reciprocal reduction in the plasma ionized calcium concentration. Hypocalcemic-induced tetany and soft tissue mineralization can occur when the solubility product of calcium times phosphorous exceeds 60 to 70.

Hypophosphatemia (Table 9–4)

In the early stages of primary hyperparathyroidism and hypercalcemia of neoplasia (pseudohyperparathyroidism) hypophosphatemia may be present.

Patients with secondary nutritional hyperparathyroidism resulting from avitaminosis D or the lack of dietary calcium have a normal or decreased serum phosphorus.

Patients with diabetes mellitus compounded by ketoacidosis and hypokalemia may have hypophosphatemia. In the ketoacidotic diabetic patient, phosphorylation is depressed which causes decomposition of intracellular phosphate compounds. Inorganic phosphate moves into extracellular fluid and is excreted in urine. Hyperglycemia, polyuria, and ketonuria produce an osmotic diuresis, which enhances phosphate elimination in urine.

Respiratory alkalosis from hyperventilation causes phosphate to move into intracellular space, resulting in hypophosphatemia.

About one third of the dogs with hyperadrenocorticism have hypophosphatemia.

Hypophosphatemia also accompanies eclampsia, hypomagnesemic tetany in ruminants, parturient paresis in cattle, malabsorption, starvation, canine Falconi-like syndrome, and insulin administration.

In the horse, hypophosphatemia may occur in association with chronic renal failure as well as vitamin D intoxication, pseudohyperparathyroidism, and after insulin administration.

TABLE 9–4. Disorders Causing Hypophosphatemia

Primary hyperparathyroidism (early stages before renal calcinosis)
Hypercalcemia of neoplasia (early stages before renal calcinosis)
Lack of dietary calcium
Hypovitaminosis D
Dogs and cats with diabetes mellitus and ketoacidosis
Respiratory alkalosis due to hyperventilation
Hyperadrenocorticism (about one third of dogs with disorder)
Eclampsia
Hypomagnesemic tetany of ruminants
Parturient paresis in cattle
Malabsorption or starvation
Canine Fanconi-like syndrome
Chronic renal failure in horse
Vitamin D intoxication
After insulin administration in diabetics
Enteral alimentation
Pseudohyperphosphatemia (associated with myeloma paraprotein)

THYROID GLAND

Thyroid Hormones and Their Regulation

Iodine and tyrosine (part of thyroglobulin) are the predominate substrates in the synthesis of the main thyroid hormones, tetraiodothyronine (T_4) and triiodothyronine (T_3). These active hormones are stored in abundance as a colloid within the acinar lumen. Their release involves a series of steps that translocates them through the follicular cell with cleavage from the thyroglobulin. The majority of T_3 formation results from the subsequent deiodination of T_4 in the skeletal muscle, liver, and kidney. A type of T_3 referred to as reverse T_3 (rT_3) is also formed but it has little biologic activity. Thyroxine-binding protein is the primary carrier of T_4 and T_3 in the dog. It is absent in the cat. Albumin and thyroxine-binding prealbumin (transthyretin) also transport thyroid hormones, the latter specific for T_4. Most of the thyroid hormone is protein-bound with only about 0.1% existing as free T_4 (fT_4) in the dog. The fT_4 is the biologically active component and enters the cells of the target tissues. This equilibrium is easily influenced, *e.g.*, estrogen shifts it to the bound form. In contrast to most hormones that have a circulating half-life of seconds to minutes, T_4 has a circulating half-life of 6 to 7 days in the dog. This is probably due to the high proportion that is protein-bound which "protects" it from degradation. In the cat it is 6 to 8 hours.

Thyroid stimulating hormone (TSH) regulates thyroid activity. Its release from the anterior pituitary is facilitated by thyrotropin releasing hormone (TRH) from the hypothalamus. The release of TSH and TRH are regulated by negative feedback inhibition from the thyroid hormones (Fig. 9–4). Glucocorticoids, androgens, and growth hormone can suppress TSH secretion.

Hypothyroidism

Hypothyroidism in the dog is manifested clinically by lethargy, mental dullness, weight gain, and symmetric endocrine alopecia. Neuromuscular dysfunction and reproductive problems occur less commonly. An uncommon but dramatic clinical presentation is a syndrome comprised of myxedema, stupor, and coma. There is an immune-mediated mechanism involved in the pathogenesis of hypothyroidism. Consequently, other endocrinopathies that can be immunologically mediated, diabetes mellitus and primary hypoadrenocorticism, may occur concurrently.

Diagnosis of hypothyroidism is problematic due to the nondescript clinical signs and the reduction of serum thyroid hormone concentrations secondary to concurrent nonthyroidal disease. A careful history and physical examination are essential to identify underlying disease. The signalment is helpful. There is a higher incidence in middle-aged, medium to large breeds such as golden and Labrador retrievers, Doberman pinscher, Irish setter, miniature schnauzer, and cocker spaniel. Preliminary laboratory findings can include the following: a mild normochromic, normocytic, nonregenerative anemia-leptocytes (target cells) may be present, (~30%), hypercholesterolemia (~70%), and raised serum alkaline phosphatase and creatine kinase activities (~30% and ~15%, respectively). Previous observations and reports suggested an association between hypothyroidism and acquired von Willebrand's dis-

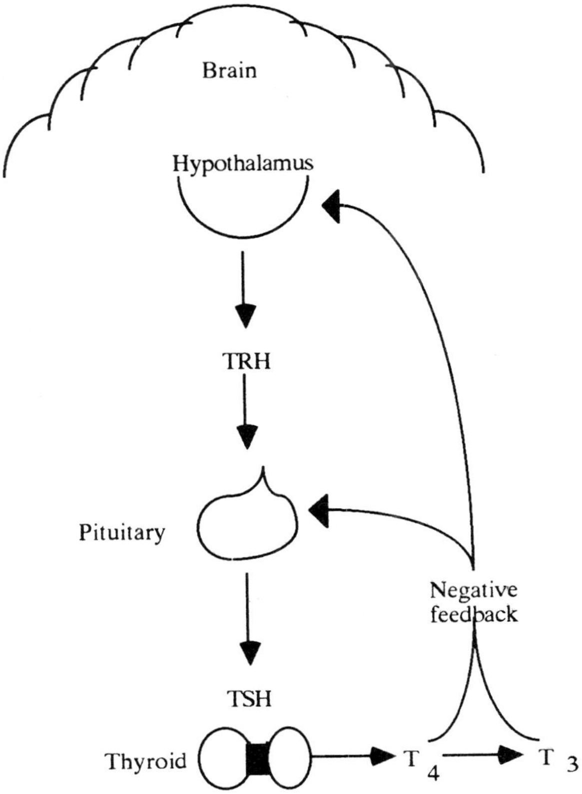

FIGURE 9-4. A simplified regulatory mechanism is illustrated for the hypothalamic-pituitary-thyroid axis. Thyrotropin-releasing hormone (TRH) stimulates the pituitary gland to release thyroid-stimulating hormone (TSH) which initiates thyroid hormone (T_4, T_3) release. Both T_3 and T_4 inhibit the pituitary gland and hypothalamus.

ease in dogs. Recent studies that have critically examined this relationship indicate that hypothyroidism does not reduce the plasma von Willebrand factor antigen concentrations nor does it predispose to a hemorrhagic tendency. The perceived relationship is likely due to the frequent coincidental occurrences of both diseases in the same breeds.

The measurement of the serum thyroid hormones should be used to support a high index of clinical suspicion of hypothyroidism and for the assessment of treatment. Their value is undermined when used as a nonspecific screening test. The measurement of the serum T4 and fT_4 concentrations and assessing the response of the thyroid gland subsequent to TSH is the diagnostic cornerstone. The measurement of fT_4 is not essential but can contribute useful information. It is important to understand that the reference range for T_4 is problematic at the lower concentrations due to overlap for dogs with hypothyroidism, euthyroid dogs with concurrent disease, and even healthy dogs. Serum T_4 and fT_4 concentrations in the upper part of the reference range are not compatible with hypothyroidism. An exception is the presence of antithyroid hormone antibodies in which case the reported values may be within or above the reference range depending on assay. Autoantibodies are suspected when there is a high index of suspicion of hypothyroidism but the value does not "fit" the patient, *i.e.*, the clinical signs are not consistent with increased thyroid activity. The presence of autoantibodies do not affect the measurement of fT4 if measured by the dialysis assay; it is inappropriately raised when measured by the analog assay. Autoantibodies are reported to be more common for T_3 than for T_4. Autoantibody formation against the thyroid hormones is preceded by the formation of antithyroglobulin antibodies. The presence of these antibodies is suggestive of immune-mediated destruction of the thyroid gland. These antibodies are present in a small percentage of clinically unaffected dogs. If the serum T_4 and fT_4 concentrations are below the reference range, the clinical findings are appropriate, and extrathyroidal disease is not present, then a trial treatment period for hypothyroidism is warranted. Concurrent disease can cause one or both of the components to be reduced. The long-term use of trimethoprim/sulfamethoxazole in dogs has been shown to reduce the serum T_4 concentration.

When there is a discordance between the two measurements, the serum T_4 concentration is "borderline," and/or the patient has not responded to a therapeutic trial, the TSH or TRH stimulation tests are used to assess the hypofunctional thyroid gland. TSH is the more reliable of the two provocative tests. There are a variety of protocols using intravenous, subcutaneous, or intramuscular routes of administration. Only one example is given to illustrate the concept. TSH is given intravenously at a dose of 0.1 IU/kg (5 IU maximum per dog). The serum T_4 concentration is measured in a pretreatment sample and another sample obtained at 6 hours postadministration. A 6-hour value of greater than 3 μg/dL (40 nmol/L) or a rise of at least 2 μg/dL (25 μmol/L) is not compatible with hypothyroidism. TRH is given intravenously at a total dose of 0.2 mg per dog. The serum T_4 concentration is measured in a pretreatment sample and another sample obtained at 4 hours postadministration. A 4-hour value of greater than 2 μg/dL (25 nmol/L) or a rise of at least 0.5 μg/dL (7 μmol/L) above the pretreatment value is not compatible with hypothyroidism. A recent study indicates that the TRH stimulation test does not separate dogs with hypothyroidism from dogs with reduced serum T4 concentrations and dermatologic signs suggestive of hypothyroidism. The recent validation of an immunoassay for canine TSH should prove helpful in the differential diagnosis of suspected cases of hypothyroidism.

When TSH is not available for stimulation testing, measurement of the serum TSH concentration (by a validated assay for the dog) is another way to assess the pituitary-thyroid axis. Measurement of both the fT_4 (by equilibrium dialysis, the 'gold standard' methodologically, or comparable method) and the serum TSH concentration provide a high degree of positive predictive value, especially when combined with an appropriate history, a predisposed breed, findings on physical examination, and other clinicopathologic changes. As a consequence of the conversion of fT_4 to T_3, there should be a corresponding rise in the plasma TSH concentration. Therefore, if the T_4 is reduced along with a reduction of the fT4 and a rise in the serum TSH concentrations, the findings are consistent with primary hypothyroidism. If the fT_4 and serum TSH concentration is reduced, secondary hypothyroidism is indicated. During the initial screening, finding a serum T_4 (total) concentration within the reference range makes the probability of hypothyroidism unlikely. It is emphasized that a variety of extra-thyroidal diseases and drugs such as glucocorticoids, phenobarbital, and sulfa combinations can alter the tests to assess the thyroid. Lastly, we now recognize breed differences in the reference ranges for the thyroid tests. The greyhound has lower values than that of other breeds and could be mistakenly classified as hypothyroid. The laboratory should be contacted for breed-related reference ranges.

A predictive formula using the serum free T_4 concentration and the serum cholesterol concentration initially showed promise as an objective diagnostic "tool." Unfortunately, it has not withstood the rigors of clinical evaluation.

Hyperthyroidism

Functional adenomatous hyperplasia (sometimes indicative of adenoma) of the thyroid gland results in feline hyperthyroidism. Bilateral involvement of thyroid gland occurs in approximately 70% of the cases. Weight loss, polyphagia, vomiting, polydipsia/polyuria, and hyperactivity are the more common clinical signs. Hematologically, findings include a high normal or slightly raised hematocrit and mean cell volume (MCV). Biochemically, one or more of the activities of alanine aminotransferase, aspartate aminotransferase, and alkaline phosphatase are raised commonly. The total bilirubin concentration is raised in a smaller percentage of hyperthyroid cats. Raised concentrations of serum urea nitrogen and creatinine are relatively common. The serum T_4 concentration is raised in most (~98%) hyperthyroid cats. Fluctuation of the basal serum T_4 concentration occurs in both cats and dogs and is of no biologic importance. However, in mildly hyperthyroid cats, the value may "fluctuate" into the reference range and should be repeated about a week later. Extrathyroidal disease may blunt the magnitude of rise of the T_4 in a cat with hyperthyroidism. Preliminary findings indicate that the measurement of the basal free thyroxine (fT_4) has at least similar to enhanced diagnostic value as T4 for the diagnosis of feline hyperthyroidism.

For problematic cases, there is both a T_3 suppression test and a TSH stimulation test developed for cats. Both testing protocols have similar diagnostic value. For the T_3 suppression test, serum is harvested initially and frozen for the measurement of T_4 and T_3. Oral T_3 is given the next morning at a dose of 25 µg per cat, three times each day for two days. A final seventh dose is given the third morning and serum is harvested 2 to 4 hours later. T_4 and T_3 are measured in both the pretreatment and posttreatment sera. The serum T_4 concentration does not suppress in hyperthyroid cats but is dramatically reduced ($\geq$50%) in cats with extrathyroidal disease (as well as in healthy cats). Why measure the T_3? The raised T_3 concentrations in the posttreatment serum sample ensure that the medication was properly administered. An equation has been developed that uses the pre- and posttreatment serum T_4 concentrations:

$$D \text{ value} = \text{posttreatment } T_4 \text{ (nmol/L)} - 0.5 \times \text{pretreatment } T_4 \text{ (nmol/L)}.$$

A value greater than 8 is diagnostic of hyperthyroidism. Euthyroid cats have a value less than 2. Interpretation of the suppression test should give the same result using either approach.

The TRH stimulation test reduces the testing period to 4 hours but is associated with transient ptyalism, vomiting, defecation, and tachycardia. Serum T_4 concentrations are measured before and 4 hours following the intravenous administration of TRH. A rise of less than 50% is indicative of hyperthyroidism. Euthyroid cats have a rise of 60% or more. Another way to assess the measurements is to use an equation:

$$D \text{ value} = 2.2 \times \text{pre-TRH } T_4 \text{ (nmol/L)} - \text{post-TRH } T_4 \text{ (nmol/L)}.$$

A value greater than 30 is indicative of hyperthyroidism (euthyroid cats have a value < 20).

Thyroid carcinoma is the primary cause of hyperthyroidism in dogs. The majority of the thyroid carcinoma are nonfunctional (>90%), *i.e.*, euthyroid, and are discovered as large neck masses that may be compromising respiration or causing dysphagia. The functional tumors cause signs of hyperthyroidism (polydipsia/polyuria, polyphagia, mild weight loss) which usually results in their earlier discovery. The serum T_4 concentration is raised as a consequence of the functional thyroid tumor.

A fine needle aspiration is valuable in differential diagnosis of neck masses. Cytologic examination can initially differentiate inflammation from a noninflammatory mass and, if the latter, differentiate between a nonneoplastic mass and neoplasia. The aspiration of a thyroid tumor usually contains a relatively large amount of blood with small islands or sheets of epithelial cells with cell borders that are poorly defined. Anisocytosis, anisokaryosis, and mitotic activity may not be remarkable even in malignant tumors.

Conversion factors:

T4 (nmol/L to μg/dL); 0.078. (μg/dL to nmol/L); 12.87
fT4 (pmol/L to ng/dL); 0.078. (ng/dL to pmol/L); 1287
T3 (nmol/L to ng/dL); 64.9. (mg/dL to nmol/L); 0.0154

ADRENAL GLANDS

Physioanatomy

The adrenal glands are endocrine organs that are composed of two distinct functional structures. The medulla is derived from neuroectoderm and is notable for its secretion of the catecholamines in response to the stimulation of the sympathetic nervous system. Hypoglycemia and "stress" (*e.g.*, an acute reduction in the blood pressure) are the two most prominent stimuli. The cortex, which enrobes the medulla, is comprised of three distinct cellular layers (zones). The outer layer (zona glomerulosa) produces aldosterone, a mineralocorticoid that orchestrates sodium and potassium balance and contributes to the regulation of blood pressure. The middle and inner layers (zona fasciculata and zona reticularis, respectively) produce glucocorticoids, notably cortisol. Figuratively speaking, the adrenal cortex can be viewed as two functionally distinct endocrine organs, one that secretes aldosterone and another that secretes cortisol. Cortisol and aldosterone are synthesized from cholesterol and only a hydroxyl group on C-17 of the cortisol structure differentiate the two resulting in an overlap in their biologic activity. However, the potency for glucocorticoid or mineralocorticoid activity is greatest for cortisol and aldosterone, respectively. Cortisol is transported in the blood by corticosteroid-binding globulin (transcortin) and to a lesser extent by albumin. Approximately 10% is unbound (free). Aldosterone is transported predominantly by albumin with approximately 40% unbound.

Cortisol Metabolism and its Regulation

Glucocorticoids play a major role in glucose metabolism. Hepatic gluconeogenesis (conversion of amino acids to glycogen) is stimulated and the effects of glucagon and epinephrine are enhanced. To support this activity, glucocorticoids inhibit protein synthesis and, in excess, cause protein catabolism with subsequent breakdown and release of amino acids. The loss of mass of the abdominal muscles contributes to the "pot-bellied" appearance of dogs with cortisol excess secondary to hyperadrenocorticism. Glucocorticoids have an "anti-insulin" effect, *i.e.*, interfere with glucose uptake and metabolism by skeletal muscle and adipose tissue. Cortisol excess should be considered in a patient with diabetes mellitus when insulin regulation is problematic. Glucocorticoid excess commonly causes excessive glycogen storage in the canine liver and abnormal hepatic enzyme tests (see Chapter 7).

The hypothalamic-pituitary-adrenal triad regulates cortisol secretion by a negative feedback loop (Fig. 9–5). Corticotropin-releasing hormone (CRH) from the hypothalamus stimulates the release of adrenocorticotropic hor-

FIGURE 9–5. A simplified regulatory mechanism for the hypothalamic-pituitary-adrenal axis. Corticotropin-releasing hormone (CRF) stimulates the pituitary to release ACTH, which stimulates cortisol release. Glucocorticoids inhibit both the pituitary and the hypothalamus.

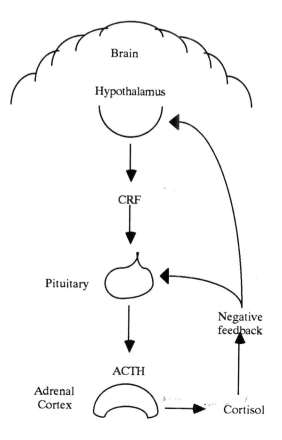

mone (ACTH) from the pituitary which then travels to the adrenal cortex to cause the secretion of cortisol. An increase in the plasma cortisol concentration impairs the release of CRH and ACTH. The administration of exogenous glucocorticoids for medical use will inhibit the release of ACTH. If the medication is abruptly discontinued prior to the hypothalamic-pituitary-adrenal triad establishing its function, clinical signs of lethargy and weakness may be manifested. Glucocorticoids facilitate water diuresis by enhancing the glomerular filtration rate and interfering with the activity of vasopressin (antidiuretic hormone) on the distal tubule. This is manifested clinically as polyuria. It is also a common, annoying side-effect of the medical use of glucocorticoids. A well-known stimulus of hypothalamic-pituitary-adrenal triad is stress. In the dog, for example, a hematologic reflection of the hypercortisolemia is a change in the differential white blood cell count referred to as the corticosteroid or "stress" leukogram (see Chapter 4). "Stress" in the form of extra-adrenal disease can complicate the interpretation of the function tests designed to evaluate the hypothalamic-pituitary-adrenal triad.

Aldosterone Metabolism and its Regulation

Aldosterone secretion is regulated through a complex interaction with the kidney (see Fig. 10–4). Briefly, a reduction in the blood pressure is sensed by the juxtaglomular apparatus, which responds by producing renin. It initiates an enzymatic chain reaction in which angiotensinogen is converted to angiotensin I, which is hydrolyzed by angiotensin converting enzyme to angiotensinogen II. In addition to causing vasoconstriction, it stimulates the release of aldosterone. The macula densa may also be involved in renin release. A decrease in the sodium concentration stimulates the release of renin. The potassium concentration is an important regulator of aldosterone release because it occurs independently of the renin-angiotensin activating cascade. A rise in the potassium concentration causes a secretion of aldosterone while a reduction is inhibitory.

Hyperadrenocorticism

Hypercortisolemia in the dog is caused by a pituitary tumor secreting excess ACTH in more than 80% of the cases. Bilateral adrenal hyperplasia occurs as a consequence of the chronic stimulation by ACTH. The remainder are due to an autonomously functioning adrenal tumor. The classic signs of hypercortisolemia are polyuria/polydipsia, polyphagia, endocrine alopecia, pot-bellied appearance, and panting. Hematologically, there may be a glucocorticoid-type of leukogram—neutrophilia, lymphopenia, and eosinopenia. Raised serum hepatic enzyme activities and cholesterol concentration may be measured and lipemia may be observed. A slight rise in the sodium and reduction in the potassium concentrations may be detected. These changes may be amplified by concurrent vomiting or diarrhea. The urine specific gravity is often less than 1.010 but, with judicious water deprivation, it can rise into the 1.020s or 1.030s. Normal renal-concentrating ability is restored following the establishment of the medullary concentrating gradient. Prolonged hypercortisolemia predisposes to infections and bacterial cystitis may be detected by the urinalysis. Chronic hypercortisolemia frequently suppresses TSH secretion and changes the metabolism of the thyroid hormones resulting in reductions in the plasma T_4, fT_4, and T_3 concentrations.

A variety of testing protocols have been developed to assess adrenal hyperfunction based on the measurement of plasma cortisol concentrations before and following the administration of ACTH to stimulate the adrenal glands or dexamethasone to suppress them. Examples of protocols will be given to illustrate their interpretive use. A convenient screening test to eliminate the possibility of hypercortisolemia takes advantage of the appearance of excess cortisol in the urine. One urine sample is collected by the owner in the dog's home environment in order to reduce the influence of stress. Cortisol and creatinine are measured in the urine and a ratio is calculated. A cortisol to creatinine ratio within the reference range indicates that hypercortisolemia is not present. An increased ratio has low specificity for pituitary-dependent hyperadrenocorticism because any extra-adrenal disorder can cause sufficient stress to increase the cortisol concentration in the urine.

The serum alkaline phosphatase (ALP) is raised in most dogs secondary to endogenous hypercortisolemia or the exogenous administration of glucocorticoids. An isoenzyme referred to as corticosteroid-induced alkaline phosphatase (CIALP) commonly contributes to the increased total serum ALP activity. Measurement of this isoenzyme has been investigated for use as a screening test for hyperadrenocorticism. However, this isoenzyme has been shown to be present in high serum activity in association with a variety of extra-adrenal diseases. Consequently, it is not recommended as a screening test. If it is measured routinely as part of a biochemical profile, its absence would make a diagnosis of glucocorticoid excess unlikely.

A positive ACTH stimulation test is indicative of hyperadrenocorticism in most cases that are pituitary dependent (80 to 85%). The plasma cortisol concentrations are measured before and 2 hours following the intramuscular administration of aqueous gelatin ACTH (1.0 IU/lb, 2.2 IU/kg). Using synthetic ACTH administered intramuscularly (0.25 mg per dog, 1 vial), the plasma cortisol concentrations are measured before its administration and 1 hour later. A poststimulation plasma cortisol concentration of 22 μg/dL or greater ($\geq$610 nmol/L) supports a diagnosis of hyperadrenocorticism. Poststimulation plasma cortisol concentrations between 17 (470 nmol/L) and 22 μg/dL ($\geq$610 nmol/L) are considered to be in a "gray zone." Approximately two thirds of the dogs with functioning adrenal tumors have an abnormal ACTH stimulation test. A baseline plasma cortisol concentration that is low-normal or below the reference range and does not rise appreciably following the administration of ACTH is suggestive of an exogenous glucocorticoid suppressive effect (iatrogenic Cushing's syndrome).

A reduced dose of synthetic ACTH (0.125, 1/2 vial) administered intramuscularly is used in cats. The plasma cortisol concentrations are measured before its administration and 30, 60, and 90 minutes later. The use of the ACTH gelatin formulation appears to give inconsistent results in cats and is not recommended.

The low-dose dexamethasone suppression test (LDDS) is used to diagnose hyperadrenocorticism and to differentiate pituitary-dependent hypercortisolemia from adrenal tumor cortisol-secreting autonomy. Dexamethasone is not measured in the assay for cortisol. The plasma cortisol concentrations are measured before and 4 and 8 hours following the intravenous administration of dexamethasone (0.01 mg/kg). Healthy, non-stressed dogs usually have cortisol values of less than 1.0 μg/dL (28 nmol/L). Pituitary-dependent hyperadrenocorticism is indicated if the 4-hour cortisol value is <50% of the basal concentration (or <1.4 μg/dL, 39 nmol/L) and the 8-hour value is $\geq$1.4 μg/dL, 39 nmol/L). Suppression at the 4-hour time point with "escape" occurs in only approximately 1/3 of the patients with the majority lacking appropriate suppression at both the 4- and 8-hour time points. A lack of suppression can occur if exogenous glucocorticoids (e.g., prednisolone, topical hydrocortisone) have been administered since they will be measured as cortisol in the assay. Use of the high-dose testing strategy is less reliable for distinguishing between pituitary-dependent and adrenal tumor hyperadrenocorticism. A 4- and 8-hour value that is <50% of the basal plasma cortisol concentration or <1.4 μg/dL (39 nmol/L) is supportive of pituitary-dependent disease. The high-dose dexamethasone suppression test is only used in dogs that do not have a 4-hour suppression in the low-dose testing protocol. Abdominal ultrasonography and the measurement of the plasma ACTH concentration are valuable procedures in patients suspected of tumor hyperadrenocorticism. In contrast to hypercortisolemia present in dogs, cats, and horses with hyperadrenocorticism, the disease in ferrets is associated with excessive secretion of androgens and estrogens. Determination of basal cortisol and ACTH-stimulated plasma cortisol concentrations are of no diagnostic value. There does not appear to be a consistent increase of one steroid hormone in ferrets with hyperadrenocorticism. Consequently, plasma analysis of steroid hormones should include androstenedione, 17-hydroxyprogesterone, and estradiol at a minimum.

Dogs with hepatic encephalopathy secondary to congenital portosystemic shunts or acquired secondary to chronic hepatic inflammation/cirrhosis have a functionally abnormal pituitary-adrenal relationship. The urinary cortisol to creatinine ratio can be increased. The basal plasma cortisol concentration can be increased and it may rise into the "gray zone" following ACTH stimulation. However, it does suppress with the LDDS test. Notably, the plasma free cortisol concentration (the biologically active component) can be increased due to a reduction in the plasma concentration of the cortisol-binding globulin. This suggests that clinical signs attributed to hypercortisolemia could develop with the basal plasma cortisol concentration within the reference range. The plasma ACTH and α-melanocyte-stimulating hormone (MSH) concentrations can be increased. In addition, the osmotic threshold of vasopressin (ADH) release is abnormally raised, which may be a consequence of prolonged hypercortisolemia. This may contribute to the development of the polyuria/polydipsia that occurs in some dogs with portosystemic shunts.

Horses with pituitary pars intermedia dysfunction ("equine Cushing's") develop abnormal hair coats (hirsutism), laminitis, polyuria/polydipsia, loss of muscle mass, raised respiratory rate, and excess sweating (hyperhidrosis). Hyperglycemia, often insulin resistant, can be present. An overnight dexamethasone suppression test is used for assessing the pituitary-adrenal relationship. Dexamethasone (40 μg/kg or 2 mg/100 lb) is administered intramuscularly between 5:00 and 6:00 PM. Plasma is harvested for cortisol measurements before and 19 hours after dexamethasone administration. A plasma cortisol concentration following the administration of dexamethasone that is greater than 1 μg/dL is consistent with the diagnosis.

Hypoadrenocorticism

Primary hypoadrenocorticism is usually a consequence of bilateral adrenal atrophy and fibrosis resulting in a deficiency of both glucocorticoids and mineralocorticoids. Occasionally, a deficiency of CRH or ACTH develops that results in only a glucocorticoid deficiency subsequent to the bilateral atrophy of the adrenal cortices responsible for their production. This rare failure of hypothalamic or pituitary function due to neoplasia or inflammation is referred to as secondary hypoadrenocorticism. Iatrogenic secondary hypoadrenocorticism is commonly associated with the prolonged use of exogenous glucocorticoids which suppress the production of CRH and ACTH.

Primary hypoadrenocorticism often causes a vague history of poor appetite, weakness, trembling, weight loss, vomiting, diarrhea, and regurgitation associated with megaesophagus. Dehydration and depression are often the only findings noted from a physical examination. Occasionally an adrenal "crisis" is manifested by hypotensive shock, collapse, and bradycardia—the latter finding a dichotomy in association with hypotension.

Hematologically, there is mild normocytic, normochromic anemia about 25% of the time; its magnitude may not be readily apparent due to the dehydration. A relative erythrocytosis is present in about 15%.

There are multiple biochemical abnormalities. There is the expected hyperkalemia and hyponatremia resulting in a sodium to potassium ratio of less than 27 in most dogs (approximately 90%). The basal plasma cortisol concentration is less than the reference range and does not rise appreciably following the administration of ACTH.

Indicators of renal insufficiency are commonly abnormal. The serum urea nitrogen (BUN), creatinine, and phosphorus concentrations are raised in approximately 80%, 65%, and 65% of the cases, respectively. Noteworthy is that the urine specific gravity is less than 1.030 in slightly more than 50%; a *non*

TABLE 9–5.   Causes of a Reduced Sodium to Potassium Ratio (<27)[a]

- Hypoadrenocorticism
- Renal disease
- Repeated drainage of effusions (pleural and peritoneal)
- Diarrhea associated with trichuriasis (whipworms)
- Diabetic ketoacidosis

[a]The sodium or potassium value can be within reference range. Generally, the lower the ratio, the more likely hypoadrenocorticism is the cause of the electrolyte abnormality. Because the clinical signs of hypoadrenocorticism are often nonspecific and of the common development of azotemia secondary to prerenal insufficiency, a mis-diagnosis of primary renal disease may occur initially. The measurement of the plasma cortisol concentration before and after ACTH stimulation is prudent in cases with renal insufficiency and an abnormal sodium to potassium ratio, especially young to middle-aged female adult dogs of a predisposed breed (standard poodle, Great Dane, rottweiler, West Highland white terrier, Wheaton terrier, leonberger, and Portuguese water dog).

sequitur in a dehydrated, azotemia dog. Approximately 30% of the dogs have hypercalcemia. The serum total CO_2 and chloride concentrations are decreased in about 40% of the cases. There is hypoglycemia about 15% of the time. The serum hepatic enzyme activities and bilirubin concentration are increased in 20 to 30% of the dogs (Case 9–1). Interestingly, the persistent increase in serum aminotransferase activities has been reported in humans to be associated with subclinical hypoadrenocorticism. Table 9–5 lists the other possible causes of a reduced sodium to potassium ratio.

Additional Reading

Calcium and Phosphorus Metabolism

Altura BT, Burack JL, Cracco RQ, et al: Clinical studies with the NOVA ISE for I Mg^{2+}. Scand J Clin Lab Invest 1994;54:53–67.

Clemens TL, Fagin JA: Parathyroid hormone-related protein: New insights into its normal biology. Endocrine 1994;2:871–873.

Dart AJ, Snyder JR, Spier SJ, et al: Ionized calcium concentration in horses with surgically managed gastrointestinal disease: 147 cases (1988–1990). J Am Vet Med Assoc 1992;201:1244–1248.

Elin RJ: Magnesium: The fifth but forgotten electrolyte. Clin Chem 1994;102:616–622.

Ferguson DC: Update on diagnosis of canine hypothyroidism. Vet Clin North Am 1994;24:515–540.

Gerloff BJ, Swenson EP: Acute recumbency and marginal phosphorus deficiency in dairy cattle. J Am Vet Med Assoc 1996;208:716–719.

Graves TK, Peterson ME: Diagnostic tests for feline hyperthyroidism. Vet Clin North Am 1994;24:567–576.

Kristensen AT, Klausner JS, Weiss DJ, et al: Spurious hyperphosphatemia in a dog with chronic lymphocytic leukemia and an IgM monoclonal gammopathy. Vet Clin Pathol 1991;20:45–48.

Jaggy A, Oliver JE, Ferguson DC, et al: Neurological manifestations of hypothyroidism: A retrospective study of 29 dogs. J Vet Intern Med 1994;8:328–336.

McLoughlin MA, DiBartola AP, Birchard SJ, et al: Influence of systemic nonthyroidal illness on serum concentration of thyroxine in hyperthyroid cats. J Am Anim Hosp Assoc 1993;29:227–234.

Messer NT, Johnson PJ, Refsal KR, et al: Effect of food deprivation on baseline iodothyronine and cortisol concentrations in healthy, adult horses. Am J Vet Res 1995;56:116–121.

Meyer HP, Rothuizen J: Increased free cortisol in plasma of dogs with portosystemic encephalopathy (PSE). Domest Anim Endocrinol 1994;11:317–322.

Moreau R, Squires RA: Hypercalcemia. Comp Cont in Educ Pract Vet 1992;14:1077–1087.

Oren S, Feldman A, Turkot S, et al: Hyperphosphatemia in multiple myeloma. Ann Hematol 1994;69:41–43.

Potts JT: Non-traditional actions of parathyroid hormone: An overview. Miner Electrolyte Metab 1995;21:9–12.

Rothuizen J, Biewenga WJ, Mol JA: Chronic glucocorticoid excess and impaired osmoregulation of vasopressin release in dogs with hepatic encephalopathy. Domest Anim Endocrinol 1995;12:13–24.

Waters CB, Scott-Montcrieff CR: Hypocalcemia in cats. Comp Contin Educ Pract Vet 1992;4:497–505.

Zaidi M, Shankar VS, Huang LH, et al: Molecular mechanisms of calcitonin action. Endocrine 1994;2:459–467.

Thyroid

Broussard JD, Peterson ME, Fox PR: Changes in clinical and laboratory findings in cats with hyperthyroidism from 1983–1993. J Am Vet Med Assoc 1995;206:302–305.

Frank LA: Comparison of thyrotropin-releasing hormone (TRH) to thyrotropin (TSH) stimulation for evaluating thyroid function in dogs. J Am Anim Hosp Assoc 1996; 32:481–487.

Hall IA, Campbell KL, Chambers MD, et al: Effect of trimethoprim/sulfamethoxazole on thyroid function in dogs with pyoderma. J Am Vet Med Assoc 1993;202:1959–1962.

Kaptein EM, Moore GE, Ferguson DC, et al: Effects of prednisolone on thyroxine and 3,5,3′-triiodothyronine metabolism in normal dogs. Endocrinology 1992;130:1669–1679.

Kemppainen RJ, Young DW, Behrend EN, et al: Autoantibodies to triiodothyroxine and thyroxine in a golden retriever. J Am Anim Hosp Assoc 1996;32:195–198.

Larsson MG: Determination of free thyroxine and cholesterol as a new screening test for canine hypothyroidism. J Am Anim Hosp Assoc 1988;24:209–217.

Muth Beale K, Halliwell REW, Chen CL: Prevalence of antithyroglobulin antibodies detected by enzyme-linked immunosorbent assay of canine serum. J Am Vet Med Assoc 1990;196:745–748.

Panciera DL: Hypothyroidism in dogs: 66 cases (1987–1992): J Am Vet Med Assoc 1994;204:761–767.

Panciera DL, Johnson GS: Plasma von Willibrand factor antigen concentration and buccal mucosal bleeding time in dogs with experimental hypothyroidism. J Vet Intern Med 1996;10:60–64.

Paradis M, Page N: Serum free thyroxine concentrations measured using chemiluminescence in hyperthyroid and euthyroid cats. J Am Anim Hosp Assoc 1996;32: 489–494.

Peterson ME, Broussard JD, Gamble DA: Use of the thyrotropin releasing hormone stimulation test to diagnose mild hyperthyroidism in cats. J Vet Intern Med 1994; 8:279–286.

Peterson ME, Grave TK, Gamble DA: Triiodothyroxine (T3) suppression test. J Vet Intern Med 1990;4:233–238.

Thacker EL, Refsal KR, Bull RW: Prevalence of autoantibodies to thyroglobulin, thyroxine, or triiodothyronine and relationship of autoantibodies and serum concentrations of iodothyronines in dogs. Am J Vet Res 1992;53:449–453.

Williams DA, Scott-Montcrieff C, Bruner J, et al: Validation of an immunoassay for canine thyroid-stimulating hormone and changes in serum concentration following induction of hypothyroidism in dogs. J Am Vet Med Assoc 1996;209:1730–1732.

Adrenal Glands

Boulton R, Hamilton MI, Dhillon AP, et al: Subclinical Addison's disease: A cause of persistent abnormalities in transaminase values. Gastroenterology 1995;109:1324–1327.

Couetil L, Paradis MR, Knoll J: Plasma adrenocorticotropin concentration in healthy horses and in horses with clinical signs of hyperadrenocorticism. J Vet Intern Med 1995;10:1–6.

Dybdal NO, Hargreaves KM, Madigan JE, et al: Diagnostic testing for pituitary pars intermedia dysfunction in horses. J Am Vet Med Assoc 1994;204:627–632.

Feldman EC, Nelson RW, Feldman MS: Use of the low- and high-dose dexamethasone tests for distinguishing pituitary-dependent from adrenal tumor hyperadrenocorticism in dogs. J Am Vet Med Assoc 1996;209:772–775.

Goossens MMC, Meyer HP, Voorhout G, et al: Urinary excretion of glucocorticoids in the diagnosis of hyperadrenocorticism in cats. Domest Anim Endocrinol 1995;12: 355–362.

Grooters AM, Biller DS, Theisen SK, et al: Ultrasonographic characteristics of the adrenal glands in dogs with pituitary-dependent hyperadrenocorticism: Comparison with normal dogs. J Vet Intern Med 1996;10:110–115.

Henry CJ, Clark TP, Young DW, et al: Urine cortisol:creatinine ratio in healthy and sick cats. J Vet Intern Med 1996;10:123–126.

Kaplan AJ, Peterson ME, Kemppainen RJ: Effects of disease on the results of diagnostic tests for use in detecting hyperadrenocorticism in dogs. J Am Vet Med Assoc 1995;207:445–451.

Lifton SJ, King LG, Zerbe CA: Glucocorticoid deficient hypoadrenocorticism in dogs: 18 cases (1986–1995). J Am Vet Med Assoc 1996;209:2076–2081.

Mack RE: Screening tests used in the diagnosis of canine hyperadrenocorticism. Semin Vet Med Surg 1994;9:118–122.

Peterson ME, Greco DS, Orth DN: Primary hypoadrenocorticism in ten cats. J Vet Intern Med 1989;3:55–58.

Peterson ME, Kemppainen RJ: Dose-response relation between plasma concentrations of corticotropin and cortisol after administration of incremental doses of cosyntropin for corticotropin stimulation testing in cats. Am J Vet Res 1993;54:300–304.

Peterson ME, Kemppainen RJ, Orth DN: Effects of synthetic ovine corticotropin-releasing hormone on plasma concentrations of immunoreactive adrenocorticotropin, alpha-melanocyte-stimulating hormone, and cortisol in dogs with naturally acquired adrenocortical insufficiency. Am J Vet Res 1992;53:421–425.

Peterson ME, Kintzer PP, Kass PH: Pretreatment clinical and laboratory findings in dogs with hypoadrenocorticism: 225 cases (1979–1993). J Am Vet Med Assoc 1996;208:85–91.

Rosenthal KL, Peterson ME: Evaluation of plasma androgen and estrogen concentrations in ferrets with hyperadrenocorticism. J Am Vet Med Assoc 1996;209:1097–1102.

Sadek D, Schaer M: Atypical Addison's disease in the dog: A retrospective survey of 14 cases. J Am Anim Hosp Assoc 1996;32:159–163.

Smiley LE, Peterson ME: Evaluation of a urine cortisol:creatinine ratio as a screening test for hyperadrenocorticism in dogs. J Vet Intern Med 1993;7:163–168.

10

Assessment of Renal Function, Urinalysis, and Water Balance

We are constantly misled by the ease with which our minds fall into the ruts of one or two experiences.
—Sir William Osler, M.D.

The functional unit of the kidney is the nephron, which consists of the glomerulus containing a vascular bed, and the tubule which modifies the filtrate (Figs. 10–1, 10–2, and 10–3). The end product of multiple hormonally mediated biochemical processes is urine.

URINALYSIS

Urine can be collected by cystocentesis, catheterization, and free catch (voided). Midstream (voided) collections are adequate for examination if results are negative. Interpretation of cell counts, protein, and culture of these specimens may lead to misleading results. Abnormal findings should be reaffirmed by a second specimen collected by cystocentesis or catheterization.

Urinalysis should be completed on freshly collected urine; refrigerated specimens are acceptable for up to 6 hours.

Physical Properties

Appearance

The color and transparency of urine should be recorded. The normal yellow color of urine is a result of urochromes. Dark yellow urine usually indicates a concentrated specimen, whereas dilute samples are often colorless. The presence of blood or hemoglobin produces a red urine that changes to brownish discoloration on standing.

Urine is transparent except in the horse, in which the thick and cloudy appearance is a result of mucus and calcium carbonate crystals. Cloudy

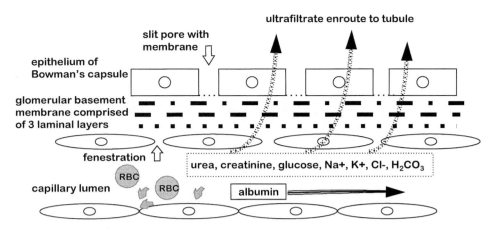

FIGURE 10–1. The glomerular capillary wall is the multilayered structure across which ultrafiltration occurs. It selectively filters out proteins with a molecular weight of greater than approximately 40,000. The meshwork of type IV collagen is involved in size selectivity. The glomerular basement membrane is composed of glycosaminoglycans; heparin sulfate is the predominant one and constitutes the anionic sites. The polyanionic constituents of the glomerular basement membrane render it hydrophilic and protect it from being clogged by albumin. The overall effect is to create an "electric field" that repels negatively charged plasma macromolecules.

urine may be observed if cells, bacteria, fat, crystals, or mucus is present in a large concentration. The cause of cloudy urine can be determined by microscopic examination of sediment.

Specific Gravity

Specific gravity is the ratio of the mass of a solution compared with the mass of an equal volume of water. It is not a direct measurement of the number of solute particles, as is osmolality. However, the two determinations are related, and the specific gravity is a clinically useful test since loss of concentrating ability is one of the first signs of renal tubule disease. The specific gravity of the glomerular filtrate is between 1.008 and 1.012. A urine specific gravity above 1.012 or below 1.008 requires tubular cell function. The specific gravity can range from 1.001 to 1.060 and reflects the hydration status of the animal (Fig. 10–4). A specific gravity greater than 1.030 in the dog and 1.035 in the cat suggests adequate concentrating ability (Case 7–1). Evaluation of the specific gravity should *always* be made with a *concurrent* serum urea nitrogen and/or creatinine value as outlined in Fig. 10–5. It is emphasized that these are only general guidelines, and the patient's history and other clinicopathologic findings should be taken into consideration. Although renal disease is one cause of low specific gravity (see Case 10–1), other factors such as excessive fluid intake, diuretic therapy, and the administration of fluids must be considered.

Chemical Examination

Chemical examination of urine routinely includes assay for pH, protein, glucose, ketones, occult blood, and bilirubin.

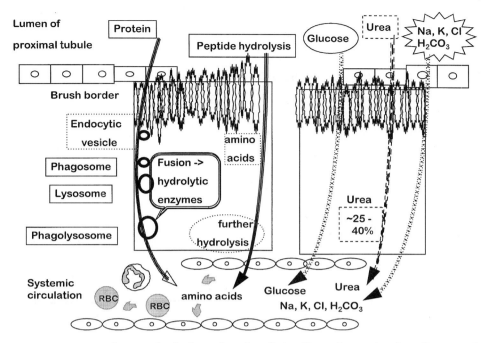

FIGURE 10–2. The renal tubule reabsorbs all the filtered proteins (insulin, growth hormone), glucose (up to ~200 mg/dL), and the electrolytes (see Figs. 10–3 and 10–4). The reabsorbed proteins are metabolized by a catabolic process that involves incorporation into endocytic vesicles (endosomes), their fusion with lysosomes, hydrolysis of the proteins to amino acids by the lysosomal enzymes, and return to the systemic circulation. Some small peptides (8 to 10 amino acids) in the ultrafiltrate are hydrolyzed at the luminal surface of the brush border. The reabsorption of abnormally large quantities of peptides or small proteins can cause tubular damage. Multiple myeloma is one example in which the large quantity of filtered light chain immunoglobulins can precipitate (perhaps in combination with Tamm-Horsfall protein) and cause tubular obstruction and damage. The condition is referred to as "light chain cast nephropathy."

pH

Urine pH is a crude reflection of the acid-base state and is influenced by the diet. Herbivorous animals have an alkaline pH, and carnivores and omnivores will vary from acid to alkaline depending upon the amount of animal protein in the diet. Increased urine acidity may result from starvation, fever, metabolic or respiratory acidosis, prolonged muscular exercise, or the administration of acid salts such as ammonium chloride. Increased urine alkalinity may accompany metabolic or respiratory alkalosis, bacterial cystitis, and the ingestion of sodium bicarbonate.

Protein

A small quantity of protein passes the glomerular filter but is reabsorbed by the renal tubules. Consequently, normal urine is usually negative when tested for protein. In concentrated urine trace to 1+ reactions may be normal. A slight transitory proteinuria may be associated with fever, muscular exercise, and seizures. A false positive may occur with an alkaline urine (pH > 8.5).

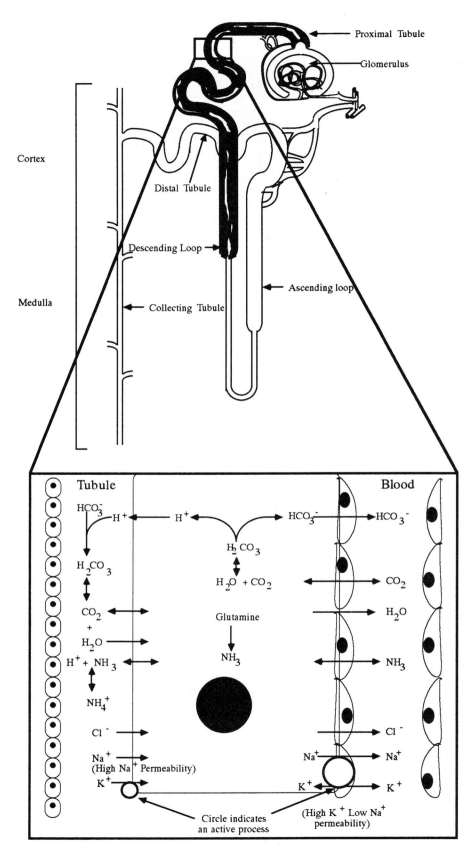

FIGURE 10–3. *See legend on opposite page.*

Proteinuria must be interpreted in association with urine specific gravity and urine sediment. A slight proteinuria in urine of low specific gravity is more significant than the same quantity of protein in concentrated urine. The significance of protein loss through the kidney can be determined by calculating the urine protein to urine creatinine ratio (UP/UCr) as follows:

$$\frac{\text{Urine protein (mg/dL)}[\text{g/L} \div 10]}{\text{Urine creatinine (mg/dL)}[\mu\text{mol/L} \div 84 \div 100]} = \frac{\text{UP}}{\text{UCr}} \text{ ratio.}$$

A $\dfrac{\text{UP}}{\text{UCr}}$ ratio greater than 1.0 for the dog or greater than 0.7 for the cat indicates renal disease or urinary tract inflammation.

The detection of proteinuria should prompt several differential considerations. *Renal proteinuria* occurs as a result of abnormal glomerular permeability. Glomerulonephritis and renal amyloidosis are the most common causes of altered glomerular permeability. In addition to albumin, other proteins can escape through the diseased glomeruli. Antithrombin 3 (62,000 MW) is of clinical interest because of its role in neutralizing thrombin, which normally becomes activated intravascularly from prothrombin during thrombus formation. Reduced plasma concentrations predispose to thrombotic disorders. Because its measurement is not readily available, a correlation to the plasma albumin concentration appears to be a useful marker. A serum albumin concentration of approximately less than 2.0 g/dL due to glomerular disease appears to be associated with an increased incidence of thromboembolism. A slight proteinuria can occur in association with canine hyper-

←——————————————————————————————————

FIGURE 10–3. The glomerulus filters creatinine and urea nitrogen from the blood but retains albumin. Decreased glomerular blood flow (prerenal) or disease involving the glomerulus (renal) can be recognized by azotemia (increased urea nitrogen and/or creatinine). In addition, certain types of glomerular injury permit albumin to escape into the filtrate, resulting in proteinuria. Tubular function can be reflected crudely by determining the urine specific gravity. Consequently, determination of serum urea nitrogen/creatine plus the urine specific gravity can be used to screen nephron function. The renal tubular cell plays a pivotal role in maintaining acid-base and electrolyte homeostasis. Hydrogen ions (H^+) are secreted into the tubular fluid, whereas bicarbonate ions (HCO_3^-) are transported to the blood; for every mol of acid secreted, 1 mol of bicarbonate appears in the blood. Chloride (CL^-) reciprocates with HCO_3^- as the major anion as needed. Similarly, when acid (H^+) is secreted a sodium (Na^+) ion is exchanged to maintain cationic electrical neutrality. In addition, the secretion of potassium (K^+) and H^+ are inversely related. Consequently, metabolic alkalosis can develop (or be perpetuated) if there is a potassium deficiency, since H^+ is secreted preferentially into the urine in order to conserve K^+. Aldosterone (secreted by the zona glomerulosa of the adrenal glands in response to the plasma potassium concentration, as well as angiotensin II) acts on the distal tubule and collecting ducts to increase K^+ secretion into the urine and conserve Na^+. Ammonia (NH_3), formed primarily from glutamine, diffuses into the tubular fluid where it combines with H^+, facilitating the conservation of Na^+. One can readily appreciate that with renal disease these complex interrelationships are disrupted and can result in metabolic acidosis, hyperkalemia, and accelerated loss of Na^+ in the urine. Interestingly, hypokalemia appears to develop initially in cats during the early stages of chronic renal failure for unknown reasons. Aldosterone is mentioned in this discussion on renal physiology because a deficiency of the hormone (hypoadrenocorticism) results in a combination of hyperkalemia, hyponatremia, and prerenal azotemia secondary to vomiting, which can mimic renal failure clinicopathologically.

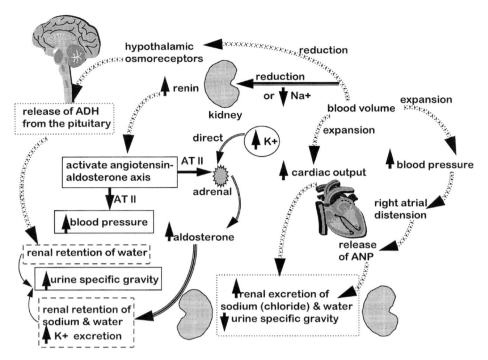

FIGURE 10–4. The kidney plays a pivotal role in the regulation of the blood volume. The urine specific gravity is a simplified reflection of the complex hormonal interactions involved in maintenance of an appropriate hydration status. A reduction of the blood volume is recognized by stretch receptors in the atria and by baroreceptors in the carotid sinus and aortic arch (which are also activated by a rise in the plasma osmolality). The hypothalamic osmoreceptors are activated, which stimulate the pituitary to release antidiuretic hormone (ADH, vasopressin, arginine vasopressin, AVP). ADH promotes the reabsorption of solute-free water in the renal distal tubules and collecting ducts. It is the predominant hormone involved in the regulation of water balance. Insufficient secretion of ADH (central) or a renal tubular resistance (nephrogenic) to its action result in diabetes insipidus. Polyuria and the resultant polydipsia are the prominent features of the clinical syndrome. When water intake becomes inadequate to compensate for the loss, dehydration, hyperosmolality, hypernatremia, and azotemia develop in concert with an inappropriately low urine specific gravity. The constellation of clinical signs and laboratory findings can mimic primary chronic renal failure. With the judicious use of the water deprivation test and limiting dehydration to 5% of the body weight with frequent monitoring of the serum urea nitrogen and creatinine concentrations, the urine specific gravity will usually rise within 24 hours with central diabetes insipidus but will not change appreciably in nephrogenic diabetes insipidus. Modifications of this procedure are detailed in internal medicine texts. It is emphasized that diabetes insipidus is uncommon and the other common causes of polyuria/polydipsia should be ruled out before attempts are made to confirm its diagnosis. Conversely, inappropriate hypersecretion of ADH results in hyponatremia with plasma hypo-osmolality. It is a rare syndrome and the reader is referred to internal medicine texts.

The expansion of the blood volume causes two cardiac effects. There is an increase in cardiac output which increases the glomerular filtration rate and formation of urine. An increase in the distention of the right atrium stimulates the myocardial release of a hormone referred to as atrial natriuretic peptide (ANP, atrial natriuretic factor, ANF, atriopeptin). It reduces the tubular sodium (Na^+) reabsorption and increases the glomerular filtration resulting in natriuresis and water loss. ANP is also a vasorelaxant and inhibits renin and aldosterone secretion through mechanisms that are not completely understood. *Legend continued on opposite page.*

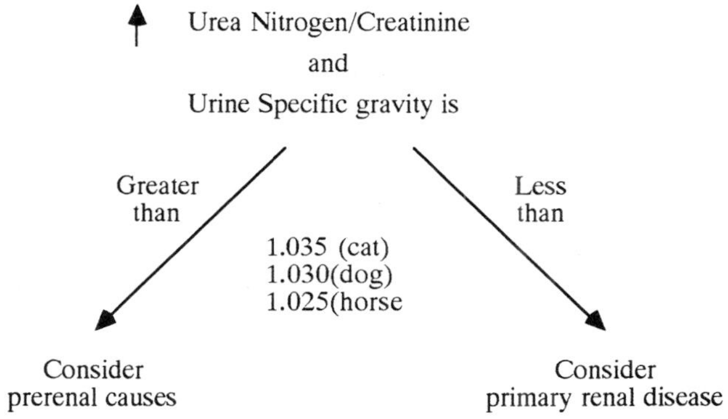

Urea Nitrogen/Creatinine

and

Urine Specific gravity is

FIGURE 10–5. Relationship of urine specific gravity to serum urea nitrogen, and creatinine values.

Greater than

Less than

1.035 (cat)
1.030(dog)
1.025(horse

Consider
prerenal causes

Consider
primary renal disease

adrenocorticism, perhaps due to hypertension-induced glomerulosclerosis. *Postrenal proteinuria* occurs when there is inflammation of the lower urinary tract. It is usually accompanied by hematuria or pyuria or both. The most common cause of postrenal proteinuria is cystitis. A midstream urine sample may also contain protein secondary to prostatitis, urethritis, and vaginal or preputial discharges.

Proteinuria also occurs when low-molecular-weight proteins (light chain immunoglobulins) pass through the glomerulus. A plasma cell tumor is the most common cause. One characteristic of finding these Bence Jones proteins is that the pad on the test tape remains negative, but the sulfosalicylic acid (Bumintest*) test is usually positive. Both *hemoglobinuria* and *myoglobinuria* may cause a positive protein reaction.

Tubular proteinuria is a consequence of injury to the tubular epithelium that impairs their ability to reabsorb and catabolize the proteins in the glomerular ultrafiltrate. The presence of these relatively small proteins such as α_1-microglobulin (30,000 MW), β_2-microglobulin (12,000 MW), lysozyme (14,000 MW), retinol-binding protein (21,000 MW) in the urine are relatively early indicators of tubular damage. They can be identified in the urine with protein electrophoretograms. Drugs (aminoglycoside antibiotics, cyclosporin A), heavy metals (lead), analgesics (nonsteroidal anti-inflammatory drugs),

---

*See Algorithms 11 and 12.

A reduction in the blood volume reduces the renal perfusion pressure which in turn stimulates the release of renin from the juxtaglomerular cells associated with the afferent arteriole. A reduction in the plasma sodium concentration can also stimulate the release of renin. Renin transforms the plasma α_2-globulin synthesized in the liver, angiotensinogen, to angiotensin I. The angiotensin-converting enzyme (ACE) present throughout the vascular endothelium converts angiotensin I to angiotensin II (AT II). It stimulates the adrenals to release aldosterone which effects renal retention of sodium and water by the collecting ducts and excretion of potassium (K^+). A rise in the plasma potassium concentration is another important effector of aldosterone release. Angiotensin II is a potent vasoconstrictor; it directly raises the systemic blood pressure and, consequently, the renal perfusion pressure. It also stimulates the renal production of the vasodilatory prostaglandins E_2 and I_2 which act to counterbalance the pressor effect.

ischemia, and metabolic diseases (Fanconi's syndrome) are examples of causation. Because the glomerular filtration function is normal, albuminuria (66,000 MW) is not present (Figs. 10–1 and 10–2).

Enzymuria

γ-Glutamyltransferase (GGT), *N*-acetyl-β-D-glucosaminidase (NAG), and alkaline phosphatase (ALP) are enzymes that are present in relatively high activity in the renal tubular epithelial cells. The measurement of their 24-hour excretion is a relatively sensitive and early marker of tubular injury in dog, horse, and sheep. The determination of an enzyme to creatinine ratio from a spot urine sample makes the test clinically applicable (Table 10–1). Tubular damage, *e.g.*, aminoglycoside toxicity, is associated with an increase in the enzyme to creatinine ratio prior to a change in the serum creatinine concentration, endogenous creatinine clearance, urine protein to creatinine ratio, and change in the urine specific gravity. The validity of the ratio is affected by a reduction in glomerular filtration rate and urinary inflammation (hematuria, pyuria).

Glucose

Glucose passes the glomerular filter and is completely reabsorbed by tubule cells; therefore, glucose is not detected in normal urine. The usual method of testing urine for glucose is the enzyme (glucose oxidase) reagent strip. False negative reactions may occur in urine containing a large quantity of ascorbic acid. Because dogs synthesize variable amounts of ascorbic acid, an alternative method should be used to detect glucosuria. A commercial tablet

TABLE 10–1. Markers of Renal Tubular Injury

Casts

Type of Cast	Possible Cause/ Association	Interpretation
Hyaline	Proteinuria (renal or extrarenal)	Mild to severe pathology
Epithelial	Ischemia, nephrotoxins	Acute, severe injury
Granular, fatty, waxy	Ischemia, nephrotoxins	Combination of Tamm-Horsfall protein plus degenerated epithelial cells or leukocytes (chronic)
Leukocyte	Inflammation	Infection involving tubules
Erythrocyte	Hemorrhage	Bleeding in the kidney
Broad	Tubular obstruction/ dilatation	Renal disease (failure)

Enzyme/Creatinine Ratios[a]

Species	GGT/creatinine	NAG/creatinine
Dog	0.39 ± 0.18	0.06 ± 0.04
Horse	10.52 ± 4.78	
Sheep	0.015 ± 0.008	$1.5 \times 10^{-3} \pm 6 \times 10^{-4}$

[a]Enzyme (U/L) divided by creatinine (mg/dL). Expressed as the mean ± SD.
GGT, γ-glutamyltransferase; NAG, *N*-acetyl-β-D-glucosaminidase.

(Clinitest*) that detects reducing substances can be used. Cats with cystitis may also give a false positive reaction with the reagent strip method.

Renal Glucosuria

When the plasma glucose concentration is normal, renal glucosuria is a component of the Fanconi-like syndrome caused by an inability of tubules to reabsorb urine constituents. It has been reported in several breeds of dog including basenji, Norwegian elkhound, Shetland sheepdog, and miniature schnauzer. Affected patients also have an aminoaciduria. Primary renal glucosuria has been reported (as an isolated finding) in Scottish terriers, Norwegian elkhounds, and mixed breeds. It is not apparently associated with clinical disease and should not be confused with diabetes mellitus.

Ketones

Excessive ketone formation results from accelerated oxidation of fatty acids as an energy source. Slight ketonuria can be seen in malnourished dogs and cats. It frequently accompanies advanced cases of canine diabetes mellitus. If the predominant ketone is β-hydroxybutyrate, ketonuria will not be detected because the reagent strip is insensitive to this ketone. Ketonuria in ruminants is also associated with abnormal carbohydrate metabolism. Acetoacetate and β-hydroxybutyrate predominate with a lesser amount of ketone.

Occult Blood

A positive reaction indicates erythrocytes, free hemoglobin, or myoglobin. A positive reaction must be interpreted in light of the urine sediment findings. After centrifugation, a positive test in the supernatant suggests hemoglobinuria, red blood cell (RBC) lysis in hypotonic urine, or myoglobinuria. Myoglobinuria and hemoglobinuria can be differentiated crudely using an ammonium sulfate precipitation test. Ammonium sulfate (2.8 mg) is added to 5 mL of urine, mixed well, and centrifuged. If the supernatant fluid remains dark, myoglobin is probable. Myoglobinuria may be supported by finding an increase in serum creatine kinase (CK) activity. Hematuria reflects hemorrhage in the urinary tract, and hemoglobinuria suggests intravascular destruction of erythrocytes.

Bilirubin

Conjugated bilirubin appears in urine if there is an increase in the plasma concentration (see Fig. 7–12 and Cases 7–1 and 7–3). Dogs have a low renal threshold for bilirubin, and a trace or 1+ reaction in urine with a specific gravity greater than 1.020 is insignificant. A stronger ($\geq$3+) reaction suggests hepatic disease and the need for a more sensitive liver function test if the patient is not jaundiced since bilirubinuria precedes bilirubinemia in the dog (see Fig. 7–12). Bilirubinuria may be also detected in dogs with hemoglobinemia secondary to increased erythrocyte destruction.

---

*Ames Company, Elkhart, IN.

Urobilinogen

Urobilinogen lacks diagnostic utility.

Microscopic Sediment

Urine collected by cystocentesis normally contains sparse numbers of cells and other formed elements from the urinary tract. The method for examining urine sediment should be consistent; 5 mL is sedimented to provide a uniform semiquantitation. We recommend the examination of unstained sediment, since stain precipitate and bacteria and yeasts introduce erroneous findings. It is important to *rack* the condenser down when examining urine sediments. Altering the light in this fashion emphasizes urine particulate constituents.

Leukocytes

Zero to 3/hpf leukocytes are normally present in urine collected by cystocentesis. Increased numbers of leukocytes (pyuria) support the presence of an inflammatory process. The sample should be cultured even if bacteria are not seen.

Erythrocytes

Normal urine has a few erythrocytes (0 to 3/hpf). An increased number of RBCs in urine is an indication of inflammation or hemorrhage. If the RBCs are in a cast, renal hemorrhage is suggested. Hematuria may be associated with uroliths, neoplasia, bacterial infections, trauma, sterile cystitis, nephritis, nephrosis, urinary parasites, and thrombocytopenia. Leukocytes and/or erythrocytes in urine collected midstream may reflect hemorrhage/inflammation in the genital tract.

Epithelial Cells

Epithelial cells may appear in small numbers in urine, but the number may be increased in animals with cystitis, neoplasia, or inflammation of the urinary tract. In a patient with persistent hematuria and stranguria, cytologic examination of the urine is a useful screening procedure for neoplasia. A small drop of sediment is spread on a glass slide, air dried, and stained similarly to a blood smear. Neoplastic cells can be more readily identified in this type of preparation.

Casts

Urinary casts reflect tubular luminal events and represent its shape. Casts rapidly disintegrate in the urine specimen, so it is best to look for them in a freshly voided sample. There is usually less than 1 cast/hpf normally present; hyalin or fine granular. Hyalin, fine granular, coarse granular, and waxy (see Case 10–1) casts represent a continuum of formation. The trapping of erythrocytes, leukocytes, or exfoliated tubular epithelial cells within the protein matrix of the cast results in casts containing these elements representative of the pathologic renal process. The protein matrix is formed by the Tamm-Horsfall protein. It is a membrane-associated renal glycoprotein that is formed in the distal nephron; predominantly the thick ascending limb of the loop of Henle. The most notable physiochemical feature of this glycoprotein, named after the two individuals that originally isolated it from human urine in 1950, is an extremely high content of half-cysteine residues. In its epithelial surface location it has a rapid metabolic turnover; approximately 9 hours. The role of the Tamm-Horsfall protein in renal physiology may be related to its ability to alter the passive tubular diffusion of water. The thick ascending loop of Henle uses an active chloride transport mechanism to reabsorb a large fraction of the sodium chloride in the ultrafiltrate. The very limited permeability to water in this segment of the tubule may be due to the association of the aggregated form of the glycoprotein within the lateral intercellular space. A tubular fluid that is hypotonic to plasma consequently is formed on its journey to the distal convoluted tubule. This contributes to the maintenance of the medullary concentration gradient in support of the countercurrent multiplier system.

Increasing physiologic concentrations of Tamm-Horsfall protein or electrolytes or hydrogen ion in the glomerular ultrafiltrate results in a molecular aggregation of a gel-like consistency. The gel-forming property appears to be related to the carbohydrate side chains and is reversible. Microscopically we recognize it when we observe hyaline casts in the urine for which it is the primary constituent. Because of the elements associated with increasing its viscosity, clinical conditions resulting in acidosis, dehydration (see Case 7–1), and oliguria facilitate their formation. Under pathophysiologic conditions, Tamm-Horsfall protein may interact with other substances such as hemoglobin, myoglobin, Bence Jones protein, and radiographic contrast media and contribute to their adverse renal effects.

Bacteria

Bacteria are not present in normal urine collected by cystocentesis but may be present in varying numbers in catheterized or midstream collections. Bacteria in urine collected by cystocentesis indicate an infectious process.

Yeast and Fungi

These organisms are usually contaminants that occur during collection. Urine sediment stains may become contaminated with yeast as well as bacteria.

Crystals

Certain crystals are of diagnostic significance. Ammonium biurate suggests hepatic insufficiency (see Case 7–4); cystine crystals may be associated with cystine uroliths; calcium oxalate monohydrate (hippuric acid–appearing) crystals occur with ethylene glycol (antifreeze) toxicity as well as the more common Maltese cross variety.

Sperm

Sperm are found in about one fourth of urine samples taken by cystocentesis from intact males and in recently bred females.

RENAL FUNCTION TESTS—BLOOD CHEMISTRY

Renal function tests are crude markers of glomerular function. Sequential evaluation is useful for monitoring treatment and disease progression.

Urea Nitrogen

Urea is formed by the liver and represents the principal product of protein catabolism in carnivorous and omnivorous species (see Fig. 7–8). Urea passes through the glomerular filter, and 25 to 40% of filtered urea is reabsorbed as it passes through the tubules. Increased filtrate flow diminishes urea reabsorption while slow flow rates facilitate reabsorption. Urea nitrogen levels may be increased (carnivores and omnivores) with a dietary increase in protein, catabolic breakdown of tissue, and hemorrhage into the gastrointestinal tract (Table 10–2). The creatinine concentration is minimally affected.

Azotemia

Prerenal Azotemia

It is caused by decreased blood flow through the kidney secondary to dehydration (see Cases 7–1 and 7–2) and cardiac insufficiency. Prerenal azotemia should be accompanied by an increased urine specific gravity ($\geq$1.030 in dog; $\geq$1.035 in cat) if there is no concurrent primary renal disease.

TABLE 10–2. **Causes of Azotemia (Increased Urea Nitrogen and/or Creatinine)**

Classification	Cause
Prerenal	Dehydration Cardiovascular disease Shock (septic or traumatic) High-protein diet (urea-nitrogen increase only) Hemorrhage into gastrointestinal tract (urea-nitrogen increase only)
Renal	Renal diseases causing two thirds to three fourths of nephrons to be destroyed
Postrenal	Obstruction of urinary tract Rupture of urinary tract

Primary or Renal Azotemia

Primary azotemia occurs with glomerular damage; proteinuria may also be present (see Case 10–1).

Postrenal Azotemia

Postrenal azotemia occurs with urethral obstruction or subsequent to rupture of the urinary bladder.

Creatinine

Creatinine is formed during skeletal muscle metabolism (see Fig. 7–18). As with urea nitrogen, the serum creatinine is a crude index of glomerular filtration. Serum creatinine is not markedly influenced by diet or intestinal hemorrhage. Severe muscle wasting will reduce the quantity of creatinine formed. As with urea nitrogen a reduced glomerular filtration rate (GFR) causes a rise in the serum concentration of creatinine. In contrast to urea nitrogen, it is not reabsorbed by the tubules. Therefore, a slightly raised serum urea nitrogen concentration in association with a serum creatinine concentration within the reference range is an initial finding of dehydration due to a reduction of the filtrate flow in the tubules. As the hypovolemia becomes more severe, the glomerular filtration rate is sufficiently reduced to cause a rise of both analytes in the plasma. If the renal tubules are functioning properly, there is a concurrent increase in the specific gravity of the urine. The same prerenal, renal, and postrenal factors that influence urea nitrogen also affect the serum creatinine concentration.

Other Blood Chemistry Determinations

Because kidneys play an important role in the elimination and conservation of many chemical components of the blood, renal disease may alter their serum values. These are summarized in Table 10–3.

TABLE 10–3. Electrolyte and Nonelectrolyte Changes in Advanced Renal Disease

	Renal Alteration	Result
Electrolytes		
Sodium	↑ Fractional excretion	Hyponatremia
Potassium	↓ Fractional excretion	Hyperkalemia
Bicarbonate	↓ Conservation	Acidemia
Phosphate	↓ Excretion	Hyperphosphatemia (dog and cat)
Calcium	↑ Excretion as phosphate ↑	Hypocalcemia
Nonelectrolytes		
Blood pH	↓ Removal of H^+ and acid products, bicarbonate loss	Acidemia
Serum proteins	Persistent proteinuria	Hypoalbuminemia

The following discussion will be directed toward alterations observed in renal disease.

Potassium. Potassium is filtered and is actively excreted. The quantity of potassium handled by the kidneys reflects potassium intake. Patients with acute renal disease may retain potassium and hyperkalemia will develop. In contrast, hypokalemia will develop in most cats and approximately 25% of dogs with chronic renal failure.

Sodium. The ability to retain sodium is frequently lost in renal disease. The measurement of the fractional clearance (FC) of sodium (%) is a good indicator of renal insufficiency ($FC_{Na} > 1$) and it is helpful in defining prerenal azotemia ($FC_{Na} < 1$).

Chloride/Bicarbonate. The chloride composition of the body varies inversely with the bicarbonate concentration. Bicarbonate deficiencies may occur with advanced renal disease.

Phosphate. Hyperphosphatemia occurs in dogs and cats with a decreased GFR (see Case 10–1).

Calcium. There are usually no changes in serum calcium in acute renal disease, but hypocalcemia may be observed with chronic renal disease. Hypercalcemia frequently occurs in *horses* with advanced renal disease and has been reported in dogs occasionally.

Blood pH. Metabolic acidosis is relatively consistent in patients with renal failure. Reduced renal function affects H^+ removal from the blood as well as the capacity to remove acid products of metabolism. This reduced ability is compounded by a deficiency to conserve bicarbonate.

Lipids. Hyperlipidemia is a common association with the nephrotic syndrome (proteinuria, hypoalbuminemia, edema) (see Case 10–1). Enhanced synthesis of cholesterol-containing lipoproteins by the liver is thought to be a related response to the hypoalbuminemia and/or decreased oncotic pressure.

Additional Reading

Adams LG, Polzin DJ, Osborne CA, et al: Correlation of urine protein/creatinine ratio and twenty-four-hour urinary protein excretion in normal cats and cats with surgically induced chronic renal failure. J Vet Intern Med 1992;6:36–40.

Adams R, McClure JJ, Gossett KA, et al: Evaluation of a technique for measurement of gamma glutamyltranspeptidase in equine urine. Am J Vet Res 1985;46:147–150.

Bernard A, Lauwerys RR: Proteinuria: Changes and mechanisms in toxic nephropathies. Crit Rev Toxicol 1991;21:373–405.

Cook AK, Cowgill LD: Clinical and pathological features of protein-losing glomerular disease in the dog: A review of 137 cases (1985–1992). J Am Anim Hosp Assoc 1996; 32:313–322.

Garry F, Chew DJ, Hoffis GF: Enzymuria as an index of renal damage in sheep with induced aminoglycoside nephrotoxicosis. Am J Vet Res 1990;51:428–432.

Grauer GF, Greco DS, Behrend EN, et al: Estimation of quantitative enzymuria in dogs with gentamicin-induced nephrotoxicosis using urine enzyme/creatinine ratios from spot urine samples. J Vet Intern Med 1995;9:324–327.

Heiene R, Biewenga WJ, Koeman JP: Urinary alkaline phosphatase and gamma glutamyltransferase as indicators of acute renal damage in dogs. J Small Anim Prac 1991;32:521–524.

Hoyer JR, Seiler MW: Pathophysiology of Tamm-Horsfall protein. Kidney Int 1979;16: 279–289.

Lulich JP, Osborne CA: Interpretation of urine protein-creatinine ratios in dogs with glomerular and nonglomerular disorders. Comp Contin Educ Small Anim Pract 1990;12:59–71.

Norden AGW, Fulcher LM, Lapsley M, et al: Excretion of beta 2-glycoprotein I (apo-lipoprotein H) in renal tubular disease. Clin Chem 1991;37:74–77.

Ortega TM, Feldman EC, Nelson RW, et al: Systemic arterial blood pressure and urine protein/creatinine ratio in dogs with hyperadrenocorticism. J Am Vet Med Assoc 1996;209:1724–1729.

Rivers BJ, Walter PA, O'Brien TD, et al: Evaluation of urine gamma-glutamyltrans-peptidase-to-creatinine ratio as a diagnostic tool in an experimental model of aminoglycoside-induced acute renal failure in the dog. J Am Anim Hosp Assoc 1996; 32:323–336.

Schultze AE, jensen RD: Sodium dodecyl sulfate polyacrylamide gel electrophoresis of canine urinary proteins for the analysis and differentiation of tubular and glomerular diseases. Vet Clin Pathol 1990;18:93–97.

Waller KV, Ward KM, Mahan JD, et al: Current concepts in proteinuria. Clin Chem 1989;35:755–765.

Weber MH: Proteinuria: Causes, forms and methods of determination. Clin Diagn Lab Med 1988;1:49–55.

Electrolyte, Acid-Base Homeostasis and Disturbances

When we try to pick out something by itself, we find it hitched to everything else in the universe.

—John Muir

Approximately 60% of an adult's body weight is water; 40% is intracellular, and 20% is extracellular (5% plasma plus 15% interstitial). The young animal has a higher per cent of body weight in water. Vomiting, diarrhea, and polyuria are the most frequent causes of altered water and electrolyte balance. The major factors that determine the plasma solute concentration and water content are shown in Figure 11–1. The input and output are normally maintained in a steady state. An abnormality will develop if the homeostatic mechanisms balancing input and output are altered. Since a number of physiologic mechanisms are involved in plasma solute homeostasis, function tests and hormone measurements are often necessary to define the nature of the disturbance.

Sodium is the principal cation in the *extracellular* fluid, and potassium is the principal *intracellular* cation. The plasma sodium concentration contributes to the maintenance of the osmotic pressure of the extracellular fluid. It influences the extracellular fluid volume, since the intravascular water flux tends to parallel changes in plasma sodium concentration. Intracellular osmolality is determined predominantly by potassium. Large potassium losses associated with chronic vomiting, diarrhea, or hypersecretion of aldosterone cause cells to shrink as intracellular water is lost. The principal anion within the cells is phosphate, whereas chloride and bicarbonate predominate in the extracellular fluid. Active transport mechanisms located in the cell membrane are responsible for maintaining the large solute gradient difference.

The maintenance of plasma volume is illustrated in Figure 11–2. Albumin is the principal protein that contributes to oncotic (osmotic) pressure because of its low molecular weight and high concentration. Despite the influence of albumin, sodium is the main determinant of plasma volume. As a consequence, the albumin concentration has to fall by at least 50% before

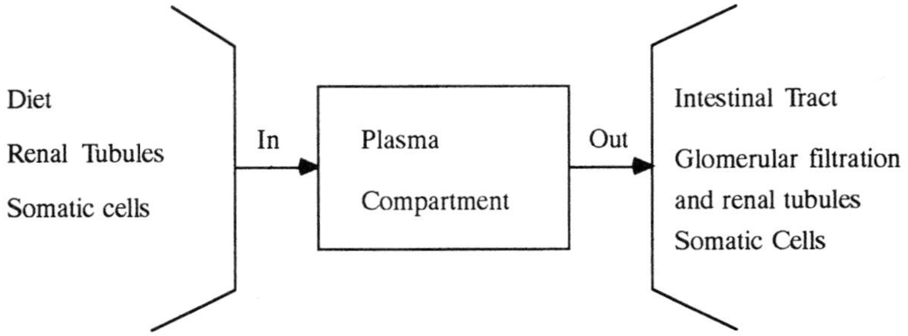

Diet

Renal Tubules — In → | Plasma
                         Compartment | → Out

Somatic cells

Intestinal Tract

Glomerular filtration
and renal tubules

Somatic Cells

FIGURE 11–1. Factors that determine plasma solute concentration and water content.

effecting a change in plasma oncotic pressure (manifested clinically as edema). Disturbances in osmolality are adjusted by the water intake or excretion. Dehydration stimulates thirst and stimulates the posterior pituitary to secrete *antidiuretic hormone (ADH)*, which promotes renal tubular reabsorption. Overhydration inhibits thirst and the release of ADH (see Fig. 10–4).

ELECTROLYTES

Sodium Disturbances

Plasma sodium is filtered by the glomerulus, and the majority is reabsorbed by the proximal and distal renal tubules. The distal tubular exchange of sodium and potassium is accelerated by *aldosterone*, promoting sodium retention and potassium excretion (Figs. 10–3 and 10–4).

Hyponatremia occurs with gastrointestinal loss (vomiting and diarrhea). If severe enough, a metabolic acidosis can develop which contributes to electrolyte shifts that mimic those associated with hypoadrenocorticism. Notably, plasma electrolyte changes suggestive of hypoadrenocorticism are associated with canine trichuriasis (referred to as trichuriasis-associated pseudohypoadrenocorticism). However, the plasma aldosterone concentration is not reduced and the adrenocorticotropin hormone (ACTH) stimulation test is not indicative of hypoadrenocorticism. Other causes of hyponatremia include uroperitoneum ("third space" loss), congestive heart failure, diuretic administration, and diabetes mellitus. Some dogs with adrenal insufficiency have only a glucocorticoid deficiency and may have a hyponatremia with a normokalemia (see Chapter 9). The development of hyponatremia con-

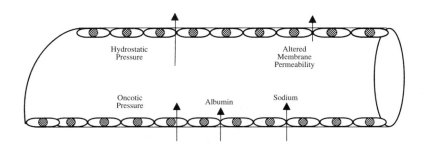

Hydrostatic
Pressure

Altered
Membrane
Permeability

Oncotic
Pressure

Albumin

Sodium

FIGURE 11–2. Maintenance of plasma volume.

TABLE 11–1. **Disorders Associated with Hyponatremia**

Gastrointestinal loss (vomiting, diarrhea)
Congestive heart failure (edema)
Hypoadrenocorticism (glucocorticoid deficiency)
Diuretic treatment
Administration of hypotonic fluid (*e.g.*, 5% dextrose in water)
Third space loss (pancreatitis, peritonitis, uroperitoneum)
Diabetes mellitus
Renal disease (polyuric acute renal failure, horse)
Factitious
Ptyalism (horse)
Cellulitis (horse)
White muscle disease (horse)
Drug-induced (nonsteroidal anti-inflammatory, intraoperative use of nafcillin)
Chylothorax

current with the use of medications can occur. Postoperative azotemia and hyponatremia is reported in association with the intraoperative use of nafcillin in dogs, and the use of ibuprofen in elderly humans can cause hyponatremia.

Facetious hyponatremia (pseudohyponatremia) may result when a lipemic sample is measured by flame photometry or indirect potentiometry. This may also occur with severe hyperglobulinemia. The falsely decreased sodium value does not occur if an ion-selective electrode is used for the electrolyte determination. A more detailed list of disorders associated with hyponatremia is presented in Table 11–1.

Hypernatremia is associated with dehydration secondary to inadequate water intake or excessive pure water loss. This is especially prominent in diabetes insipidus if the patient is not allowed free access to water. An increased sodium concentration may occur with cirrhosis and be exaggerated by the osmotic catharsis used in the management of hepatic encephalopathy. Hypernatremic hypovolemia may develop in patients with chronic renal failure and inadequate water intake. A more detailed list of the causes of hypernatremia is presented in Table 11–2.

Potassium Disturbances

Hypokalemia results from decreased intake, excessive loss, extracellular to intracellular shift, and dilution. The use of potassium-poor intravenous fluids may enhance the renal loss plus dilute further the marginal plasma potassium in an anorectic animal, resulting in hypokalemia. Gastrointestinal loss (vomiting and diarrhea) is a common cause of hypokalemia, often exacerbated by inadequate dietary intake. Excess loss will also occur with hyperaldosteronism (hypernatremia is also present) and renal tubular acidosis (hyperchloremic acidosis is present). Diuretics also enhance renal loss of

TABLE 11–2. Disorders Associated with Hypernatremia

Diabetes insipidus
Increased insensible water loss (fever, high environmental temperature)
Gastrointestinal loss (vomiting, diarrhea)
Inadequate intake
Renal failure (acute and chronic)
Diabetes mellitus (following insulin treatment)
Diuretic treatment
Increased salt intake or intravenous administration
Hyperaldosteronism
Artifact caused by improper sample handling (allowing evaporation of serum)

potassium. The administration of furosemide to horses results in sufficient total body cation depletion to cause the formation of echinocytes. Erythrocytic dehydration is probably a consequence of the rapid reduction in the serum sodium, potassium, and erythrocyte potassium concentrations that occurs subsequent to furosemide treatment. The use of insulin in the management of the ketoacidotic diabetic patient will carry potassium into the cell (along with glucose). Table 11–3 contains a more detailed list of disorders associated with hypokalemia.

Hyperkalemia develops secondary to increased intake, decreased secretion (kidney dependent), or a shift from the rich intracellular store to the extracellular fluid. Life-threatening hyperkalemia most frequently occurs secondary to adrenal insufficiency or renal failure (both represent decreased excretion). A sodium to potassium ratio of less than 27:1 with an abnormal ACTH stimulation test (decreased response) confirms the diagnosis of hypoadrenocorticism (see Chapter 9).

Since cells are rich in potassium, there is a potential for its shift to the extracellular fluid to cause hyperkalemia. With acidosis the cell helps maintain acid-base balance by exchanging intracellular potassium for the extracellular hydrogen ion. The kidney can usually increase potassium excretion blunting this effect unless there is concomitant organ dysfunction that facil-

TABLE 11–3. Disorders Associated with Hypokalemia

Gastrointestinal loss (vomiting, diarrhea)
Intravenous administration of potassium-poor fluids
Bicarbonate therapy
Diuretic treatment
Hyperaldosteronism
Renal tubular acidosis
Chronic renal failure (especially cats)
Insulin treatment of ketoacidotic diabetic
Alkalosis (translocation)
Prolonged anorexia (horse)
Excessive sweating (horse)
Factitious (hyperlipidemia, improper sample handling)
Reduced dietary intake (rarely the sole cause)

TABLE 11–4. Disorders Associated with Hyperkalemia

Hypoadrenocorticism
Renal failure (including urethral obstruction)
Diffuse cell death secondary to shock; circulatory stasis, chemotherapy
Acidosis
Rhabdomyolysis (horse)
Periodic paralysis (horse)
Uroperitoneum
Chylothorax
Factitious
   Hemolysis
   Delayed separation of clotted blood (Akita breed, herbivores, excessive
     leukocytosis of thrombocytosis)[a]
   Collection in potassium heparin
   Collection from intravenous tube when potassium administered

[a]Markedly raised leukocyte or platelet counts are associated with raised serum potassium concentrations due to cell leakage during the clotting process for harvesting the serum. This artifact is avoided by using plasma for its measurement.

itates the development of hyperkalemia. Diffuse cell necrosis or altered membrane permeability allowing potassium leakage may accompany shock, circulatory failure, crush-type injury, chemotherapy, and rhabdomyolysis. Hyperkalemia occurs in humans treated with trimethoprim/sulfamethoxazole. Mechanistic studies in rats indicate that trimethoprim (an organic anion) blocks the apical membrane sodium channels in the mammalian renal distal tubule which inhibits the secretion of potassium.

Factitious hyperkalemia (pseudohyperkalemia) may occur secondary to a delay in separating serum from blood with extreme leukocytosis or thrombocytosis, cellular elements rich in potassium. A breed peculiarity has been noted in the Akita dog wherein delayed separation of the clotted specimen can result in an increased potassium value. The Akita's erythrocyte apparently has more potassium than that of other breeds. Hemolysis may also result in an abnormal potassium determination in horses and cattle. A more detailed list of disorders with hyperkalemia is presented in Table 11–4.

Chloride Changes

Chloride is the extracellular anion in highest concentration. Since it cannot accept the hydrogen ion at physiologic pH, it cannot act as a buffer. Because of electrochemical neutrality, chloride varies inversely with bicarbonate. Its measurement provides the least clinical information of the electrolytes. It is

TABLE 11–5. Reference Ranges of Fractional Clearance (%) of Urinary Electrolytes

	Dog	Cat	Horse	Cow	Sheep
Sodium	0–0.7	0.24–0.1	0.02–1.0	0.2–1.43	0–0.071
Potassium	0–20	6.7–23.9	15–65	15–63	80–180
Chloride	0–0.8	0.41–1.3	0.04–1.6	0.4–2.3	0–4.7
Phosphate	3–39	17–73	0–0.2		0–0.53

TABLE 11–6. Disorders Resulting in Metabolic Acidosis and Normal or Increased Anion Gap

Increased anion gap (chloride normal or decreased)
  Diabetic ketoacidosis
  Uremia
  Shock, anoxia, exercise (overproduction of acid, *e.g.*, lactate)
  Grain overload in cattle (>lactic acid)
  Ethylene glycol toxicity
  Salicylate toxicity
Normal gap (increased chloride)
  Severe diarrhea
  Chronic vomiting
  Renal tubular acidosis
  Diuretics (carbonic anhydrase inhibitors)
  Oral acidifying agents

helpful for determining the anionic gap. Hyperchloremia is associated with dehydration and renal tubular acidosis. Pseudohyperchloremia refers to the artificially raised serum chloride concentration measured in patients treated with bromide salts. Decreased concentrations occur in metabolic acidosis and prolonged vomiting (hypokalemic, hypochloremic metabolic alkalosis).

Electrolytes in the Urine

The excretion of electrolytes in the urine is influenced by the diet, fluid therapy, production endogenously, and renal function. The values measured should be compared to a "control" population due to the numerous variables that abruptly affect their appearance in the urine. The measurement of electrolytes and minerals in the urine of grazing cattle and sheep can provide information on the dietary deficiencies or excesses. The measurement of urinary sodium is useful in the differential diagnosis of acute renal failure and hyponatremia in humans but is less useful in veterinary medicine.

The direct measurement of an electrolyte in the urine is not reliable due to the variability of the urine volume in response to water balance. The fractional clearance (FC) or fractional excretion rate (FE) of an electrolyte (E) in the urine (U) can be determined by the use of an equation that uses creatinine (Cr) as a benchmark substance of the glomerular filtration rate. A single

TABLE 11–7. Disorders Resulting in a Metabolic Alkalosis

Vomiting (acute, gastric contents only)
Gastric (abomasal) sequestration
Small intestine obstruction
Cecal volvulus (cattle)
Excess use of potassium-depleting diuretics
Excess administration of sodium bicarbonate
Endurance competition (horse)
Excessive sweating (horse)
Ptyalism (horse, cow)

TABLE 11–8. Disorders Resulting in Respiratory Acidosis (Depressed Respiration)

Central (respiratory center)
  Drugs (anesthetics, narcotics)
  Trauma
  Tumor, inflammation
Impaired pulmonary function
  Pneumonia
  Pneumothorax
  Airway obstruction
  Pulmonary edema
  Hydrothorax
  Deficient diaphragm (muscle/chest wall movement)

random urine sample is collected and the serum (S) concentration of the electrolyte and creatinine concentrations are used. The FC of an electrolyte is simply a reflection of the immediate events affecting its appearance in the urine. The FC does not necessarily equate to a 24-hour quantitation of the electrolyte.

$$FC_E = \frac{U_E/S_E}{U_{Cr}/S_{Cr}}$$

The calculated value is multiplied by 100 to express it as the per cent of filtered electrolyte that is excreted. An example of its potential use follows. A relatively reliable FC_{Na} for the dog and cat is less than 1%. A value greater than 1% in a dehydrated patient with hypernatremia suggests renal failure. A value greater than 1% in a dehydrated patient with hyponatremia suggests excess renal sodium loss due to diuretic treatment or hypoadrenocorticism. The FC for potassium in the urine is used to investigate the association of hypokalemia, diet, azotemia, and renal failure in cats. Table 11–5 lists reported FC reference ranges.

ACID-BASE BALANCE

The metabolism of fats, carbohydrates, and proteins for energy results in the formation of large quantities of CO_2. Although CO_2 forms a weak acid (H_2CO_3) in plasma, the process is reversed in the lung, and CO_2 is eliminated rapidly. Incomplete oxidation of metabolites results in the formation of non-

TABLE 11–9. Disorders Causing Respiratory Alkalosis

Central (stimulation of respiratory center)
  Anxiety
  Pain
  Pathologic lesions
Hypoxemia
  Severe anemia (with hyperventilation)
  Congestive heart failure
Excessive mechanical ventilation

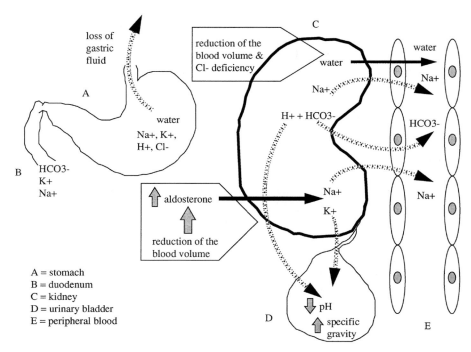

loss of
gastric
fluid

reduction of the
blood volume &
Cl- deficiency

C

water

water

Na+

Na+

A

H+ + HCO3-

HCO3-

water
Na+, K+,
H+, Cl-

B   HCO3-
K+
Na+

aldosterone

Na+

Na+

K+

reduction of the
blood volume

A = stomach
B = duodenum
C = kidney
D = urinary bladder
E = peripheral blood

pH
D   specific
gravity   E

FIGURE 11–3. *A*, Gastric fluid is comprised of water which contains high concentrations of H^+ and Cl^- and smaller concentrations of Na^+ and K^+. Vomiting initially causes dehydration due to the inability to replace the lost fluids. Prolonged loss of only gastric fluid, often secondary to pyloric outflow obstruction, causes a more severe dehydration and the development of the expected metabolic alkalosis and electrolyte imbalances (hypochloremia, hypokalemia) as well as an unexpected finding, aciduria. The loss of H^+ generates the formation of HCO_3^- by the parietal cell which causes a rise of the extracellular fluid's pH. The pathophysiologic process is referred to as alkalosis and the rise of the pH of the extracellular fluid is referred to as alkalemia. The loss of Cl^- plays a pivotal role in the maintenance of the alkalemia. Why? Let's link the answer to the concurrent water and potassium losses and the explanation for the common occurrence of the latter.

In health, the excess plasma HCO_3^- that is generated following a meal (referred to as "alkaline tide") is excreted by the kidney resulting in a rise in the pH of the urine (alkalinuria). This process is impaired subsequent to the chronic loss of gastric fluid due to a combination of factors. Due to the importance of maintaining adequate hydration, there is enhanced renal tubular reabsorption of Na^+ in order to "drag" more water back into the extracellular fluid space. Electroneutrality is usually maintained by the concurrent movement of Cl^- in association with the active Na^+ reabsorption. The deficiency of Cl^- forces the kidney to use K^+ and H^+ as exchange ions to maintain electroneutrality. There is limited K^+ available because of its loss in the gastric fluid and its paradoxical renal excretion associated with the hypovolemic drive to maintain Na^+ (see aldosterone discussion, Fig. 10–4). Consequently, H^+ is preferentially used because of its relative greater availability. However, the use of H^+ as an exchange ion generates HCO_3^- which is reabsorbed and, ironically, amplifies the alkalemia. Thus, the excretion of H^+ in order to conserve Na^+ (water) is the cause of the paradoxical aciduria in the presence of alkalemia. This is one example of why the urine pH should be used cautiously as the sole indicator of the systemic acid-base status. Because of chloride's role in the maintenance of metabolic alkalosis, it must be an integral component of the fluid therapy. Normal saline (0.9% NaCl) with the appropriate potassium supplementation is a logical replacement fluid in the management of hypochloremic, hypokalemic, metabolic alkalosis. *Legend continued on opposite page.*

volatile acids which rely on the kidney for excretion. When tissues are subjected to oxygen deficiency (anoxia, inadequate perfusion) the H^+ is incompletely transferred to O_2 to form water, and acidosis develops.

Normal blood pH is maintained between 7.35 and 7.45. Several buffer systems are utilized in the regulation of blood pH. The bicarbonate/carbonic acid buffer system is the most important one because of the rapidity with which CO_2 can be eliminated by the lung after the conversion from H_2CO_3. The rate of CO_2 elimination depends upon the rate and depth of respiration. The hemoglobin buffer system and phosphate buffer system also contribute to maintenance of normal blood pH but are not used clinically in assessing acid-base disturbances.

An abnormal blood pH occurs when the HCO_3^- (metabolic)/P_{CO_2} (respiratory) ratio deviates from 20:1 (based on the Henderson-Hasselbalch equation). As we mentioned, the lung can respond rapidly (hours) to changes by blowing off CO_2, whereas the kidney takes 12 to 24 hours to respond and days for complete metabolic compensation. Base excess is a measurement used to assess metabolic changes. A positive base excess (increased HCO_3^-) indicates an excess of base (metabolic alkalosis), and a negative value (decreased HCO_3^-) indicates a base deficiency (metabolic acidosis). Conversely an increase in P_{CO_2} (which actually causes the $[H_2CO_3]$ to increase) is referred to as a *respiratory acidosis*, and a decrease is called *respiratory alkalosis*. Since the body is well endowed with buffering systems, compensation (an attempt to correct the acid-base disturbance) is seen clinically. Thus a pure metabolic/respiratory acidosis/alkalosis is uncommon. The primary acid-base disturbance is usually indicated by determining blood pH (acidemia or alkalemia) and the respiratory (P_{CO_2}) and metabolic (HCO_3^-) components. The one that deviates greater from normal suggests the primary disturbance. For example, if the blood pH is below the normal range; the HCO_3^- is decreased (base deficit) and shows a greater deviation from normal than the decreased P_{CO_2}, a metabolic acidosis would be suggested.

Some of the most common causes of acidosis and alkalosis are summarized in Tables 11–6, 11–7, 11–8, and 11–9. The chronic loss of gastric fluid illustrates the complexity of systemic events that occur in the development of metabolic alkalosis and multiple electrolyte abnormalities (Fig. 11–3). The paradigm can be applied to vomiting in the dog and cat, left displacement of the abomasum and abomasal volvulus in the ruminant, and, in the horse, gastric reflux and sequestration of a large quantity of fluid secondary to a high obstruction or anterior enteritis.

B, The above model of only gastric fluid loss is useful for examining the complex interactions of maintaining acid-base and electrolyte balance. However, metabolic acidosis is the more common disturbance subsequent to persistent vomiting. Why? In addition to the loss of gastric fluid, there is often concurrent loss of duodenal fluid which has a high bicarbonate concentration (from the pancreatic fluid). The acidemia (reduction in the extracellular pH) can be amplified by prerenal azotemia and lactic acidosis that are a consequence of dehydration; a reduction of the glomerular filtration rate and perfusion of skeletal muscle, respectively. In addition, the gastric fluid has a relatively reduced amount of H^+ in the fasted state (pH $\sim$ 5.0 to 7.0), which lessens the impact of its loss compared to the magnitude of the HCO_3^- loss. In contrast, when there is pyloric outflow obstruction (*A*), gastric distention causes the release of gastrin, which promotes acid secretion and net acid loss.

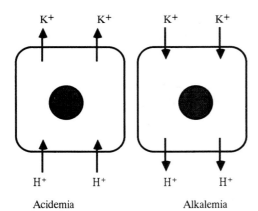

FIGURE 11-4. Cellular movement of H^+ and K^+ with acidemia and alkalemia.

The biochemical profile often contains a measurement referred to as total CO_2 (CO_2 content). Since most of the total CO_2 is comprised of bicarbonate, it gives a reasonable indication of the acid-base status.

Anion Gap

The term *anion gap* refers to difference between the measured cations and measured anions:

$$\text{Anion gap} = (Na^+ + K^+) - (Cl^- + HCO_3^-)$$

The normal range is 12 to 18 mEq/L (mmol/L) and represents the gap or unmeasured anions. These include phosphate, sulfate, and lactate. Ketones, ethylene glycol metabolites, and salicylate are examples of unmeasured anions not normally present in the blood. The anion gap can facilitate the classification of metabolic acidosis. If the total $[HCO_3^-]$ is not available, the total CO_2 value can be substituted.

There is a relationship between acid-base status and potassium transcellular flux (see Fig. 11-4). This concept is of particular importance when therapeutically approaching the management of metabolic acidosis. The acidemia shifts the potassium extracellularly and is then excreted by the kidney, thus depleting the total body potassium. The more chronic the disorder, the greater the potassium depletion. When managing the disorder (thereby correcting the acidemia), the extracellular potassium returns into the cell, precipitating abrupt hypokalemia. The serum potassium concentration (which is a poor reflection of the total body stores) should be monitored frequently when managing disorders in Tables 11-7, 11-8, and 11-9.

Additional Reading

Electrolyte and Acid-Base Homeostasis and Disorders

Autran de Morais HS, Chew DJ: Use and interpretation of serum and urine electrolytes. Semin Vet Med Surg 1992;7:262–274.

DiBartola SP, Johnson SE, Davenport SJ, et al: Clinicopathologic findings resembling hypoadrenocorticism in dogs with primary gastrointestinal disease. J Am Vet Med Assoc 1985;1987:60–63.

Dow SW, Fettman MJ: Chronic renal disease and potassium depletion in cats. Semin Vet Med Surg 1992;7:198–201.

Graves TK, Schall WD, Refsal K, et al: Basal and ACTH-simulated plasma aldosterone concentrations are normal or increased in dogs with trichuriasis-associated pseudohypoadrenocorticism. J Vet Intern Med 1994;8:287–289.

Greenberg S, Reiser IW, Chou SY, et al: Trimethoprim-sulfamethoxazole induces reversible hyperkalemia. Ann Intern Med 1993;119:291–296.

Nijsten MWN, deSmet BJGL, Dofferhoff ASM: Pseudohyperkalemia and platelet counts. N Engl J Med 1991;325:1107.

Pascoe PJ, Ilkiw JE, Kass PH, et al: Case-control study of the association between intraoperative administration of nafcillin and acute postoperative development of azotemia. J Am Vet Med Assoc 1996;208:1043–1047.

Rault RM: Case report: Hyponatremia associated with nonsteroidal antiinflammatory drugs. Am J Med Sci 1993;305:318–320.

Spier SJ, Carlson GP, Harrold D, et al: Genetic study of hyperkalemic periodic paralysis in horses. J Am Vet Med Assoc 1993;202:933–938.

Valazquez H, Perazella MA, Wright FS, et al: Renal mechanism of trimethoprim-induced hyperkalemia. Ann Intern Med 1993;119:296–301.

Weiss DJ, Geor R, Smith CM, et al: Furosemide-induced electrolyte depletion associated with echinocytosis in horses. Am J Vet Res 1992;53:1769–1772.

Whitehair KJ, Haskins SC, Whitehair JG, et al: Clinical applications of quantitative acid-base chemistry. J Vet Intern Med 1995;9:1–11.

Willard MD, Fossum TW, Torrence A, et al: Hyponatremia and hyperkalemia associated with idiopathic or experimentally induced chylothorax in four dogs. J Am Vet Med Assoc 1991;199:353–358.

12

Examination of Cerebrospinal Fluid

Cerebrospinal fluid (CSF) is a clear, colorless ultrafiltrate of the plasma which bathes the exterior of the brain and spinal cord. Pathology of the outer surfaces of these structures may cause changes in the CSF whereas pathologic changes deeper in the nervous tissue usually do not. Evaluation of the CSF minimally should include a nucleated cell count, cytologic examination, and protein determination. Other biochemical measurements which can be performed include glucose, creatine kinase, lactic dehydrogenase, protein electrophoresis, and specific immunoglobulin quantification. These measurements are usually restricted to use by clinical investigators at this time.

There are certain visually recognizable changes in the CSF. Turbidity implies abnormal numbers of nucleated cells (pleocytosis). A pink to red color indicates the presence of erythrocytes, and a yellow discoloration (xanthochromia) suggests the prior (days to weeks) presence of erythrocytes (hemorrhage) in the nonicteric patient.

ENUMERATION AND DIFFERENTIAL OF NUCLEATED CELLS

The normal CSF is devoid of erythrocytes and contains less than five to eight nucleated cells per microliter. Because of the low cell numbers, counts cannot be done on an automated counter but must be performed by directly loading a hemacytometer. The condenser of the microscope should be lowered to enhance the silhouette of the cells and aid in differentiating erythrocytes (anuclear with irregular, crenated surface) and nucleated cells. The cells in the nine large squares of the Neubauer-ruled chamber are counted and the nucleated and erythrocyte counts each multiplied by 10/9 to yield the cell number per microliter.

The microscopic examination of the cellular component must be performed soon after collection (preferably within 1 hour) to avoid the artifact of cell deterioration. Refrigeration (4° C) of the specimen will delay cell deterioration by several hours. All CSF specimens should be examined cytologically even if the total nucleated cell number is normal. A concentration procedure is necessary so that sufficient nucleated cells are present for cytologic examination. The use of a cytocentrifuge provides a cell preparation of uniform quality with good preservation of cell morphology. Although the expense of the equipment limits its widespread availability in veterinary practices, most medical facilities and commercial laboratories have a unit. Simplified sedimentation chambers have been adapted for use with CSF for economic reasons. These concentration methods can provide adequate cell preparations for those experienced with the procedure. Membrane filtration techniques also yield acceptable cytologic preparations, but special training or prior experience is recommended.

Cell Types

Small to medium mononuclear (mature lymphocytes and monocytoid cells) monopolize the normal CSF microscopically. A lymphoplasmacytic pleocytosis is associated with certain viral infections and granulomatous meningoencephalitis. Macrophages may also be prominent in the latter pathologic process. A neutrophilic pleocytosis is most frequently associated with septic and certain sterile inflammatory processes. Suppurative, nonseptic disorders include immune-mediated disease, rickettsial infection, feline infectious peritonitis, cryptococcosis, trauma and myelographic procedures, and neoplasia (which have not exfoliated cells into the CSF). Lymphoma is the most commonly diagnosed neoplasm of the central nervous system cytologically. Much less frequently other types of neoplastic cells, often associated with metastatic lesions, are detected. Occasionally small clumps of epithelial-like cells will exfoliate from the choroid plexus and ependymal lining. These uniform cell clusters should not be confused with neoplastic cells.

BIOCHEMICAL DETERMINATIONS

Protein

Quantification of the total protein requires a dye-binding or turbidimetric procedure because of the small, milligram concentrations normally present. The reference range for normal values varies depending on the procedure used, usually it is less than 20 mg/dL (200 mg/L) or less than 40 mg/dL (400 mg/L). It is essential to know the normal range for the laboratory use. A urine reagent strip may be used to get a rapid estimate of the protein concentration. A 1+ to 3+ relates to a mild to marked protein increase, respectively. A simple precipitation procedure, the Pandy test, which is selective for globulins, may also be used in a practice setting. Three to four drops of CFS are mixed with 1.0 mL of Pandy reagent (1.0 g of carbolic acid crystals [phenol] in 10 mL of distilled water) and the degree of precipitation (cloudiness) graded from slight to marked. Increased protein concentrations are associated with a variety of pathologic processes, with or without pleocytosis.

Glucose

The glucose concentration of CSF is 60 to 80% of plasma and may be measured by the same methodology. Hypoglycorrhachia, low CSF glucose, may be associated with hypoglycemia or bacterial meningitis.

Suppurative *Versus* Nonsuppurative Disease

Examination of the CSF is an adjunct to the neurologic examination and should minimally include a nucleated cell count, cytologic evaluation, and determination of the protein concentration. A positive finding may assist in the differential diagnostic considerations, especially between nonsuppurative and suppurative conditions. The latter often show fever, cervical rigidity, and vertebral pain.

A sterile, suppurative, corticosteroid-responsive meningitis appears to be a relatively common disease in large, young adult dogs. Certainly the observation of bacteria dictates a septic meningitis and the need for antibiotic treatment.

Neutrophils predominate (with occasional eosinophils) in the CSF infected with *Cryptococcus neoformans*. The organisms are recognized readily. A prominent eosinophilic pleocytosis has been described in young to young adult dogs, the golden retriever apparently overrepresented. An etiology was not determined. Eosinophils also predominate in central nervous system infections with *Toxoplasma gondii* and *Neospora caninum*. Serologic titers should be measured for these agents.

Granulomatous Meningoencephalitis

In granulomatous meningoencephalitis the protein is increased, and lymphocytes, monocytes, and macrophages predominate with lesser numbers of neutrophils and plasma cells. Affected dogs are commonly young adult small breeds with an acute onset in the disseminated form and a more insidious onset in the focal form. Clinical signs reflect the form present, head signs that progress to signs reflecting involvement of the caudal fossa as well as changes in mental status.

Canine Distemper

Young, unvaccinated dogs are common candidates for distemper. The disease is usually multisystemic with progressive multifocal central nervous system involvement. Older dogs may develop a more insidious form with gradual loss of mentation and progressive posterior paresis. Changes in the CSF, when present, include an increase in protein and slight lymphocytic pleocytosis.

Rickettsial Infections

Rickettsial infections may also involve the central nervous system. The dogs usually show systemic signs of illness, a nonregenerative anemia and thrombocytopenia, and a neutropenia (ehrlichiosis) or neutrophilia (Rocky Mountain spotted fever). A lymphocytic pleocytosis may be noted. Serologic titers are required to confirm the diagnosis.

Feline Infectious Peritonitis

In this disease the protein is markedly increased, and neutrophils and monocytes/macrophages predominate.

Neoplasia

Dogs with brain tumors may show an increased protein with normal to mild pleocytosis with variable cell types.

Disc Disease

Dogs with intervertebral disc disease have normal CSF and radiographic findings.

Additional Reading

Bailey CS, Higgins RJ: Comparison of total white blood cell count and total protein content of lumbar and cisternal cerebrospinal fluid of healthy dogs. Am J Vet Res 1985;46:1161–1165.

Bailey CS, Higgins RJ: Characteristics of cisternal cerebrospinal fluid associated with primary brain tumors in the dog: A retrospective study. J Am Vet Med Assoc 1986; 188:414–417.

Furr MO, Bender H: Cerebrospinal fluid variables in clinically normal foals from birth to 42 days of age. Am J Vet Res 1994;55:781–784.

Green EM, Constantinescu GM, Kroll RA: Equine cerebrospinal fluid: Physiologic principles and collection techniques. Contin Educ Pract Vet 1992;14:229–238.

Jamison EM, Lumsden JH: Cerebrospinal fluid analysis in the dog. Methodology and interpretation. Semin Vet Med Surg 1988;3:122–132.

Lane SB, Kornegay JN, Duncan JR, et al: Feline spinal lymphosarcoma: A retrospective evaluation of 23 cats. J Vet Intern Med 1994;8:99–104.

Rand JS, Parent J, Jacobs R, et al: Reference intervals for feline cerebrospinal fluid: Cell counts and cytologic features. Am J Vet Res 1990;51:1044–1048.

Rand JS, Parent J, Jacobs R, et al: Reference intervals for feline cerebrospinal fluid: Biochemical and serologic variables, IgG concentration, and electrophoretic fractionation. Am J Vet Res 1990;51:1049–1054.

Rand JS, Parent J, Percy D, et al: Clinical, cerebrospinal fluid, and histological data from twenty-seven cats with primary inflammatory disease of the central nervous system. Can Vet J 1994;35:103–110.

Rand JS, Parent J, Percy D, et al: Clinical, cerebrospinal fluid, and histological data from thirty-four cats with primary noninflammatory disease of the central nervous system. Can Vet J 1994;35:174–181.

Smith-Maxie LL, Parent JP, Rand J, et al: Cerebrospinal fluid analysis and clinical outcome of eight dogs with eosinophilic meningoencephalitis. J Vet Int Med 1989; 3:167–174.

Vandevelde M, Spano JS: Cerebrospinal fluid cytology in canine neurologic disease. Am J Vet Res 1977;38:1827–1832.

Welles EG, Tyler JW, Sorjonen DC, et al: Composition and analysis of cerebrospinal fluid in clinically normal adult cattle. Am J Vet Res 1992;53:2050–2056.

Widner WR, DeNicola DB, Blevens WE, et al: Cerebrospinal fluid changes after iopamidol and metrizamide myelography in clinically normal dogs. Am J Vet Res 1992;53:396–401.

13

Evaluation of Effusions

Pleural, Peritoneal, Pericardial*

Evaluation of body cavity fluids is often diagnostically rewarding. It may provide an etiologic diagnosis or a general classification of the underlying disorder.

CELLULAR EVALUATION

Collection of fluid is usually done using a 20- to 22-gauge needle and a 10- to 12-mL syringe. After surgical preparation of the skin, the needle with syringe attached is placed into the subcutaneous tissue and slight negative pressure applied as the needle is advanced at an angle. Fluid will appear in the syringe as soon as the needle penetrates the lining of the cavity. Angling the needle helps prevent fluid from potentially leaking from the cavity into the surrounding tissue. A small drop of fluid is layered thinly on a glass slide. About three fourths of the way down the slide any excess fluid is *left on* the slide and allowed to *flow back* and dried with a hair blower. Such a two-part slide provides for an estimate of the cell count from the thin area, and the concentrated area can be searched for cell clumps or organisms. The remaining fluid should be placed in an EDTA tube (purple top) to prevent any potential clotting and the fluid used for cell counts and other biochemical parameters that may need to be determined at a later date.

TRANSUDATES AND EXUDATES

Analysis of fluid in the pericardial, pleural, and peritoneal cavities includes the measurement of certain physiochemical properties and a description of cells present on stained smears. Evaluation of the cell component includes an absolute and differential nucleated cell count. Fluids with very low cell counts are concentrated by routine centrifugation or with a cytocentrifuge. Fluids are generally classified as a transudate, modified transudate, or an exudate. Special classifications will be noted (Table 13–1).

---

*See Algorithm 20.

TABLE 13–1. Guidelines for Characterizing Effusions Other Than Hemorrhagic

	Transudate	Modified Transudate	Exudate
Total protein (g/dL)	<2.5	>2.5	>2.5
Nucleated cell count/μL	<1000	<5000	>5000
Horse	<5000	<10,000	>10,000
Predominant nucleated cell type	Mesothelial/ macrophage	Mesothelial/ macrophage	Neutrophil/ macrophage
Horse	Up to 60% may be neutrophils	Up to 60% may be neutrophils	>60% are neutrophils
More common causes	Portal hypertension secondary to liver insufficiency	Ascites secondary to right-sided cardiac insufficiency	Inflammatory Septic Nonseptic
	Severe hypoalbuminemia	Intestinal disorder (equine)	Intestinal disorder (equine)

Transudates

Transudates are characterized by a protein concentration that is *less than 2.5 g/dL*, and *modified transudates* are characterized by a protein concentration *greater than 2.5 g/dL* (25 g/L), an important biochemical parameter to measure. The transudate and modified transudate have low nucleated cell counts, the predominant cell type is the large mononuclear cell (mesothelial cells). The mesothelial cell may be either the reactive form or the macrophage type.

The pathophysiologic event leading to the formation of a transudate or modified transudate *ascitic fluid* can be related to an increase in the hydrostatic pressure, a decrease in the oncotic, or an alteration in the integrity of the vascular wall (Fig. 13–1). Knowledge of the difference in protein concentration in the different locations of the lymphatic system is helpful in linking a transudate or modified transudate to the pathophysiologic event responsible for its formation. The lymph vessels within the hepatic parenchyma have a relatively *high protein lymph*. The lymphatic vessels associated with the intestinal tract have a relatively *low-protein lymph* (Fig. 13–2). A disease process that involves area 1 (in Fig. 13–2) will cause hepatic congestion and

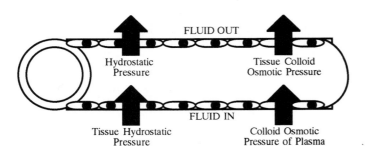

FIGURE 13–1. Diagram of a capillary.

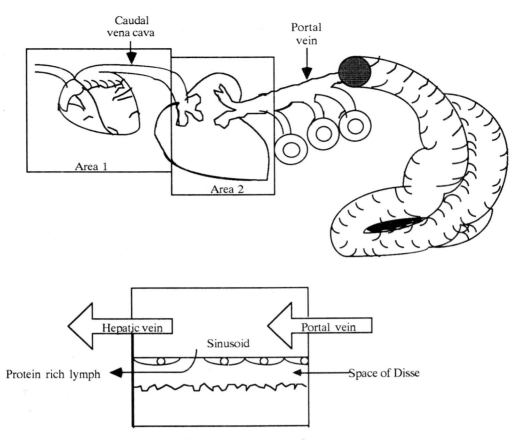

FIGURE 13–2. Normal vascular and lymphatic drainage of the abdominal cavity. *Bottom section* shows microscopic view of sinusoidal blood flow and lymph formation. (From Greene CE: Diagnostic and therapeutic considerations. Comp Contin Educ Small Anim Pract 1979;1:712–719, with permission.)

leakage of the high-protein lymph from the hepatic parenchyma into the abdominal cavity. This will result in a *modified transudate*. The most common cause is right-sided heart failure. A less common cause is lesions that constrict the caudal vena cava. The important point to remember is that when an ascites is classified as a modified transudate one should direct diagnostic efforts toward area 1. Modified transudates may also occur in association with a sterile inflammation.

The portal circulation drains the entire gastrointestinal tract and delivers the blood to the liver by the porta hepatis. A disease process that interferes with the blood flow through or to the liver will cause *portal hypertension* and leakage of low-protein lymph into the abdominal cavity, yielding a *transudate*. The most common pathology involving area 2 (in Fig. 13–2) which results in portal hypertension is hepatic cirrhosis. A less common cause is a constrictive lesion at the porta hepatis where the portal vessels enter the liver. Once again the important point to remember is that when an ascites is classified as a transudate the differential diagnostic focus should be toward area 2. Severe hypoalbuminemia (1.0 g/dL [10 g/L]) can also predispose to the formation of an ascitic transudate without the presence of portal hypertension.

Exudates

An exudate is characterized by a protein concentration of greater than 3.0 g/dL (30 g/L) and an increased nucleated cell count composed primarily of *neutrophils* with lesser numbers of macrophages and lymphocytes. Infectious and noninfectious inflammatory causes of an exudate may be distinguished usually by the microscopic examination and biochemical determinations. *Septic exudates* are defined by the identification of bacteria in the fluid. Some bacteria contain potent toxins which cause neutrophils to undergo nuclear karyolysis giving the nuclei a mushy (unhappy) appearance. When these neutrophils are identified in an exudate, an extensive search for bacteria should be made using the oil objective. The neutrophil and not the macrophage is the primary cell involved in phagocytosis of bacteria. Consequently, microscopic examination of neutrophils is the preferential cell when looking for bacteria.

Feline infectious peritonitis (FIP) is one example of a nonseptic exudate that can involve the pleural or peritoneal cavities. Immune complex deposition within vessels causes two pathophysiologic events to occur: (1) altered vascular permeability, allowing protein to leak into the fluid; and (2) neutrophil chemotaxis. This results in an exudate with a particularly high protein concentration, sometimes becoming close to that of the plasma, and numerous numbers of "happy" neutrophils with lesser numbers of macrophages present. *Electrophoresis* of effusions resulting from FIP virus infection reveals that globulins predominate. An A:G ratio of less than 0.81 in an *effusion* from a cat is highly suggestive of FIP virus infection and may be used to supplement the cytologic examination.

Irritant substances may also cause a *nonseptic exudate*. Examples include bile from a ruptured gallbladder and urine from a ruptured urinary bladder. An irritant process may initially cause an effusion with a protein that is less than 2.5 g/dL (25 g/L) but with increased cell numbers comprised predominantly of neutrophils. This type of *modified transudate* should direct one's thinking toward an irritant process as discussed previously. We have also seen this type of effusion in association with *neoplasia* within the cavity.

EQUINE ABDOMINAL FLUID

The normal equine abdominal fluid is different from that of the dog and cat with regard to the normal total nucleated cell counts and the differential cell types. This takes on diagnostic importance when evaluating the equine patient for abdominal disorders. The nucleated cell count is approximately 5000/μL although some report up to 9000 nucleated cells/μL as normal. The most important difference from a diagnostic standpoint is that the *neutrophil* may comprise up to 60% of the nucleated cells. This physiologic phenomenon creates increased diagnostic frustration when examining equine abdominal fluid. Total cell numbers as well as neutrophil morphology take on greater importance when evaluating equine abdominal fluid (see Table 13–1).

OPAQUE EFFUSIONS

White opaque fluid initially conjures a differential diagnosis of a chylous effusion. However, other types of effusion may have a similar physical appearance, emphasizing the importance of appropriately examining the fluid.

A *chylous effusion* (peritoneal or pleural) is associated with a ruptured thoracic duct and reflects its components, that is, triglyceride-rich chylomicrons and small to medium lymphocytes. This type of fluid is very irritating to the serosal surface, and within days to weeks increased exfoliation of mesothelial cells and an influx of neutrophils may even give the effusion an exudative appearance. The reader should also remember that lipid will cause the total protein on the refractometer to appear *factitiously* increased, and one could be misled into suspecting an inflammatory exudate. Therefore in the differential approach to a fluid that is suspected of being a chylous effusion the determination of the triglyceride concentration becomes critical. A specimen of the fluid and of the serum from the patient can be sent to a commercial laboratory for a quantitative triglyceride determination. A fluid value that is greater than the serum triglyceride concentration is supportive of a diagnosis of a chylous effusion. Any fluid for which an etiology cannot be determined or, in case of pleural effusions, recurs after symptomatic management should be examined for triglyceride concentration. It should be emphasized that in a patient who is not eating, the amount of chylomicrons being generated will be decreased and will result in a lower triglyceride value in the effusion. Consequently it is best to obtain a specimen after an animal has had a meal if the value obtained in the fluid is very close to that in the serum.

Lymphosarcoma involving the body cavity may also have an opaque fluid associated with it. Microscopic examination will reveal that the predominant cell type is a medium to large, sometimes blastic appearing lymphocyte characteristic of a lymphoid neoplasm. Since the neoplastic process may involve the lymphatic system it is not surprising that occasionally a chylous effusion may develop coincidentally.

Lastly, an opaque pleural effusion has been described in cats with *congestive cardiomyopathy*. The cell types include macrophages, small lymphocytes, and occasionally neutrophils; however, the triglyceride concentration of these fluids is less than serum, indicating a nonchylous effusion. In these patients the next diagnostic approach would be the echocardiographic examination of the heart.

Tests such as fat stains (Sudan) and ether clearance of effusions have not been discussed because they are unreliable in the differential diagnosis of chylous effusions.

NEOPLASTIC EFFUSIONS

Occasionally the microscopic examination of an effusion will reveal cell types that are not normally present in an effusion. The neoplastic cell types most commonly associated with effusion are lymphosarcoma and carcinomas because of their ease of exfoliation. Exfoliation of reactive mesothelial cells in response to an irritation may be dramatic enough to cause confusion with neoplastic carcinoma cells. There are no simple guidelines for separating these confusing cell types, and the clinician is encouraged to submit these slides to a clinical pathologist for examination.

PERICARDIAL EFFUSIONS

Pericardial effusions are evaluated in the same way as are pleural or peritoneal fluids. Most pericardial effusions are bloody and contain a relatively small number of nucleated cells. It has been our experience that the cytologic evaluation of these effusions is of limited value in distinguishing between the two more common causes in the dog: neoplasia (hemangiosarcoma, heart-base tumor) and idiopathic. The cytologic examination of a "buffy-coat" prepared smear is a simple way to concentrate the nucleated cells and separate them from the blood. Determination of the pH of the fluid using a reagent strip appears to be diagnostically helpful. A pH greater than 7.0 is supportive of neoplasia and a pH less than 7.0 is more commonly associated with a benign cause.

CELLS COMMONLY SEEN IN EFFUSIONS

Mesothelial cells comprise the serious lining of the pericardial, pleural, and peritoneal cavities. Their size is variable, but their morphology is similar. They are observed singly or in hyperplastic clumps. The cell is usually oval to round; the diameter is 10 to 30 μm. The cytoplasm is basophilic without vacuoles or phagocytized material. The centrally located nucleus is round, has a prominent nuclear membrane, fine dark purple chromatic pattern, and one or two blue nucleoli. Classically the reactive mesothelial has an eosinophilic villous-like cytoplasmic membrane border, a sun burst effect. Binucleated and multinucleated forms are normally observed. Occasional mitotic figures are seen.

At the slightest irritation the mesothelial cells undergo hyperplasia and exfoliate readily. The cells enlarge and pseudogranular structures or rosettes can be observed. These reactive or basophilic mesothelial cells subsequently undergo morphologic changes reflected as vacuolization in gray-blue cytoplasm. The cytoplasm may contain numerous pink-staining granules. The nuclei stain pale, and the chromatin is more coarse.

The *pale mesothelial cells* derived from basophilic mesothelial cells have lightly basophilic abundant cytoplasm with varying degrees of vacuolization. The cytoplasm may contain pink-staining granules which at times may be very prominent. These cells are usually observed as singles or in small clusters. Similar cell types may be observed with ingested neutrophils and amorphous debris and are referred to as *macrophages*.

Additional Reading

Edwards NJ: The diagnostic value of pericardial fluid pH determination. J Am Anim Hosp Assoc 1996;32:63–67.

14

Examination of Synovial Fluid*

The cytologic examination of synovial fluid can provide clinically useful information for the identification of a number of joint disorders. Indications for obtaining synovial fluid include: (1) a swollen hot joint suggestive of an infective process; (2) radiographic findings suggestive of a degenerative joint process and a synovial fluid analysis is obtained to rule out a concomitant inflammatory process; and (3) *polyarthritis* in which the patient has a history of nondescript pain, short choppy gait, or rotating leg lameness. In this last group of disorders multiple joints are frequently involved, and synovial fluid from the carpal joint will usually reflect the inflammatory process in the other joints.

SAMPLE COLLECTION AND EVALUATION

Synovial fluid is obtained using a 23- to 25-gauge needle attached to a 3-mL syringe. The procedure is not painful. The area over the joint is clipped and surgically prepared, and the leg is alternatively flexed and extended as the joint surface is palpated until a soft spot is located. The soft part is entered with the needle, and a few drops of synovial fluid are gently aspirated. In a patient with an inflammatory process it may be possible to remove as much as 0.5 to 1.0 mL of fluid. The suction is released, the needle removed, and the specimen is used to prepare at least two slides for cytologic examination. Cytology preparations are made in the same fashion as blood films for differential counts except that the spreader slide is drawn *slowly* into the drop of fluid on the slide, the fluid is allowed to spread, and the spreader slide is moved *slowly* away from the drop. The fluid should not go off the end of the slide. The slide is air dried and, if to be analyzed in the practice, it is stained using a polychromic stain. If the slide is to be forwarded to an outside laboratory it should be dried but not stained. Care should be taken to make sure that the cytologic preparation is not too thick. Cells are difficult to eval-

---

*See Algorithm 21.

uate on thick specimens as the nuclei are rounded up, making a differential count difficult.

After the slides have been prepared, some of the remaining synovial fluid can be added to a *purple*-top tube for cell counts. If possible, several drops should be left in the sterile syringe, capped and saved for possible bacterial culture if the cytologic examination suggests an infectious process. Even if bacteria are seen, the fluid culture may be negative. If the neutrophils have been effective, ingested bacteria may be dead. Cytologic examination takes precedence over culture, and culture takes precedence over a cell count (an optional request).

The first decision to be made is whether the synovial fluid is normal or abnormal. Synovial fluid is low in cellularity (<3000 cells/μL) and usually has a lightly granular slightly eosinophilic background with small to medium mononuclear cells. These cells have a round to oval nucleus and a rim of pale blue cytoplasm. The presence of other cell types is abnormal.

Having identified an abnormal synovial fluid, the next procedure is to decide whether the fluid is inflammatory or noninflammatory. Noninflammatory disorders include hemarthrosis (hemorrhage into the joint) and degenerative joint disease.

NONINFLAMMATORY DISORDERS

Hemarthrosis is associated with trauma (which should be in the history) or coagulation deficiencies (usually found in young animals) and in patients with warfarin intoxication. Finding blood in a joint should prompt a reevaluation of the history, and a coagulation panel is indicated.

Blood can be aspirated as a contaminant during the procedure. This is suggested when clear fluid is obtained initially and then blood appears in the specimen. In such cases erythrocytes and neutrophils are present in approximately the same proportion as in peripheral blood.

Degenerative joint diseases have synovial fluid that contains macrophages with none to very few neutrophils. Macrophages are larger than the normal mononuclear cells and have a vacuolated cytoplasm and a coarse-appearing nucleus. Eosinophilic granules may be noted in the cytoplasm.

INFLAMMATORY DISORDERS

Inflammatory joint diseases are characterized by the presence of many neutrophils.

Septic arthritis is suspected if neutrophils are identified. In this case they should be examined with the oil immersion objective to look for bacteria. Some neutrophils may have a mushy chromatin. These are "unhappy" neutrophils, highly suggestive of a bacterial etiology. If such cells are identified it is prudent to submit any remaining fluid for microbiologic examination.

Nonseptic arthritis (immune mediated) is characterized by an increased number of "happy" neutrophils with a clumped chromatin, a clear cytoplasm, and no evidence of bacteria. If the inflammation has been present for some time, days to weeks, macrophages and erythrocytes may be present. When blood is present, evidence of inflammation is suggested by comparing the number of neutrophils per number of erythrocytes. If the red blood cells (RBCs) are a contaminant caused by hemorrhage during collection and the patient has a normal peripheral blood leukocyte count, the neutrophils present in the synovial fluid will be in a ratio of 1 white blood cell (WBC) for every 750 RBC. If the patient has a leukocytosis then we allow about 1 WBC for every 250 RBC. If the WBC number exceeds this ratio it indicates an increase in the WBC count in synovial fluid in addition to the presence of blood.

Nonseptic (poly)arthritis is often *idiopathic*; however, other known associated causes should be ruled out. Drugs such as trimethoprim/sulfamethoxazole will produce a nonspecific arthritis. It is thought that the sulfa component stimulates an immune-mediated process. Nonseptic arthritis is a common clinical sign of the uncommon immune-mediated disease lupus erythematosus. Patients suspected of lupus can be screened by use of an antinuclear antibody assay (ANA) (see Case 7–6). A strongly positive ANA titer is supportive of lupus. It must be remembered that lupus is a multiorgan disorder, and other organs should be evaluated for disease. For example, a marked proteinuria suggests glomerulonephritis, and hematologic aberrations such as hemolytic anemia and immune-mediated thrombocytopenia may also complicate the disease. Lupus erythematosus (LE) cells may be found in the synovial fluid of patients with systemic lupus erythematosus. These are neutrophils that contain an amorphous lump of protein. Although their presence is not common, if present they are diagnostic for lupus.

Erosive polyarthritis synovial fluid contains numerous "happy" neutrophils, and when the joints are examined radiologically there are erosive, proliferative lesions present. This immune-mediated disease is uncommon and can be verified by biopsy of the synovial membrane.

Patients with rickettsial or *Borellia* infections can be included under both noninfectious and infectious categories because cytologically when these organisms induce a polyarthritis the neutrophils are "happy." It is virtually impossible to identify any organisms in the specimen. If these infectious agents are endemic in one's geographic area, serologic tests can be used to aid in identifying the infection in the differential diagnosis of suppurative polyarthritis.

Bacterial arthritides have synovial fluid that contains few to many mushy neutrophils, and occasionally bacteria can be seen in the cytoplasm.

15

The Microscopic Examination of Tissue Specimens Obtained with Fine-Needle Aspiration Biopsy

Dr. Watson: *"And yet I believe my eyes are as good as yours."*
Sherlock Holmes: *"Quite so. You see but do not observe. The distinction is quite clear."*
—A. Conan Doyle, *Scandal in Bohemia*

The microscopic examination of the cytologic specimen is a valuable, simple, pragmatic, and financially rewarding test in veterinary medicine. The fact that it was proactively applied as a clinically useful diagnostic tool in veterinary medicine earlier than in the medical profession in this country is an endorsement of its perceived value. The popularity of cytology continues to increase due to the increased application of ultrasonography for the examination of internal organs and the availability of educational seminars. Fine-needle aspiration biopsy provides an opportunity for the aspirator to also be the interpreter. This maximizes the link between the historical information and findings on the physical examination to the interpretation of the cytologic specimen. It permits an immediate triage of the specimen to determine adequacy of the specimen and can provide immediate diagnostic information. This chapter will focus on the value and limitations of cytology for the differential diagnosis of inflammatory disorders and neoplasia.

THE MICROSCOPE AND OBJECTIVES

It is desirable to have a minimum of two microscopes in a clinical setting. A high-quality microscope is dedicated to the examination of "clean" specimens (hematology and cytology) and another of lesser quality is used for the evaluation of "dirty" specimens (fecal parasite and skin scraping examinations). The "dirty" specimens can be adequately scanned with a 10× objective and examined more closely with a 20× objective. The latter will identify most infectious agents in these types of specimens. Planachromat objectives are the recommended appendage for the high-quality microscope. The combination of 20× and 50× oil objectives are "user friendly" for most clinical applications pertaining to hematology and cytology. They permit a meaningful scan of the slide and obviate the need for cover-slipping which is required for the 40× (high-dry) objective. Inadvertent "dragging" of the 40× objective through the immersion oil is a common reason for "out of focus" appearance of specimens and contributes to the early demise of the objective. The addition of a 100× (oil) objective amplifies the ability to recognize microorganisms such as bacteria, *Hemobartonella* sp., and *Ehrlichia* sp. The 20× objective facilitates an efficient determination of the differential leukocyte count on the blood film and the recognition of the predominant cell type comprising cytologic specimens. Problematic cell types can be subsequently interrogated by the use of the higher power objective. Microscopic alignment and adjustment of the condensing system should be performed on an annual basis for maximizing the optical value of the microscope.

MANAGEMENT OF THE SPECIMEN

The quintessence of cytology can be fully appreciated only with an adequate sample that is properly prepared. The dictum "garbage in, garbage out" is well applied to the preparation of the cytology specimen. Acquisition and management of the specimen is an "art" that must be practiced like any other skill and technique. Hepatic and lymphoid tissue exfoliate easily and make excellent tissues in support of this process.

Obtaining the Specimen and Slide Preparation

The full value of the microscopic examination of cytologic specimen cannot be realized unless it is used frequently in the decision-making process in contrast to continually trying to decide when to use it. In general, body cavity fluids, cutaneous and subcutaneous masses, lymph nodes, and diffuse organomegaly lend themselves to fine-needle aspiration biopsy. Recommendations for needle and syringe sizes vary and usually reflect personal preference; use what works for you. A 20- to 22-gauge, 1-inch needle and a 6- to 12-cc syringe are useful combinations for obtaining many of these specimens. The needle and syringe can be connected with a Silastic tube used for the administration of intravenous fluids to provide greater flexibility and accommodate unexpected patient movement. A 2½-inch, 22-gauge spinal needle with stylet can be used for sampling internal organs. When using a spinal needle, the stylet is removed after the organ of interest is penetrated, a syringe attached, and suction applied. As with other aspiration techniques, the suction is gently relieved *before* the needle is removed from the tissue.

Aspiration is not always necessary for obtaining a cytologic specimen from certain tissues. A technique that is based on the principle of capillarity, referred to as "fine-needle capillary sampling," is performed by placement of a needle into the lesion without syringe attached. Cells are displaced into the cylinder of the needle by capillary action. The technique has been successfully applied to the diagnosis of cutaneous mast cell tumors and to lymph nodes for the diagnosis of lymphoma. One has the option of subsequently performing the suction technique if the initial specimen is nondiagnostic. It has the advantage of minimizing blood contamination and possibly reducing the risk of cell breakage.

To expel the specimen from the needle with either technique it may be necessary to remove the needle from the syringe, aspirate 1 to 2 cc of air into the syringe, replace the needle (while holding the tip of the needle over the glass slide), and *gently* express the specimen. Multiple slide preparations should be made when possible.

The risks associated with fine-needle aspiration biopsy include rupture of an encapsulated inflammatory process, dissemination of an infectious agent, "seeding" of neoplastic cells in the needle tract, and hemorrhage. Each risk factor must be weighed against the benefits of diagnosis and the impact on the long-term outcome of the disease process. It is probable that neoplastic cells are displaced into unaffected tissue with relative frequency during fine-needle aspiration biopsy. Clinical studies indicate that neoplastic implants are uncommon, probably as a consequence of cytotoxic mechanisms associated with the immune system and other related inflammatory response. However, despite the low risk, it is prudent to locate the needle track in the field of anticipated surgery so that it is removed along with the lesion. Similarly, when investigating a suspected infectious process involving an internal organ, surgical readiness is advisable.

The microscopic examination of a cytologic specimen of an effusion is an important test in its differential diagnosis. All specimens should be placed in an EDTA tube to prevent possible clot formation. Since cellularity varies tremendously in these specimens, both direct and sedimentation preparations should be made routinely. A conical-tipped plastic tube is ideally suited for obtaining a "cell pellet" with centrifugation. The same recommendation is made for specimens obtained by bronchoalveolar washings/lavages and urine specimens. Cytocentrifuges are available that provide concentrated cell preparations of fluids that are low in cellularity. They are cost-effective in support of high-volume use and are highly recommended for making slide preparations from cerebrospinal fluids. Several direct slide preparations should always accompany fluids that are submitted to an outside laboratory should the question of artifact arise. It is paramount that when making a direct slide preparation from a fluid specimen *all* the fluid used for making the preparation remains on the slide. The excess fluid may contain diagnostic clumps of cells that are discarded into the garbage if dragged off the end of the slide; referred to as the "edge-of-the-cliff" phenomenon. The spreader (pusher) slide should be stopped approximately 1 cm (½ inch) from the end of the specimen slide and the excess fluid allowed to flow backwards slightly (towards the start point) and allowed to dry. This technique also serves to concentrate cells in hypocellular fluids. A small hair dryer mounted on a stand facilitates the drying process, especially in geographic locations with high humidity.

Cytologic slide preparations of fluids that have a very low protein concentration (*e.g.*, transudates, cerebrospinal fluids, urine) are problematic because the cells tend to be washed off during the staining process. "Special" slides can be prepared for these types of cytologic specimens. Serum, harvested from a clotted blood specimen, is used to thinly coat a number of glass slides. Once dry, they can be used immediately or they can be labeled as serum-coated, placed in an appropriate slide-holding container (a plastic slide holder with a snapping lid is ideal), and stored in the freezer until needed. Subsequent to their removal from the freezer, the slides must be completely dry before the cytologic specimen is applied. If not, the hypotonic water condensation will lyse the cells. Because serum is a great medium for bacterial growth, one of the stored slides should be occasionally stained and examined if not used for several months.

Staining the Specimen

The staining process also requires a certain degree of "art and practice." One of the most common problems encountered in cytology is an understained specimen that is not recognized by the interpreter to be understained. This is especially true for the thicker preparations such as aspirates from lymph nodes, liver, and bone marrow. A combination of circumstances contributes to the staining deficiency. These include inadequate exposure to the staining solutions, dilution and weakening of the solutions over time, and cytologic preparations that simply are too thick. The marketing dictum "one size fits all" does not apply to the use of Romanowsky-type stains such as Diff-Quik (Baxter Scientific Products, McGraw Park, IL), *i.e.*, five dips in each solution "fits" all cytologic specimens. Modifications to the staining process are found in Table 15–1. The length of time for "dipping" in each of the solutions depends on the age of the stain and the cellularity (thickness) of the sample. The active process of "dipping" ensures exposure of the specimen to stain. Short times are adequate for hypocellular samples that have a

TABLE 15–1. Suggested Procedure for Staining Cytologic Specimens Using Diff-Quik Solutions[a,b]

Fixative: 60 to 120 seconds
Solution 1: 30 to 60 seconds
Solution 2: 5 to 60 seconds[c]
Rinse under cold tap water: 15 seconds
Examine staining adequacy using low power; eosinophilia or basophilia can be enhanced by returning to solution 1 or solution 2, respectively, followed by a rinse.
Air dry and examine

[a]Modified from Henry MJ, Burton LG, Stanley MW, Horwitz CA: Application of a modified Diff-Quik stain to fine needle aspiration smears: Rapid staining with improved cytologic detail. Acta Cytol 1987; 31:954–955, with permission.
[b]Suggested times are based on fresh stains; with time and use the stains weaken and longer times will be required. Consistently understained specimens are an indication for replenishing with fresh stain.
[c]The shortest times are suggested for hypocellular fluids that are low in protein such as transudates, cerebral spinal fluids, and urine sediments.

low protein content such as transudates while longer times are required for thick specimens. Adequate fixation of thick specimens prior to staining is important; specimens cannot be overfixed. Subsequent to staining, the preparation is washed with cold running tap water for at least 15 seconds to remove excess stain and debris. The slide is air-dried and examined with the 20× objective. Understained specimens can be placed in either solution 1 and/or 2 again. An overstained specimen can be tempered by dipping in the fixative several times, although the staining quality sometimes appears to be altered. Diff-Quik has an inherent tendency to overstain nuclear chromatin or accentuate nucleoli compared to a Wright-stained or Wright-Giemsa–stained specimen. This can be problematic for certain specimens such as bone marrow.

Sample Shipment and Identification

The glass slides must be protected by rigid plastic or Styrofoam containers when shipping or mailing. The flat cardboard or plastic slide containers that generally hold two slides are definitely not acceptable for mailing specimens. Cytology slide preparations should never be placed in the same shipping container as formalin-fixed tissues. In fact, making a cytology preparation in the same room as an open formalin container can cause sufficient cell damage to violate the diagnostic integrity of the specimen. The exposure to formalin fumes causes nucleated cell types to stain a bland, indiscriminate bluish color with indistinct cellular detail. Erythrocytes often appear greenish blue.

Glass slides with a "frosted" end should be used for all cytologic preparations. The names of the owner and patient and/or the case number and the date are placed on the frosted section using a pencil, never a felt-tipped pen. The signalment, the aspiration site, and history associated with the lesion should be included on the submission form. It is rare to hear a pathologist complain that too much information is provided with specimens. Once the reported findings are reviewed by the clinician, a subsequent phone conversation with the pathologist that provides missing or new information can sometimes facilitate a more conclusive interpretation.

EXAMINATION AND CLASSIFICATION OF THE SPECIMEN

One of the first general lessons to be learned when examining the cytologic specimen is to be able to clearly appreciate the important findings and disregard the detractors and artifact. This requires training and experience. All cytologic specimens should not be construed to have the same degree of difficulty. Just as with the histologic examination of tissue, some specimens are easier to interpret than others. The interpreter must recognize their limitations and focus on the specimens that are consistent with their knowledge base to avoid frustration. For example, when examining a thoracic fluid that contains neoplastic cells, the untrained eye sees clumps of what appear to be dark blue cellular structures of unknown identity but could be meso-thelial cells. The trained eye observes clumps of epithelial cells forming ac-inar structures consisting of variably sized cells (anisocytosis) with variable nuclear to cytoplasm ratios, variable nuclear size (anisokaryosis), surrounded by basophilic cytoplasm with variable tinctorial intensity compatible with a (adeno)carcinoma. It is from the summation of all the findings present and subsequently observed that a valid conclusion is formed.

The procedure for the microscopic examination of the cytology specimen is similar to that used for the hematology slide. The entire specimen is scanned using a low-power objective (10× or 20×) noting sample adequacy, stain quality, and unusual findings such as cell clumps or structures. Em-phasis is given to the "feathered" end of the slides made from fluid speci-mens. Once an overall impression of the specimen is attained, high-power (40× with a coverslip or 50× oil) is used to define the cell morphology. Microscopic findings should be routinely and immediately recorded; initial impressions are important to jot down on paper. These initial findings can be expanded or tempered during the detailed examination of the specimen. There are several basic statements that should be addressed for each spec-imen examined. Every cytologic description is initiated with the statement: "The predominant cell type is _____." Making a commitment to the defi-nition of cell type is a critical first step in defining the cytologic process. If definition of the predominant cell type is problematic, it may be at this point that a decision is made to seek assistance with the knowledge that the spec-imen is of adequate quality.

Anticipate the Expected, Expect the Unexpected

When a known tissue is aspirated, it should be determined if the specimen is or is not interpreted to be compatible with the expected tissue, *i.e.*, antic-ipate the expected. Defining the predominant cell type often accomplishes this responsibility. Making observations that support or deny what is cyto-logically expected is critical to proceeding in the interpretive process. For example, if the tissue aspirate is thought to be from a lymph node and the specimen is compatible with lymphoid tissue, then the subsequent observa-tions are used to classify the lymph node cytologically. However, if the tissue is not compatible with the anticipated observation of lymphoid constituents, then the specimen remains an unknown and requires additional cytologic definition. A relatively frequent example of this process is the inadvertent aspiration of the salivary gland instead of the submandibular or retropha-ryngeal lymph node. The diagnostic dilemma may be accentuated by the clinical setting; perhaps the patient has a unilateral nasal discharge or an oral mass. The importance of this example is intuitive: since a lymph node was thought to be aspirated, then the interpretation is that it has been effaced by a well-differentiated (adeno)carcinoma. An experienced cytologist would rapidly come to the conclusion that the tissue was salivary due to familiarity with salivary gland tissue and the absence of other findings consistent with a metastatic lymph node, *i.e.*, expect the unexpected. At other times, the subcutaneous mass thought to be consistent with a lymph node is actually an unexpected nonlymphoid neoplasm or inflammatory process. Again, the involvement of the interpreter in obtaining the specimen is especially valuable when dealing with problematic specimens.

WHAT IT IS

Inflammation *Versus* Noninflammation; Neoplasia *Versus* Nonneoplastic

The segmented neutrophil is an easily recognized cell as an indicator of supurative inflammation, either sterile or septic. Often it is considered a marker of acute inflammation since the attendant chemotactic factors attract the circulating neutrophils to migrate rapidly to the affected tissue. The identification of suppurative inflammation should prompt examination for microorganisms that may be located within the neutrophil (bacteria) or extracellularly (mycotic agents, filamentous bacteria). Bacteria are small, uniform coccoid, rod, or filament-shaped structures that stain a deep blue-purple with Romanowsky stains. The tinctorial property does not confer a Gram-positive finding. Only a Gram stain per se can define Gram-positive or Gram-negative. The observation of "unhappy" neutrophils (mushy nuclear chromatin) is a hint that bacteria may be present. The 50× or 100× oil objectives are used to confirm the presence of bacteria. Their visual identification is especially important in specimens, *e.g.*, synovial fluid, because the specimen may culture negatively. This can occur because of too few organisms, lysosomal degradation of the organisms, or the presence of antibiotics in the specimen subsequent to prior treatment systematically.

The nonsuppurative cell component often predominates as the suppurative processes "age" and in certain types of inflammatory processes. The *mixture* of macrophages, often foamy, and lymphocytes along with lesser numbers of neutrophils defines the chronic inflammatory process cytologically. The identification of these cellular sentinels of a different stage or type of inflammation guides the attendant differential diagnoses. At times, macrophages (histiocytes) morphologically mimic neoplastic cells. Obtaining a second opinion can be rewarding or the histologic examination of tissue may be required for the assessment of tissue architecture. Tissue cells, both mesenchymal and epithelial, can undergo hyperplasia in the presence of inflammation. These "reactive" cells can appear mild to moderately pleomorphic with more abundant, basophilic cytoplasm, and the nuclei can have coarser chromatin with prominent nucleolus. Obviously, these findings fulfill some of the criteria of malignancy. The predominating presence of the inflammatory cells should be used to temper the conclusion of malignancy. Tissues such as the nasal cavity, lung, urinary bladder, prostate, and mesothelium are notorious for undergoing notable inflammatory induced hyperplasia. Consequently, specimens from these sites should be examined judiciously when inflammation is present.

For ulcerated cutaneous lesions, obtaining multiple, deep samples is mandatory or, if inconclusive, evaluated by an excisional biopsy. It is emphasized that the two most important guidelines in dealing with these specimens are to make diagnostic preparations and to obtain professional assistance when bothersome or unidentifiable cells are observed.

Noninflammatory Lesions

The noninflammatory cytologic specimen may represent either neoplasia or nonneoplastic tissue. Epidermal cysts and adnexal (epithelial-derived) tumors, with or without cystic components, are virtually impossible to specifically identify cytologically but their benignancy is usually apparent. The possibility of a normal structure is a consideration as illustrated by the cytologic *faux pas* associated with submandibular salivary gland aspirate described earlier.

Neoplasia—Distinctive Cell Type

When a neoplastic cell population is considered, the first goal in cytology is to place the predominant cell type into a general classification (see Algorithm 22). The easiest group of tumors to define is predicated on their distinctive or "unique" morphologic features. Consequently, we prefer to use the "distinctive" term for the nomenclature of that classification. The morphologic features of lymphoma, mast cells, plasma cells, transmissible venereal cell tumors (TVT), histiocytoma, melanocytes, and lipocytes are denotative of the cell types in this classification. The histologically based term "round cell tumor" is avoided as a term for classifying some of these tumors because the neoplastic cells of epithelial derivation and poorly differentiated tumors can appear round to oval cytologically thereby obfuscating their classification. The term "discrete" has been used for the classification of some of these tumors as well. It has descriptive value since those listed in the "distinctive" classification do not have the classic cell-to-cell cohesion that is observed for epithelial tumors cytologically. However, epithelial- and mesenchymal-derived tumors also can occasionally appear as discrete (noncohesive) cell preparations cytologically. The "variable" criteria listed in Table 15–2 to assist in the definition of malignancy for epithelial and mesenchymal cells have little to no value for determining malignancy for the cell types in the "distinctive" classification.

Mast cell neoplasia is defined by the presence of predominantly mast cells. Occasionally, lesser numbers of eosinophils may be observed in the mast cell tumor of the dog. The vibrant tinctorial properties of the mast cell make descriptive terminology banal. The numerous metachromatic granules that fill the relatively voluminous cytoplasm often obscure the underlying round, light-blue nucleus. The scattered granules in the background from ruptured cells give the appearance of bacteria or stain artifact. The Diff-Quik stain does not reliably stain the granules of mast cells. The mast cell then has the

---

TABLE 15–2. Morphologic Variables of Epithelial and Mesenchymal Neoplasms Suggestive of Malignancy

Variable cell sizes (anisocytosis)
Variable cell forms (pleomorphism)
Variable cytoplasmic staining intensity
Variable nuclear sizes (anisokaryosis)
Variable nucleolar sizes and shapes (may be multiple)
Variable nuclear to cytoplasm ratio

---

microscopic appearance of a discreet epithelial-like cell. The new methylene blue stain or a Wright-Giemsa stain can be used to highlight the granules.

Neoplasia—Epithelial and Mesenchymal Cell Types

A neoplasm that lacks the criteria for inclusion into the distinctive classification is placed into the epithelial or mesenchymal category. Epithelial cells are generally oval to polygonal and tend to form variably sized sheets and clumps. The cells are linked to one another by membrane structures (referred to as cell-to-cell cohesion) that can be observed by careful examination. The mesenchymal classification includes connective tissue, skeletal tissue, and vessels (blood and lymphatic). The cell types are stellate to spindle to ovoid in shape. Eosinophilic ribbons of amorphous material (intercellular matrix) may be observed swirled among the cells. The definitive nomenclature of a neoplasm placed into one of these two categories is more difficult and should have lesser importance *per se*. The initial objective cytologically is to differentiate between benign and malignant. Histologic examination to assess architecture is often required for a specific diagnosis, especially for neoplasms of mesenchymal derivation. The "variables" listed in Table 15–2 are supportive of this exercise.

Malignant tumors of neuroendocrine origin often do not demonstrate morphologic variation. Thyroid, adrenal, and pancreatic tumors show similar morphologic characteristics. One often observes a relatively uniform cell population often containing free nuclei from ruptured cells due to their fragility. The banal-appearing cells often stain blandly and appear to lack well-delineated cell borders. The apocrine gland adenocarcinoma of the anal sac have a similar nonaggressive appearance even when found in a metastatic site such as the sublumbar lymph node.

DIAGNOSTIC APPLICATION

> *Another source of fallacy is the vicious circle of illusions which consist on the one hand of believing what we see and, on the other, seeing what we believe.*
> —Sir Clifford Allbutt

The more common indications for the use of fine-needle aspiration biopsy are listed in Table 15–3.

TABLE 15–3. Indications for the Use of Cytology

Effusions—thoracic and abdominal
Urine sediments, urinary bladder washing
Vitreous/aqueous infiltrates
Prostate—direct aspirate, washing
Pulmonary/nasal lesion—direct aspirate, bronchoalveolar/nasal washing/lavage
Lymphadenopathy—focal, generalized
Cutaneous/subcutaneous mass, ulcerative lesion
Diffuse organomegaly—liver, spleen, kidney
Unidentified abdominal mass
Evaluation of a mass or lesion discovered intraoperatively

Effusions

Cytology plays a pivotal role in the differential approach for evaluating effusions (see Chapter 13). The cytologic findings can segregate inflammatory from noninflammatory from neoplasia and can often suggest the cell type of the latter. This provides valuable information in determining therapeutic management for some of the more common neoplasms identified in effusions such as lymphoma and carcinomas. As alluded to earlier, inherent to the examination of effusions is the cytologic incubus of the mesothelial cell. This chameleon of cells can take on a variety of morphologic appearances that mimic immature basophilic clumps of epithelial cells, pale-staining vacuolated epithelial cells, and even individual, immature basophilic large lymphoblasts. When the decision-making cytologic process is obfuscated by their presence in a possible neoplastic effusion, it is always prudent to get a second opinion. There are times when even the most experienced cytopathologist must acquiesce to indecision. It is emphasized that this potentially problematic cell type in effusions should not cause one to circumvent its cytologic examination.

Lymphoid Tissue

Fine-needle aspiration biopsy can be effectively applied for the evaluation of lymphadenopathy. The most common use is for the differentiation of lymphoid hyperplasia (reactive) and neoplasia (lymphoma). In addition to the identification of the predominant cell type, i.e., lymphoid, it is critical to characterize the predominant type of lymphocyte. When the small lymphocyte comprises the majority (>50%) and variably sized lymphocytes (medium, large, blast-form) constitute the remaining population, hyperplasia is defined. Observing a relatively uniform (monotonous) population of predominantly (>50%) medium, large, or blastic lymphocytes supports a cytologic diagnosis of lymphoma. To semiquantitate the cell type proportions, 10 (or more) oil fields of 10 lymphocytes are counted and the percentage of small calculated. Lymphocyte size determination is aided by the use of other cell types that may be present in the sample as micrometers. The small lymphocyte with its barely visible scant rim of cytoplasm approximates the size of an erythrocyte and is smaller than a neutrophil. Using this criterion as an example, a diagnosis of lymphoma is made if the majority of the lymphocytes from an aspirate from an enlarged lymph node are relatively monomorphic and larger than a neutrophil. There are occasions when there is a sufficiently polymorphous lymphoid picture to cause prudent indecision. The two options are to aspirate a different lymph node (if generalized lymphadenopathy is present) or submit the lymph node for the histologic examination of architecture. A similar cytologic strategy can be used to define lymphoma in aspirates from other organs such as liver, spleen, and kidney. An additional advantage for the identification of lymphoma in these organs is that large numbers of lymphocytes are not expected findings. In other words, "What is that cell type doing here?"

In contrast to the dog in which lymphoma is a relatively common differential consideration for generalized lymphadenopathy, a caveat must be realized for the cat. A syndrome of generalized lymphadenopathy, referred to as distinctive lymph node hyperplasia, develops in young adult cats with or without other clinical signs. Cytologically there can be a marked polymorphic lymphoid picture in which the small lymphocyte is in the minority and huge lymphoblasts are observed. Noteworthy is that erythrophagocytosis usually can be found by adequate scanning. There can be sufficient distortion of the architecture that even the histologic examination of the lymph node can be suggestive of lymphoma. The majority spontaneously resolve weeks to months later without subsequent development of neoplasia. Argyrophilic bacteria (silver stain positive), not visible with routine stains, have been identified in some of these cases. Exposure to the feline immunodeficiency virus also has been proposed to be a cause of this exuberant lymphoid reaction.

The examination for metastatic disease can be applied to peripheral and internal lymph nodes. Since a lymph node is cytologically comprised of lymphoid elements, it provides a useful backdrop for the identification of "alien" cells—"What is that other cell type doing here?" Slide preparations can made from either a fine-needle aspirate biopsy or touch imprints of an excised specimen. Multiple specimens should be scanned; a 20× objective is valuable for this task.

Cutaneous and Subcutaneous Lesions

Cutaneous and subcutaneous lesions lend themselves to fine-needle aspiration biopsy. A wide array of disease processes are possible, and the extent to which a decision-making "tree" illustrated by Algorithm 22 is pursued depends on the experience and philosophical approach taken by the aspirator. For some, the value of cytology may be limited to the differentiation of inflammatory and noninflammatory processes. When the latter is identified, an incisional or excisional biopsy is performed. For others, the identification of selected neoplastic cell types is diagnostic and an excisional biopsy is precluded. For the distinctive category of neoplasia, fine-needle aspiration biopsy can correctly identify them most (~90%) of the time. The histiocytoma can be a problematic mass to evaluate cytologically without considerable experience. Their morphologic variability can lead to an interpretation as a malignant mesenchymal tumor or, as lymphocytes infiltrate during their regression, give the appearance of chronic inflammation. Fine-needle aspiration biopsy of canine mammary gland enlargement is also problematic due to the mixture of tissue types and relative ease of marked hyperplasia in response to an inflammatory process. If cytology is used for the identification of neoplasia in the canine mammary gland, the absence of neoplastic cells should be interpreted with circumspection.

Liver

Hepatomegaly is the primary indication for fine-needle aspiration biopsy of the liver. Normal hepatocytes are large polygonal cells often found in cohesive clumps. The round nuclei are surrounded by abundant lightly basophilic cytoplasm that may contain specks of dark-staining bile pigment. Occasional binucleate cells may be seen. Sheets of biliary epithelium may be encountered. These tightly clumped cuboidal-shaped cells are smaller than hepatocytes with central round nuclei and scant basophilic cytoplasm. Hyperplastic hepatocytes may demonstrate slight anisokaryosis, binucleate cells, multiple nucleoli, and increased cytoplasmic basophilia. These morphologic findings are associated with nodular hyperplasia, very common in old dogs, or as a response to hepatic inflammation.

Cytoplasmic findings are common in hepatic disease. An abundance of tiny clumps of dark bile pigment is indicative of cholestasis. Thick plugs (casts) of bile pigment may be observed outlining the canalicular space on the surface of the hepatocytes. Hepatocellular vacuolation occurs secondary to lipid accumulation and is dramatic in cats with hepatic lipidosis. These distinctly round structures with clear lumen range from multiple small to a single large form that pushes the nucleus to the periphery of the cell. Lesser degrees of hepatocellular accumulation of lipid is a common sequela to both toxic and metabolic disorders that involve the liver. Glucocorticoid excess, exogenous or endogenous, causes moderate to marked glycogen accumulation in the canine liver. Microscopically, the affected hepatocytes are larger, if a normal sized hepatocyte is available for comparison, and appear to be comprised of wispy swirls of cytoplasm or the cytoplasm appears to have reduced basophilia. The nuclei usually maintain a central location.

Carcinomas, sarcomas, and tumors composed of distinctive cell types can be identified cytologically in the liver. Lymphoma and mast cell neoplasia readily exfoliate and are recognized by finding a large population of their respective cell types. Hepatocellular carcinoma can be readily defined by the use of the criteria in Table 15–2 unless it is well differentiated. Since the tumor is a large asymmetric mass, finding a relatively normal appearing hepatocyte population is suggestive of that possibility. Aspirates of bile duct neoplasia typically result in very dense clusters of epithelial cells. It is often difficult to clearly delineate cell characteristics due to the thickness of the clusters. The examination of the periphery of these clumps is fruitful. The cells may be slightly smaller to larger than hepatocytes with a very high nuclear to cytoplasm ratio and prominent nucleoli. The formation of tubular or acinar structures can be observed ("imagined") occasionally. Metastatic carcinomas and sarcomas are usually focal to multifocal and are detected and sampled ultrasonographically. Malignant histiocytosis frequently involves the liver in dogs and cats. The morphology of the cell type is described under the section on lung.

Inflammatory disease is difficult to identify with fine-needle aspiration biopsy. Touch imprints made from an excisional biopsy can be used to quickly determine the presence of a suppurative inflammatory process. The cytologic examination of bile is also valuable for the identification of a suppurative process consistent with cholecystitis or for the identification of fluke ova. Extramedullary hematopoiesis does develop in the liver, and bone marrow elements may be detected in a touch imprint. These cell types are associated commonly with nodular regeneration in older dogs.

Spleen

Splenomegaly is the primary indication for fine-needle aspiration biopsy of the spleen. The aspirate from a nondiseased spleen often contains peripheral blood cells. Occasionally, a few monomorphic spindle cells representing fibrocytes or endothelial cells are seen. The predominate nucleated cell population is lymphoid and their assessment is made using the criteria established for the lymph node. Small lymphocytes predominate with a lesser population of prolymphocytes and lymphoblasts. Occasional plasma cells, macrophages, and mast cells can be seen. Increased numbers of prolymphocytes, lymphoblasts, and plasma cells are seen in reactive spleens especially in association with gastrointestinal inflammation. A marked plasmacytosis, resembling multiple myeloma, can be observed in canine ehrlichiosis and feline immunodeficiency infections.

Neoplasms comprised of lymphocytes, plasma cells, mast cells, and myeloid cells readily exfoliate. Lymphoma is characterized by a monomorphic population of lymphoid cells; the criteria are discussed with the lymph node section. Extraskeletal plasma cell tumors can occur in both the spleen and the liver. These are characterized by a uniform population of plasma cells with eccentric nuclei, clumped "cartwheel" chromatin, deeply basophilic cytoplasm, and a perinuclear clear area. Binucleate and multinucleate plasma cells can be observed. Sometimes these "classic" descriptors of the plasma cell are not expressed morphologically and the cell type is suggestive of a lymphoma or histiocytic tumor. Splenic mast cell tumors are common, particularly in cats where they comprise approximately one third of the splenic lesions. Myeloproliferative disease involving any of the cell lines can involve the spleen. Generally, it is characterized by a relatively monomorphic population of predominantly immature myeloid elements. Concurrent evaluation of peripheral blood and bone marrow is necessary to fully characterize the neoplastic process. Myeloproliferative disease must be differentiated from extramedullary hematopoiesis which is a relatively common finding in the spleen, especially in association with anemia. The erythroid series and megakaryocytes with normal morphology are seen most frequently.

The use of ultrasonography for the identification of focal, cavitational lesions is valuable for the characterization of hemangiosarcomas which are the most common splenic neoplasia in the dog. Splenic hemangiosarcoma is difficult to diagnosis with aspiration cytology. The specimens are often comprised of peripheral blood elements. Examination of a buffy coat preparation from such a specimen can enhance the probability of finding atypical mesenchymal cells that have spontaneously exfoliated into a blood-filled cavity of the neoplasm. The cells will have a spindle to elliptical shape with indistinct cytoplasmic borders and wispy "tails" and demonstrate the criteria of malignancy. The possibility of the fragile neoplastic tissue leaking and "seeding" the abdomen or blatantly rupturing is a high risk and the procedure is discouraged. If performed, the hematocrit and plasma protein should be subsequently monitored for 4 to 6 hours.

Gastrointestinal Tract

The cytologic examination of scrapings of gastrointestinal tract taken via endoscopy or from touch imprints of the biopsy specimen can be diagnostic or provide preliminary information. The specimen will represent the surface of the lesion and may not accurately reflect deeper pathology. The expected cell type is a monomorphic-appearing cuboidal to columnar epithelial cell. The presence of other cell types can be suggestive of either inflammation or neoplasia. The predominance of a lymphocytic-plasma cell mixture or eosinophils are indicative of their respective disease syndromes. Fungi that cause histoplasmosis, candidiasis, and zygomycosis (phycomycosis) and algae that cause protothecosis can be readily identified. Cytology is useful in detecting spiral-shaped organisms in gastric samples. The initial examination of a fecal specimen cytologically can be diagnostic for some of these diseases. A small amount of fresh feces is mixed with saline to form a specimen that has the consistency of thick blood. Multiple slide preparations are made, air-dried, stained, and examined microscopically. It is prudent to change the staining solutions or use a staining setup that is dedicated for fecal examination because of the rich bacterial population. The bacteria are easily eluded from the slide, especially if the smear is not completely dry, and contaminate the stain. They can adhere subsequently to sterile specimens and give the impression of a septic process, a potential diagnostic disaster.

Lymphoma and mast cell tumors readily exfoliate and are more easily identified than epithelial or mesenchymal tumors of the gastrointestinal tract. Exfoliation of the latter two cell types is enhanced by aggressive scraping. Inflammatory cells are frequent "neighbors" of the tumor cells when the neoplasm is ulcerated. Epithelial cell hyperplasia is readily stimulated by inflammation which can obfuscate its separation from an inflamed epithelial neoplasm. The examination of a fine-needle aspiration biopsy of a lymph node(s) in the region of the gastrointestinal lesion can provide the needed information if neoplastic cells are observed. Mesenteric lymph nodes frequently demonstrate moderate to marked hyperplasia, especially when the gastrointestinal tract is diseased. It should be noted that aggregates of lymphoid nodules, often hyperplastic, are located along the small intestine, notably the ileum.

Prostate

Prostatomegaly and/or the finding of hematuria and pyuria in an intact, older male dog are indications to investigate the prostate cytologically. Infection/inflammation of the urinary tract should be placed highest on the differential diagnostic list as the more common disease. A urethral discharge that is not prepucial in origin is commonly associated with prostatic disease. Following cleansing of the prepuce, the discharge can be collected and examined. Prostatic fluid is sterile, and finding a uniform population of a bacterium (cultured at $>10^5$/mL) in a suppurative surrounding is indicative of prostatitis. Examination of an ejaculate is another approach for obtaining a cytologic specimen since more than 95% of it is contributed by the prostate. Collection of the latter part of the ejaculate provides the more diagnostically useful specimen for culture and microscopic examination.

Prostatic massage is another technique to capture a cytologic specimen. It aids in differentiating disease of the urinary bladder from prostatic disease. The urinary bladder is emptied and flushed several times with the use of a urinary catheter. An aliquot of the final wash is saved for comparison to the postmassage specimen. The urinary catheter is slowly withdrawn until, using digital palpation per rectum, the tip of the catheter is at the level of the prostate or slightly caudad. The prostate is digitally massaged per rectum for 60 to 90 seconds followed by the slow infusion of approximately 10 mL of sterile physiologic saline while digitally occluding the urethral orifice around the catheter to prevent the external escape of the fluid. At this point the process is reversed and gentle, slow, continuous aspiration is applied while slowly advancing the catheter into the urinary bladder. The remainder of the fluid is aspirated, aspiration is discontinued, and the catheter is removed. Microscopic evaluation and culture of the pre- and postmassage specimens are conducted.

Fine-needle aspiration biopsy of the prostate is conducted by use of either a perirectal or transabdominal approach. Aspiration of a suspected abscess, based on clinical, laboratory, and ultrasonographic findings is not recommended. A 2½-inch spinal needle facilitates the perirectal approach. The cytologic interpretation of abnormal-appearing epithelial must be done with caution due to the "reactive" ability of the tissue in the presence of inflammation. In addition, squamous metaplasia of the urethra or of prostate that has undergone hyperplasia can occur secondary to the influence of estrogen, endogenous or exogenous, and chronic inflammation. The presence of these cell types in different morphologic stages can contribute to the cytologic confusion associated with the examination of the prostatic specimen. Finding an epithelial cell cluster in an ultrasonographically guided fine-needle aspiration biopsy of the sublumbar lymph node is a reassuring strategy in support of prostatic carcinoma.

Kidney

Renomegaly is the primary indication for fine-needle aspiration biopsy. Ultrasonographically guided fine-needle aspiration biopsy permits the cytologic investigation of a focal lesion. To facilitate the aspiration procedure, the kidney can be restrained against the abdominal wall by digital pressure in cats and small dogs. The kidney is a fibrous organ that spontaneously yields few of its elements. Segments of tubules and epithelial and small spindle-shaped cells can be aspirated along with peripheral blood components from a nondiseased kidney. Epithelial cells from the feline kidney often contain multiple, punctate vacuoles representing areas of lipid that dissolved during the staining process. Renal carcinomas are the most common primary tumors in the dog and cat (if lymphoma is not considered primary in the cat). Extrarenal disorders associated with renal carcinomas include absolute erythrocytosis secondary to increased erythropoietin production and hypertrophic osteoarthropathy secondary to pulmonary metastases. Lymphoma is the most common renal tumor in the cat.

Renal carcinomas usually exfoliate sufficiently to provide a diagnostic specimen. Criteria of epithelial malignancy are used for their cytologic classification. The cell type with its basophilic cytoplasm can resemble a blast-type lymphoma upon superficial examination especially when areas are examined that lack cell-to-cell cohesion. However, the cells comprising the carcinoma are larger than neoplastic lymphocytes when a cell such as a neutrophil is used as a "micrometer" for the determination of cell size. Other cell types that can cause primary renal tumors include the transitional cell and clear cell. The latter cell type can give a well-differentiated "endocrine-type" cell appearance and require histopathologic examination for identification.

Urinary Bladder

The preparation of cytologic specimens of urine is covered in an earlier section. Plump transitional epithelial cells with abundant relatively clear cytoplasm line the urinary bladder and urethra. They can demonstrate remarkable morphologic changes when hyperplasia is stimulated by inflammation. Consequently, the criteria of malignancy must be applied cautiously when inflammation is present concurrently. If in doubt, medical management of the bacterial cystitis followed by a second cytologic evaluation is a reasonable option. The transitional cell carcinoma is the most common tumor of the urinary bladder in the dog and cat. It is identified by using the criteria of malignancy that are applied for the other epithelial neoplasms.

Lungs

Evaluation of the respiratory tree by transtracheal wash or bronchoalveolar lavage is used to evaluate airway-related diseases such as bronchopneumonia or allergies. Identification of neoplastic, mycotic, or protozoal diseases by examination of airway material is possible only if cells or organisms are exfoliated into the airway. Obtaining an adequate sample is crucial when using these techniques. Respiratory epithelial cells are observed in these samples. These cells are columnar to cuboidal and often ciliated. Oval nuclei with granular chromatin are situated towards the base of the cell and the cytoplasm is lightly basophilic. Goblet cells may contain eye-catching pink to mauve-colored granules. Mucus is often present in respiratory samples as ribbons of eosinophilic material. Occasionally, this material is found in tightly coiled forms referred to as Curschmann's spirals. They apparently represent mucus casts of the lower airway.

Alveolar macrophages are observed in samples from nondiseased lungs and in both acute and chronic inflammatory processes. These cells are large and often vacuolated. In chronic disease, binucleate and multinucleate forms may be seen. Increased numbers of eosinophils are associated with allergic or hypersensitivity reactions and lung worms. Healthy cats can have a higher percentage of eosinophils in their airways than other species. Even in specific pathogen-free cats, eosinophils are the second most common cell type obtained by bronchoalveolar lavage comprising approximately 20% of the cell population. Other inflammatory cell types may be seen including lesser numbers of mast cells, lymphocytes, and plasma cells.

Fine-needle aspiration biopsy of the lung parenchyma is rewarding when the interstitial disease is diffuse or when large focal lesions are identified radiographically. Both infectious and neoplastic diseases can be identified cytologically. The lung is a primary site of involvement in both systemic histiocytosis of Bernese mountain dogs and canine malignant histiocytosis. Systemic histiocytosis is a histiocytic proliferative disorder confined to Bernese mountain dogs. Malignant histiocytosis has been identified in several breeds of dogs with a suggested predisposition in Bernese mountain dogs, golden retrievers, and flat-coated retrievers. Malignant histiocytosis occurs in cats and can involve the liver, spleen and bone marrow. Malignant histiocytes are large pleomorphic discrete cells with abundant, often vacuolated, basophilic cytoplasm. Nuclei are oval to reniform with prominent nuceoli; multinucleated cells may be present. Cells may also exhibit phagocytosis of erythrocytes and leukocytes which helps to suggest a histiocytic origin. Malignant histiocytosis can be cytologically difficult to differentiate from granulomatous inflammation, large cell anaplastic carcinoma, histiocytic lymphoma, and pulmonary lymphomatoid granulomatosis. Even with histopathologic evaluation, a positive immunoreactivity to lysozyme is required in the differential diagnosis.

Occasionally samples are obtained that are not consistent with the lung or airway. Oropharyngeal contamination results in squamous epithelial cells with adherent bacteria including large *Simonsiella* colonies ("railroad-track" appearance). Inflammation and bacterial organisms attributable to dental or other oropharyngeal diseases must be considered if contamination is present. The two most common nonrespiratory cells seen with lung aspirates are mesothelial cells and hepatocytes. Sheets of mesothelial cells are seen if the lung surface is scraped during the aspiration process. The sheets are comprised of monomorphic cells with angular, cohesive borders resembling fish scales. As the cells begin to exfoliate from the sheets, they round up, become more basophilic, and begin to demonstrate the glycocalyx halo associated with more classic mesothelial cells. Aspiration of the liver occurs when the chest is entered too far caudal.

Additional Reading

Brown PH, Hopper CD, Harbour DA: Pathological features of lymphoid tissues in cats with natural feline immunodeficiency virus infection. J Comp Pathol 1991;104: 345–355.

Caniatti M, Roccabianca P, Scanziani E, et al: Canine lymphoma: Immunohistochemical analysis of fine-needle aspiration biopsy. Vet Pathol 1996;33:204–212.

Carter RF, Valli VEO: Advances in the cytologic diagnosis of canine lymphoma. Semin Vet Med Surg 1988;3:167–175.

Cowell RL, Tyler RD: Diagnostic Cytology of the Dog and Cat. Goleta, CA, American Veterinary Publishers, 1989, pp 1–259.

Else RW, Simpson JW: Diagnostic value of exfoliative cytology of body fluids in dogs and cats. Vet Rec 1988;123:70–76.

Griffiths GL, Lumsden JH, Valli VEO: Fine needle aspiration cytology and histologic correlation in canine tumors. Vet Clin Pathol 1984;13:13–17.

Leveille R, Partington BP, Biller DS, Miyabayashi T: Complications after ultrasound-guided biopsy of abdominal structures in dogs and cats: 246 cases (1984–1991). J Am Vet Med Assoc 1993;203:413–415.

Livraghi T, Damascelli B, Lombardi C, et al: Risk in fine-needle abdominal biopsy. J Clin Ultrasound 1983;11:77–81.

Mair S, Dunbar F, Becker PJ, Du Plessis W: Fine needle cytology—is aspiration suction necessary? A study of 100 masses in various sites. Acta Cytol 1989;33:809–813.

Meyer DJ: The management of the cytology specimen. Comp Contin Educ Pract Vet 1987;9:9–16.

Meyer DJ, Franks P: Effusion: Classification and cytologic examination. Comp Contin Educ Pract Vet 1987;9:123–128.

Mooney SC, Patnaik AK, Hayes AA, MacEwen EG: Generalized lymphadenopathy resembling lymphoma in cats: Six cases (1972–1976). J Am Vet Med Assoc 1987;190: 897–900.

Moore FM, Emerson WE, Cotter SM, DeLellis RA: Distinctive peripheral lymph node hyperplasia of young cats. Vet Pathol 1986;23:386–391.

O'Keefe DA, Couto CG: Fine-needle aspiration of the spleen as an aid in the diagnosis of splenomegaly. J Vet Intern Med 1987;1:102–109.

Perman V, Alsaker RD, Riis RC: Cytology of the Dog and Cat. American Animal Hospital Association, Denver, 1979, pp 1–159.

Rideout BA, Lowenstine LJ, Hutson CA, et al: Characterization of morphologic changes and lymphocyte subset distribution in lymph nodes from cats with naturally acquired feline immunodeficiency virus infection. Vet Pathol 1992;29:391–399.

Ross DL, Neely AE: Textbook of Urinalysis and Body Fluids. Norwalk, CT, 1983, pp 1–336.

Simpson RM, Meuten DJ: Development of a teaching laboratory aid for instruction of fine needle aspiration biopsy cytology technique. Vet Clin Pathol 1992;21:40–44.

Smith EH: The hazards of fine-needle aspiration biopsy. Ultrasound Med Biol 1984; 10:629–634.

Smith RF: Microscopy and Photomicroscopy: A Working Manual. Boca Raton, FL, CRC Press, 1990, 1–135.

Spangler WL, Culbertson MR: Prevalence and type of splenic diseases in cats: 455 cases (1985–1991). J Am Vet Med Assoc 1992;201:773–776.

Spangler WL, Culbertson MR: Prevalence, type, and importance of splenic diseases in dogs: 1,480 cases (1985–1989). J Am Vet Med Assoc 1992;200:829–834.

Takeda M: Atlas of Diagnostic Gastrointestinal Cytology. New York, Igaku-Shoin Medical Publishers, 1983, p 229.

Vos JH, van den Ingh TSGAM, van Mil FN: Non-exfoliative canine cytology: The value of fine needle aspiration and scrapping cytology. Vet Q 1989;11:222–231.

Part II

CASE HISTORIES

To study the phenomenon of disease without books is to sail an uncharted sea, while to study books without patients is not to go to sea at all.

—Sir William Osler, M.D.

Case 2–1

Patient: German shepherd dog, spayed female, 10 years of age.

History: Urinary incontinence began about a month ago. The referring veterinarian treated the dog with diethylstilbestrol (DES), increasing the dosage to 3 mg PO SID when the incontinence persisted. A single treatment of estradiol cypionate (ECP) of unknown dose was also given 2.5 weeks before referral. The animal was referred with a primary complaint of blood-stained perineal area.

PE: Slightly depressed with normal hydration, mucous membrane color, pulse rate, respiratory rate, and temperature. Moderate dental tartar and gingivitis were present. An open wound was present on the lateral aspect of the left stifle. Isolated ecchymotic hemorrhages were observed on the ventral abdomen.

Notable Laboratory Findings:

Hematology: HCT = 23% with normal RBC indices, platelet count = 6000/μL, neutrophil count = 500/μL, lymphocyte count = 2000/μL, monocyte count = 100/μL, eosinophil count = 0/μL, RBC morphology = 1+ echinocytosis and moderate rouleaux, lymphocyte morphology = frequently reactive.

Clinical chemistry: not done.

Bone marrow: Aspirate and core biopsies were markedly hypocellular. The marrow particles present in aspirate smears consisted primarily of reticular cells, macrophages, plasma cells and mast cells. Low numbers of erythroid precursor cells and even lower numbers of granulocytic precursor cells were present. No megakaryocytes were observed. Large amounts of stainable iron were present.

Assessment: The anemia in this dog was considered nonregenerative because no polychromasia was seen in the stained blood film. The reactive lymphocytes indicated increased antigenic stimulation, probably related to the profound neutropenia and open wound. The subcutaneous hemorrhages resulted from the thrombocytopenia. Bone marrow evaluation revealed that the pancytopenia present resulted from a lack of bone marrow precursor cells. When erythroid precursors, granulocyte precursors and megakaryocytes are markedly reduced or absent the term "aplastic anemia" is used. The lymphocyte count was normal because most lymphocytes in blood enter from lymph nodes rather than from the bone marrow. The reticular cells, macrophages, and plasma cells were considered to be normal residual cells. Mast cells are rare in bone marrow of normal animals, but are sometimes seen in aplastic bone marrow, possibly because microenvironment changes potentiate their development.

Comment: The dog was given a blood transfusion and antibiotic therapy was begun. Epistaxis began 5 days later. The HCT was 27%. A bone marrow aspirate collected at that time was again aplastic. A second blood transfusion was given. Marked hematuria occurred 3 days later and the owner decided to have the dog euthanized. The aplastic anemia in this dog resulted from the prior administration of high doses of estrogens. ECP is much more toxic to canine bone marrow than is DES. Experimental studies have indicated that aplastic anemia develops about 3 weeks after toxic doses of estrogen are given, in agreement with the time-course of this case. Only dogs and ferrets have been reported to develop estrogen-induced aplastic anemia. In addition to iatrogenic estrogen toxicity, dogs with endogenous hyperestrogenism (sertoli cell tumor, interstitial cell tumor, and seminoma of the testicle; and granulosa cell tumor of the ovary) can develop aplastic anemia, as can ferrets with protracted estrus.

References

Kociba GJ, Caputo CA: Aplastic anemia associated with estrus in pet ferrets. J Am Vet Med Assoc 1981;178:1293.

Miura N, Sasaki N, Ogawa H, et al: Bone marrow hypoplasia induced by administration of estradiol benzoate in male beagle dogs. Jpn J Vet Sci 1985;47:731.

Morgan RV: Blood dyscrasias associated with testicular tumors in the dog. J Am Anim Hosp Assoc 1982;18:970.

Case 2–2

Patient: Quarter horse, gelding, 15 years of age.

History: Intermittent unilateral epistaxis for 4 months and weight loss for 2 months.

PE: Pale mucous membranes, tachycardia, temperature = 103.8°F.

___

Notable Laboratory Findings:

Hematology: HCT = 12% with normal RBC indices, fibrinogen = 1000 mg/dL, platelets = 142,000/μL, neutrophil count = 400/μL, lymphocyte count = 2200/μL, monocyte count = 100/μL, RBC morphology = 2+ anisocytosis, lymphocyte morphology = 50% of lymphocytes were moderately large with fine nuclear chromatin and scant basophilic cytoplasm.
Urinalysis: normal.
Clinical chemistry: unremarkable.
Coggins' test: negative.
Coombs' test: negative.
Coagulation tests: PT and APTT were normal.
Platelet function tests: normal platelet aggregation and normal vWF concentration.
Bone marrow biopsy: Replacement of normal marrow cells with a monotonous population of moderately large lymphocytes with fine nuclear chromatin and scant basophilic cytoplasm similar to those present in blood. Indistinct nucleoli were visible in some cells. As expected, these neoplastic cells were peroxidase negative.

Endoscopy: Normal nasopharynx, guttural pouch and upper trachea.

Assessment: In the absence of identifiable peripheral tumors, a presumptive diagnosis of acute lymphocytic leukemia was made. The severe neutropenia and anemia were explained by the replacement of normal marrow precursor cells with neoplastic cells. The normal platelet count was unexplained, as was the long history of intermittent epistaxis. The increased fibrinogen concentration suggested the presence of concomitant inflammation.

Comment: The horse was euthanized. Multiple submucosal hematomas were present in the maxillary sinuses and mesenteric and sublumbar lymph nodes were enlarged. As in the antemortem biopsy, the bone marrow was diffusely filled with sheets of neoplastic lymphocytes. Lymphoid infiltrates were present in the spleen, liver, kidney, and lymph nodes. Moderate extramedullary hematopoiesis was present in the spleen; consequently, some of the blood platelets may have originated in the spleen. It is also possible that some bone marrow sites, not evaluated during the antemortem biopsy or necropsy, contained megakaryocytes. The necropsy findings were more supportive of a diagnosis of lymphocytic leukemia than of a diagnosis of lymphoma with secondary leukemia.

Reference

Lester GD, Alleman AR, Raskin RE, et al: Pancytopenia secondary to lymphoid leukemia in three horses. J Vet Intern Med 1993;7:360.

Case 3–1

Patient: Irish Setter dog, female, 13 years of age.

History: Weakness, anorexia, and weight loss for a week, and unable to walk at presentation.

PE: The dog was depressed, emaciated, approximately 8% dehydrated, and nonambulatory because of extreme weakness. Pale mucous membranes, ocular and nasal discharges, excessive dental tartar, otitis externa and large numbers of fleas were present. The rectal temperature was 99.6°F.

Notable Laboratory Findings:

Hematology: HCT = 11%; MCV = 52 fL; MCHC = 30 g/dL; RDW = 20%; reticulocyte count = 80,000/μL; total plasma protein = 6.8 g/dL; platelet count = 532,000/μL; band count = 3300/μL; neutrophil count = 24,800/μL; lymphocyte count = 500/μL; monocyte count = 3600/μL; eosinophil count = 0; RBC morphology = 1+ polychromasia, 2+ anisocytosis, 2+ hypochromasia.

Clinical chemistry: BUN = 29 mg/dL, creatinine = 1.0 mg/dL.

Serum iron assays: serum iron = 16 mg/dL (reference range 84 to 233 μg/dL), total iron binding capacity (TIBC) = 462 μg/dL (reference range 284 to 572 μg/dL), and ferritin = 140 μg/L (reference range 80 to 800 μg/L).

Fecal flotation: *Trichuris* eggs.

Assessment: The presence of a severe microcytic hypochromic anemia indicates the presence of chronic iron deficiency. The low serum iron, normal serum TIBC, and low-normal serum ferritin concentrations support the diagnosis of iron deficiency. Serum ferritin concentration generally correlates well with total body iron content, but ferritin is an acute phase reactant protein that increases during inflammation. Consequently, serum ferritin might have been lower in the absence of the inflammation documented in the physical examination. Iron deficiency is almost always the result of blood loss in adult animals. The massive flea infestation was believed to be the major source of blood loss in this dog. Some blood loss may have also occurred in the feces, but whipworms alone do not cause enough hemorrhage to result in iron deficiency anemia. The increased RDW indicates that there is increased variation in RBC volumes present. In iron deficiency anemia, this results from a mixture of normocytic RBCs and microcytic RBCs formed after iron becomes limiting for RBC development. The absolute reticulocyte count was not increased, indicating that decreased iron availability is limiting the bone marrow response to the anemia. The normal total plasma and serum protein concentrations in a dehydrated animal suggests that the concentration will be low-normal or decreased after rehydration. Serum proteins are synthesized more rapidly than RBCs; consequently, the total plasma protein concentration may be normal in animals with chronic blood loss. A majority of dogs with iron deficiency anemia have a thrombocytosis, as was present in this case. The neutrophilia, lymphocytopenia, monocytosis, and eosinopenia are likely the result of stress (endogenous glucocorticoid release), but the significant left-shift and the magnitude of the neutrophilia indicates a concomitant inflammatory response is also present. The slightly increased BUN concentration is probably prerenal and secondary to dehydration.

Comment: The dog was given a whole blood transfusion (two units) and treated with intravenous lactated ringers solution to correct the dehydration. The following day the HCT was 34%, total plasma protein was 6.2 g/dL, rectal temperature was 101.5°F, and marked clinical improvement was apparent. The animal was also given a flea bath and treated with an anthelmintic, and the client was instructed on appropriate flea control measures for the dog's environment. Oral iron therapy was not considered essential because of the amount of iron present in the transfused blood.

Reference

Harvey JW, French TW, Meyer DJ: Chronic iron deficiency anemia in dogs. J Am Anim Hosp Assoc 1982;18:946.

Case 3–2

Patient: Domestic short-hair cat, castrated male, 2 years of age.

History: Presented for evaluation of deformed carpus, that was present when the client acquired the cat as a stray.

PE: Deformity of carpus secondary to traumatic luxation, alopecia over pinna secondary to dermatomycosis, slightly depressed and afebrile with marked splenomegaly.

Notable Laboratory Findings:

Hematology: HCT = 13%; MCV = 86 fL; MCHC = 33%; total plasma protein = 8.3 g/dL; platelet count = normal; leukocyte counts = normal; nucleated RBCs = 1400/μL; RBC Morphology = 1+ anisocytosis, 2+ polychromasia, 4+ *Haemobartonella felis* organisms.

Clinical chemistry: Bilirubin = 0.4 mg/dL, ALT = 143 U/L, globulin = 5.8 g/dL.

Serology: FeLV = negative, FIV = positive.

Assessment: The anemia present was regenerative based on the degree of polychromasia present. Reticulocyte counts may not be accurate when high numbers of *H. felis* organisms are present. The macrocytosis and nucleated RBCs are consistent with the regenerative bone marrow response present. The increased total plasma protein concentration is the result of increased globulin concentrations and could represent an inflammatory reaction to the blood parasite. The slightly increased bilirubin concentration is attributable to the increased RBC destruction that accompanies these RBC parasites. The slightly increased ALT may reflect hypoxic injury to the liver.

Comment: Doxycycline and glucocorticoid therapy was initiated and the cat was discharged. The client was told that the *Haemobartonella* infection should respond to therapy, but that the cat would probably remain FIV positive, which would likely result in increased susceptibility to bacterial infections at a later date. Concurrent infections of *H. felis* and FeLV generally results in more severe clinical signs and more severe anemia than occurs when a cat is infected with either agent alone. In contrast, concurrent infection with *H. felis* and FIV does not appear to cause more severe anemia than does infection with *H. felis* alone. Consequently, the regenerative anemia in this cat is attributable primarily to the *H. felis* infection.

Reference

Harvey JW: Haemobartonellosis. In Greene CE (ed): Infectious Diseases of the Dog and Cat, 2nd ed. Philadelphia, W.B. Saunders, 1997, in press.

Case 4–1

Patient: Standardbred horse, female, 10 years of age.

History: Dystocia resulting in a vaginal tear and displacement of intestines into the vagina. Attempts to repair the laceration on the farm were initially unsuccessful due to hemorrhage and straining. Xylazine was administered as an analgesic and sedative, the intestines were replaced into the abdomen, and the laceration was sutured.

PE: The horse was uncomfortable, exhibiting evidence of pain, but otherwise appeared normal.

Notable Laboratory Findings (Day 1):

Hematology: HCT = 38%, total plasma protein = 6.0 g/dL, fibrinogen = 300 mg/dL, platelet count = normal, metamyelocyte count = 100/μL, band count = 600/μL, neutrophil count = 2400/μL, lymphocyte count = 600/μL, monocyte count = 200/μL, eosinophil count = 0/μL, and neutrophilic morphology = 2+ toxicity.

Clinical chemistry: AST = 506 U/L.

Abdominal fluid: HCT = 8%, protein = 4.0 g/dL, nucleated cell count = 13,100/μL, most nucleated cells present were toxic neutrophils.

Microbiology: No bacterial growth was obtained from the abdominal fluid, but antibiotic therapy may have been initiated prior to culture.

Assessment: The abdominal fluid analysis revealed evidence of hemorrhage and inflammation. The toxic left shift with low-normal neutrophil numbers in blood resulted from peritonitis with movement of neutrophils into the abdominal cavity. The absorption of endotoxin, which results in increased margination of neutrophils, may also have contributed to this leukogram. The lymphopenia and eosinopenia probably resulted from the endogenous release of glucocorticoids. The slightly decreased plasma protein concentration probably resulted from the peritonitis with protein movement into the abdominal cavity. The increased serum AST activity was attributed to tissue injury.

Comment: The abdomen was lavaged with large volumes of saline solution containing penicillin and streptomycin and the horse was treated with intravenous penicillin and intravenous fluids. Laboratory analyses were done again on day 3.

Notable Laboratory Findings (Day 3):

Hematology: HCT = 42%, total plasma protein = 7.1 g/dL, fibrinogen = 700 mg/dL, platelet count = normal, band count = 200/μL, neutrophil count = 900/μL, lymphocyte count = 300/μL, monocyte count = 200/μL, eosinophil count = 0/μL, and neutrophilic morphology = 2+ toxicity.

Clinical chemistry: AST = 795 U/L.

Abdominal fluid: HCT = 3%, protein = 2.9 g/dL, nucleated cell count = 33,800/μL, most nucleated cells present were toxic neutrophils.

Assessment: The abdominal fluid analysis revealed continued evidence of inflammation. The toxic neutropenia on day 3 resulted from peritonitis with movement of neutrophils into the abdominal cavity. The lymphopenia and eosinopenia resulted from the endogenous release of glucocorticoids. The fibrinogen increased in response to inflammation. The increased serum AST activity was attributed to tissue injury. The horse eventually made a full recovery.

Case 4–2

Patient: Himalayan cat, castrated male, 5 years of age.

History: Respiratory distress developed 3 days earlier. The referring veterinarian began treatment with an antibiotic, but the condition worsened.

PE: The cat presented with abdominal respiration and tachypnea. Harsh lung sounds were auscultated. The cat was underweight and may have been slightly dehydrated. Enlarged prescapular, axillary, and inguinal lymph nodes and splenomegaly were palpated. Papules and scabs on the head and base of the tail were believed to represent a flea-bite allergy. The rectal temperature was 102.6°F.

Notable Laboratory Findings:

Hematology: HCT = 29% with normal RBC indices, total plasma protein = 8.6 g/dL, platelet count = normal, neutrophil count = 15,600/μL, lymphocyte count = 5100/μL, monocyte count = 1200/μL, band eosinophil count = 400/μL, eosinophil count = 22,300/μL, basophil count = 2100/μL, RBC morphology = normal.

Clinical chemistry: Total serum protein = 8.1 g/dL, total globulins = 5.9 g/dL.

Exfoliative cytology: Transthoracic lung aspiration revealed histiocytic eosinophilic inflammation. Increased numbers of eosinophils were also present in splenic and lymph node aspirates that appeared to exceed those present in contaminating blood.

Histopathology: Chronic ulcerative eosinophilic dermatitis.

Parasitology: ELISA heartworm test was negative.

Thoracic Radiographs: Patchy interstitial infiltrate.

Abdominal Ultrasound: Splenomegaly and slightly thickened loops of bowel.

Assessment: Based on the magnitude of the eosinophilia and evidence of eosinophilic infiltration and injury in multiple organs, a diagnosis of hypereosinophilic syndrome was made. The etiology of this syndrome is unknown. Evidence that the overproduction of IL-5 may be involved in producing this disorder has been presented in people with hypereosinophilic syndrome. A marked left shift in the eosinophilic series is expected in cats with eosinophilic leukemia. Eosinophilic leukemia was considered unlikely in this cat, because most of the eosinophils in blood and tissues were mature. When present in animals, basophilia generally accompany eosinophilia, possibly because certain growth factors (most notably IL-5) stimulate the production of both cell types. The slight neutrophilia and monocytosis present may be associated with the inflammation recognized in several tissues. The mild nonregenerative anemia is probably the result of the anemia of inflammatory disease. The increased serum protein concentration was the result of increased globulins, further supporting the likelihood of an inflammatory reaction.

Comment: The cat was placed in an oxygen cage and treated with aminophylline (a bronchodilator) and an antibiotic pending the outcome of diagnostic tests. Once a diagnosis of hypereosinophilic syndrome was reached, glucocorticoid therapy was initiated. Clinical signs improved rapidly and the cat was discharged with a plan to taper glucocorticoid dosage as clinical signs resolved.

References

Huibregtse BA, Turner JL: Hypereosinophilic syndrome and eosinophilic leukemia: a comparison of 22 hypereosinophilic cats. J Am Anim Hosp Assoc 1994;30:591.

Swenson CL, Carothers MA, Wellman ML, et al: Eosinophilic leukemia in a cat with naturally acquired feline leukemia virus infection. J Am Anim Hosp Assoc 1993;29:467.

Weller PF, Bubley GJ: The idiopathic hypereosinophilic syndrome. Blood 1994;83:2759.

Case 5-1

Patient: Rottweiler dog, female, 2 years of age.

History: Depression, lethargy, fever, and purulent bloody vaginal discharge for several days. Vomited the day of admission.

PE: Moderately depressed, panting respiration, slightly distended abdomen, dark-pink mucous membranes, rectal temperature 102 °F.

Notable Laboratory Findings (Day 1):
Hematology: HCT = 48%, total plasma protein = 7.5 g/dL, fibrinogen = 200 mg/dL, manual platelet count = 180,000/μL, band neutrophil count = 3700/μL, neutrophil count = 57,400/μL, lymphocyte count = 7700/μL, monocyte count = 3700/μL, eosinophil count = 700/μL, basophil count = 0/μL, RBC morphology = 1+ echinocytes, leukocyte morphology = 1+ toxicity of neutrophilic cells and occasional reactive lymphocytes.
Clinical chemistry: unremarkable.
Coagulation tests: prothrombin time (PT) = 9 seconds (control = 8 seconds), activated partial thromboplastin time (APTT) = 20 seconds (control = 10 seconds), activated clotting time (ACT) = 105 seconds (reference <120 seconds), fibrin degradation products (FDP) = positive at 1:20 dilution.

Abdominal Radiographs: No abnormalities appreciated.

Abdominal Ultrasound: Large, fluid-filled uterus identified.

Assessment: The marked neutrophilia with toxic left-shift and monocytosis indicated a severe inflammatory reaction. The presence of a dilated uterus and purulent vaginal discharge indicated that the dog had pyometra. The lymphocytosis may have reflected antigenic stimulation. The decreased platelet count, prolonged APTT and positive FDP test indicated the presence of DIC. Although the PT was normal, this test appears to be less sensitive than the APTT in the diagnosis of DIC. The ACT may have been normal because the ACT is less sensitive than the APTT in revealing abnormalities of the intrinsic and common coagulation pathways. Fibrinogen is an acute-phase protein that tends to increase during inflammation; consequently, the normal fibrinogen value did not rule-out DIC.

Comment: Antibiotic and intravenous fluid therapy was begun after the first blood sample was taken. Epistaxis began on the following day and the animal became more depressed.

Notable Laboratory Findings (Day 2):
Hematology: HCT = 32% with normal RBC indices, total plasma protein = 6.4 g/dL, fibrinogen = 400 mg/dL, manual platelet count = 61,000/μL, metamyelocyte count = 800/μL, band neutrophil count = 8400/μL, neutrophil count = 65,900/μL, lymphocyte count = 2100/μL, monocyte count = 7200/μL, eosinophil count = 0/μL, basophil count = 0/μL, RBC morphology = 1+ echinocytes, leukocyte morphology = 1+ toxicity of neutrophilic cells and occasional reactive lymphocytes.

Coagulation test: ACT = 150 seconds (reference <120 seconds).

Assessment: The neutrophilia with toxic left-shift and monocytosis were more pronounced on the second day. The decrease that occurred in lymphocyte count and eosinopenia that developed suggested that increased endogenous glucocorticoid release occurred as the dog's clinical condition worsened. The decreased HCT on the second day was primarily the result of fluid therapy. The further decrease in the platelet count and the prolonged ACT suggested the continuation of DIC.

Comment: Ovariohysterectomy was performed after the blood sample was collected on the second day and the dog made an uneventful recovery.

Reference

Sevelius E, Tidholm A, Thoren-Tolling K: Pyometra in the dog. J Am Anim Hosp Assoc 1990;26:33.

Case 6–1

Patient: Cocker spaniel dog, male, 4 years of age.

History: Rear-leg lameness associated with bilateral hip dysplasia was diagnosed 2 years ago and erosive nonseptic arthritis involving the carpal and tarsal joints was recognized 4 months ago. The HCT and platelet counts were normal at that time, but the ANA test was positive at 1:100 dilution (reference <1:20). The dog has been treated with aspirin the past 4 months.

PE: The dog was depressed with pale mucous membranes. A polyarthropathy was present and all joints were painful. There were multiple raised pigmented skin lesions and small petechial hemorrhages were present on the penis and abdomen. The rectal temperature was normal.

Notable Laboratory Findings:

Hematology: HCT = 23%; MCV = 74 fL; MCHC = 33 g/dL; reticulocyte count = 184,000/μL; total plasma protein = 7.9 g/dL; fibrinogen = 400 mg/dL; manual platelet count = 8000/μL; band neutrophil count = 600/μL; neutrophil count = 12,900/μL; lymphocyte count = 700/μL; monocyte count = 2000/μL; eosinophil count = 1000/μL; nucleated RBC count = 500/μL; RBC morphology = 3+ anisocytosis, 2+ polychromasia, 3+ spherocytosis, occasional Howell-Jolly bodies, and autoagglutination of saline washed RBCs.

Clinical chemistry: Total serum protein = 8.2 g/dL and the total globulin = 5.6 g/dL.

Urinalysis: S.G. = 1.042, moderate bilirubinuria.

Joint fluid: A direct smear from a swollen joint revealed increased numbers of nondegenerate neutrophils and macrophages.

ANA test: Positive at 1:320 dilution (reference <1:20).

Skin biopsy: Histologic lesions were consistent with pemphigus foliaceous, an immune-mediated skin disorder, but direct immunofluorescence examination for IgG deposits in skin was negative.

Assessment: The presence of autoagglutination of saline-washed RBCs and spherocytosis indicates the presence of an immune-mediated anemia. The high normal MCV and slightly decreased MCHC result from the increased percentage of reticulocytes present and the absolute reticulocytosis indicates an appropriate bone marrow response to the anemia. The low number of nucleated RBCs present is suitable for the degree of reticulocytosis. The petechial hemorrhages present can be attributed to the severe thrombocytopenia. Based on the presence of an immune-mediated hemolytic anemia and a positive ANA test, the thrombocytopenia was presumed to be immune-mediated. The combined presence of immune-mediated anemia and thrombocytopenia has been termed the "Evans syndrome." The presence of high-normal numbers of eosinophils suggests that endogenous glucocorticoid release is not responsible for the neutrophilia, monocytosis and lymphopenia. The increased total globulins in serum and high-normal plasma fibrinogen concentration are consistent with inflammation, as is the mild neutrophilia with left shift and monocytosis. Bilirubinuria is common in dogs with hemolytic anemia even when bilirubinemia is not present, because of the low renal threshold for bilirubin in dogs. A presumptive diagnosis of systemic lupus erythematosus (SLE) was made based on the concomitant occurrence of immune-mediated hemolytic anemia, thrombocytopenia, nonseptic polyarthritis and positive ANA test. The skin lesion may also have been a component of this syndrome, but an immune-mediated etiology could not be confirmed.

Comment: Therapy consisted of glucocorticoid steroids and cyclophosphamide. When examined one week later, the animal appeared less painful, skin lesions were resolving, the HCT was 27%, MCV was 77 fL, and platelet count was $1.2 \times 10^6/\mu$L. The resolution of the thrombocytopenia following initiation of immunosuppressive therapy provides retrospective evidence that the thrombocytopenia was immune-mediated. It is assumed that the animal had high plasma thrombopoietin values when thrombocytopenic and that the subsequent thrombocytosis occurred as a rebound phenomenon when premature platelet destruction was reduced or eliminated by immunosuppressive therapy.

Reference

Grindem CB, Johnson KH: Systemic lupus erythematosus: literature review and report of 42 new canine cases. J Am Anim Hosp Assoc 1983;19:489.

Case 7–1

Patient: Mixed-breed dog, female, 4 years of age.

History: Showing signs of estrus, gone all night, returned the next day, vomited "garbage" two or three times, taken to the veterinarian the next day.

PE: Depressed, 6 to 8% dehydrated, fluid- and gas-filled intestinal tract

Radiology: Unremarkable.

Notable Laboratory Findings:
Hematology: Hct = 49%, plasma protein = 7.7 g/dL, neutrophil count = 18,800/μL, lymphocyte count = 600/μL, platelet count = 220,000/μL.
Chemistries: ALT = 1340 U/L, AST = 655 U/L, ALP = 155 U/L, urea nitrogen = 41 mg/dL, creatinine = 2.1 mg/dL, total bilirubin = 1.1 mg/dL, total protein = 7.1 g/dL albumin = 4.1 g/dL, amylase and lipase within reference range.
Urinalysis: specific gravity = 1.045, moderate bilirubinuria, hyalin casts (0–2/hpf).

Assessment: The changes of the Hct, plasma protein, total protein, albumin, urea nitrogen, creatinine, urine specific gravity, and hyalin casts are a consequence of dehydration. The neutrophilia and lymphopenia are indicative of "stress." The raised serum ALT (moderate) and AST (marked) activities indicate acute, severe, hepatocellular injury. The hyperbilirubinemia (with bilirubinuria) and raised serum ALP activity indicate a cholestatic component; the minimal increase of the ALP further supports an acute timeline. The raised serum urea nitrogen and creatinine concentrations coincident with a concentrated urine specific gravity indicate prerenal azotemia secondary to dehydration.

Comment: Supportive medical management was instituted. During the third day, spontaneous bleeding was noted from the venepuncture sites, the dog appeared stuporous, and was referred.

PE: Semicomatosed, pale mucous membranes, scleral icterus, abdominal fluid.

Notable Laboratory Findings:
Hematology: Hct = 12%, plasma protein = <2 g/dL, schistocytes present, platelet count = 5000/μL, slightly reddish yellow discolored plasma, prothrombin time = prolonged-20 seconds, activated partial thromboplastin time = prolonged-33 seconds, fibrin degradation products (+, >1:40).
Chemistries: ALT = 102 U/L, AST = 93 U/L, ALP = 41 U/L, glucose = 45 mg/dL, urea nitrogen = 4 mg/dL, creatinine = 1.5 mg/dL, total bilirubin = 3.1 mg/dL, total protein = 1.1 g/dL, albumin = 0.6 g/dL, ammonia = 125 μg/dL (reference <40 μg/dL).
Abdominocentesis: red-colored fluid, cytologically consistent with blood.

Assessment: The Hct and plasma protein indicate blood loss, in this case there is no external hemorrhage, therefore internal bleeding. The reduced serum albumin concentration cannot be due to liver disease because its plasma half-life is approximately 2 weeks. The hemolyzed plasma, schistocytes, thrombocytopenia, prolonged coagulation tests, and presence of fibrin degradation products indicates a coagulopathy (disseminated, intravascular, DIC). The precipitous reduction of the serum ALT and AST activities is suggestive of inadequate hepatocellular mass to maintain their increase; in part, an indirect reflection of the absence of a critical hepatic structural mass to support the regeneration/reparation process subsequent to injury. The reduced serum glucose concentration, urea nitrogen concentration (with a normal creatinine), and the absence of a further increase in the serum ALP activity (in fact, a reduction) despite the presence of a cholestasis lends further support to inadequate hepatic tissue for their production. Both the hemolytic component of DIC and cholestatic process contribute to the raised serum total bilirubin concentration. The hyperammonemia confirms the presence of hepatic encephalopathy.

Comment: The dog died 6 hours later. Histologically, there was virtually no viable hepatocellular tissue observed. Numerous pigment-filled macrophages replaced most of the parenchymal tissue. No etiology was apparent. These findings are consistent with an acute toxic insult to the liver. Drugs such as mebendazole and trimethoprim/sulfa combinations can cause similar hepatic histopathologic findings. Fulminant hepatic failure is likely the cause of the coagulopathy.

Case 7–2

Patient: American quarter horse mare, 8 years of age.

History: Acute onset of lethargy, inappetence, head-pressing, circling. She had a 2-month-old foal and had been given tetanus antitoxin at the time of parturition.

PE: Lethargy, stuporous, jaundice, self-inflicted facial skin lesions.

Notable Laboratory Findings:

Hematology: Hct = 58%, plasma protein = 8.0 g/dL, icteric plasma.

Chemistries: total bilirubin = 12 mg/dL, AST = 1966 U/L, SD = 445 U/L, CK = 1105 U/L, GGT = 135 U/L, total bile acid = 55 μmol/L, plasma ammonia concentration = 25 μg/dL (reference <40 μg/dL), total protein = 7.6 g/dL, urea nitrogen = 48 mg/dL, creatinine = 3.1 mg/dL.

Assessment: The polycythemia, raised plasma protein concentration, serum urea nitrogen, and creatinine concentrations indicate dehydration. Acute hepatocellular injury is indicated by the raised SD and AST activities. The slightly raised serum CK activity indicates muscle injury, probably associated with the trauma. The raised serum GGT activity indicates a cholestatic component to the hepatic pathology. Fasting results in hyperbilirubinemia; in this case, cholestasis may be contributing to the raised total bilirubin concentration as well because of the raised serum total bile acid concentration which indicates hepatic dysfunction, consistent with signs of hepatic encephalopathy. The plasma ammonia concentration was within the reference range; not surprising since it is labile and dependent on the ingestion of protein.

Comment: The histopathologic findings of a needle biopsy of the liver included severe hepatocellular degeneration and parenchymal collapse (predominantly zone 3) with canalicular/bile ductular casts and mild bile duct hyperplasia. The histopathologic findings of relatively acute hepatocellular injury involving zone 3 are consistent with the disease termed "serum hepatitis."

Case 7–3

Patient: Doberman pinscher, female, spayed, 8 years of age.

History: Persistent, mildly increased serum hepatic enzyme tests for 1 year. Treatment with prednisolone for 1 month resulted in no change of the serum ALT activity, an increase in serum ALP activity, and severe polydipsia/polyuria. The client declined further treatment. The dog was active and eating well during this entire time. One month prior to referral, polydipsia/polyuria developed; 2 weeks prior, she developed a distended abdomen, and was observed to drool frequently and have intermittent head-shaking and act disoriented.

PE: Alert, ascites present

Notable Laboratory Findings:

Hematology: Hct = 40%, MCV = 58 fL, platelets adequate, prothrombin time = normal, activated partial thromboplastin time = prolonged-8 seconds (24 hours after two subcutaneous treatments with vitamin K_1 it returned to normal).

Chemistries: albumin = 2.2 g/dL, ALT = 155 U/L, ALP = 242 U/L, (fasting) total bile acid = 235 μmol/L. During an episode of abnormal neurologic behavior: ammonia = 160 μg/dL (reference <40 μg/dL), (fasting) total bile acid = 226 μmol/L, 24 hours after treatment with neomycin and lactulose, ammonia 21 μg/dL and total bile acid = 240 μmol/L.

Urinalysis: specific gravity = 1.025, bilirubinuria 2+.

Abdominal fluid: total protein <2.5 g/dL, low cell count, predominantly mesothelial cells with a small number of neutrophils and lymphocytes.

Ultrasound: Abdominal fluid, small liver with irregular surface and variable echogenic density. An attempt to obtain a needle biopsy was not successful.

Assessment: The findings are consistent with hepatic insufficiency resulting in hepatic encephalopathy, reduced albumin and coagulation factor (activated) production, and portal hypertension causing ascites (transudate). The ammonia and total bile acid measurements demonstrate the different value in assessing the different components of hepatic function. The microcytosis, sometimes accompanied by a mild anemia, is observed in association with portosystemic shunts (congenital and acquired) for reasons that are poorly understood.

Comment: After 3 days of vitamin K_1, neomycin, and lactulose treatment, a laparotomy was used to obtain a hepatic biopsy from a small liver with multiple, variably sized and colored (tan to dark brown) nodules. Multiple portocaval shunts were prominent near the left kidney. The descriptive histopathologic findings included nodules of hepatocytes often vacuolated, cholangiohepatitis, bile duct proliferation, and lipogranulomas (fatty cysts), the findings initially suggestive of cirrhosis. Reassessment following reticulin and trichrome stains demonstrated multiple nodules that compressed the existing hepatic tissue into the portal tract areas. These areas consisted of condensed reticulin tissue, mixed inflammatory cell infiltration, extramedullary hematopoiesis comprised of myeloid precursors giving the additional appearance of inflammation, and bile duct proliferation. There was minimal increase in the connective tissue to warrant a classification of cirrhosis. The findings were interpreted as marked nodular proliferation (hyperplasia) with nonspecific secondary changes (Kelly, 1993). The differentiation from cirrhosis is important because the pathology is not "driven" by a necroinflammatory process. The patient with hepatic insufficiency secondary to nodular hyperplasia can be managed more favorably with supportive management than the cirrhotic patient. The polydipsia and polyuria may be associated with an abnormal "setting" of the pituitary-adrenal axis. It has been found that dogs with either congenital or acquired portosystemic shunts often have raised basal plasma cortisol and ACTH concentrations (dexamethasone suppressible) and abnormal vasopressin regulation with a consequent reduced urine specific gravity (Rothuizen et al, 1995).

References

Kelly WR: The liver and biliary system. In Jubb KVF, Kennedy PC, Palmer N (eds): Pathology of Domestic Animals, 4th edition, vol II. San Diego, Academic Press, 1993, p 349.
Rothuizen J, Biewenga WJ, Mol JA: Chronic glucocorticoid excess and impaired osmoregulation of vasopression release in dogs with hepatic encephalopathy. Domest Anim Endocrinol 1995;12:13–24.

Case 7–4

Patient: Persian, female, 6 months of age.

History: Mellow personality, occasional exaggerated chewing movements (like something stuck in its mouth), appears occasionally ataxic, seizured twice, presented semicomatosed.

PE: Small for age, semicomatosed, aware of surroundings but could not be aroused.

Notable Laboratory Findings:

Hematology: Hct = 28%, MCV = 36 fL, normochromic erythrocytes with moderate numbers of poikilocytes.

Chemistries: ALP = 125 U/L, urea nitrogen = 8 mg/dL, creatinine = 1.5 mg/dL, ammonia = 340 μg/dL (reference <40 μg/dL), fasting total bile acid = 78 μmol/L.

Urinalysis: ammonium biurate crystals.

Assessment: Hepatic encephalopathy is confirmed by the hyperammonemia; the reduced serum urea nitrogen concentration in combination with a normal serum creatinine concentration and the raised serum total bile acid concentration are also consistent with hepatic insufficiency. The underdeveloped physical status and neurologic signs plus the abnormal hepatic function tests and ammonia biurate crystalluria are indicative of a congenital portosystemic shunt. A microcytic anemia, sometimes with irregularly spiculated erythrocytes, also is noted occasionally in this disorder for reasons that are poorly understood. The raised serum ALP activity is probably due to an increased activity of the bone isoenzyme associated with growth.

Comment: 48 hours after neomycin and lactose medical management the cat was alert and the ammonia was 35 μg/dL, the (fasting) total bile acid was 75 μmol/L. The reduction of the plasma ammonia concentration with an unchanged serum total bile acid concentration demonstrates the value of using different "types" of tests for the evaluation of hepatic function. A single extrahepatic portocaval shunt was identified with contrast portography and ligated. Two weeks after surgery the plasma ammonia concentration was 15 μg/dL and the fasting serum total bile acid concentration was 4 μmol/L.

Case 7–5

Patient: Thoroughbred foal, 4 months of age.

History: Small for age, clumsy, observed occasionally head-pressing and circling, poor appetite.

PE: Poorly developed muscle mass, dull, depressed, unresponsive to the menace response, staggering, slightly ataxic gait, scleral icterus.

Notable Laboratory Findings:
Hematology: Hct = 34%, MCV = 34 fL, normochromic erythrocytes.
Chemistries: total bilirubin concentration = 6.5 mg/dL, ammonia = 150 μg/dL (reference <40 μg/dL), total bile acid concentration = 76 μmol/L.

Assessment: The Hct and MCV are appropriate for the age of the animal. Hepatic encephalopathy is confirmed by the hyperammonemia. The raised serum total bile acid concentration is also indicative of liver insufficiency. The neurologic signs in a young animal with liver insufficiency is compatible with a congenital portosystemic shunt and "rule out" a primary central nervous system disease as the cause of the clinical signs. The hyperbilirubinemia is probably secondary to inappetence; it does not interfere with bile acid kinetics.

Comment: Jejunal vein contrast portography was used to identify a portocaval shunt.

Case 7-6

Patient: Golden retriever, male, 3 years of age.

History: Reluctant to chase the Frisbee for 3 weeks, walks stiff legged, remains alert and has a good appetite. At least two previous episodes during the past 3 months that resolved within 1 week with aspirin treatment.

PE: Alert, has a short, choppy gait, no neck pain, manipulation of the stifle joints causes discomfort.

Notable Laboratory Findings:
   Hematology: neutrophil count = 17,430/μL.
   Chemistries: AST = 178 U/L (ALT normal); based on these results a CK was requested from the same sample; CK = 1253 U/L.
   Synovial fluid: samples from both stifle and both carpal joints were examined cytologically. Specimens from all joints had slightly to markedly increased nucleated cell numbers (estimated to be 10,000/μL to >50,000/μL) comprised predominantly of neutrophils, no bacteria were observed.

Assessment: The neutrophilia indicates an inflammatory process. The raised serum CK activity and neutrophil infiltration of the joints are indicative of myositis and synovitis, respectively.

Comment: Radiographs of the joints were unremarkable. Multiorgan disease is suggestive of an immune-mediated process. An antinuclear antibody (ANA) tests was 1:640 (reference <1:20), supportive of an immune-mediated disease. The dog was successfully managed with prednisolone. Nonerosive polyarthritis is generally found in large-breed dogs. The concurrence of myositis is uncommon.

Case 8–1

Patient: Domestic Long Hair, female, spayed, 7 years of age.

History: Vomiting 2 to 3 times a day on most days for the past 6 weeks. Most of the time the vomitus is yellow-green fluid or is slightly thicker and is the color of the canned food that it eats. Hair balls are occasionally observed. There are days when the cat does not act hungry. The stools have been poorly formed on occasion during the past 2 weeks. Slight weight loss has occurred.

PE: The body weight is 1.5 pounds less than it was 8 months earlier when seen for its annual vaccinations. The cat is tense and difficult to examine.

Notable Laboratory Findings:
   Hematology: neutrophil count = 16,590/μL.
   Chemistries: ALT = 155 U/L; ALP = 99 U/L; glucose = 368 mg/dL.
   Urinalysis: glucosuria (+1).

Radiology: Examination of the abdomen is unremarkable.

Assessment: The neutrophilia and hyperglycemia (and resultant glucosuria) may be the result of stress. The findings could also be consistent with a stressed cat with diabetes mellitus (type I or type II). The raised ALT and ALP activities suggest liver disease; either primary or possibly secondary to diabetes mellitus (lipidosis). The measurement of the serum bile acid and fructosamine concentrations are suggested along with ultrasonography to evaluate for acute pancreatitis (the measurement of serum amylase and lipase activities are not diagnostically useful in the cat; the measurement of the serum TLI activity by methodology specific for the cat is an alternative). The owner is reluctant to pay for more tests at this time. The amount and frequency of its usual oral treatment for hair balls is increased and metoclopramide hydrochloride is dispensed for one week.

Examination 2 weeks later (did not show up for its one week evaluation):
   There was a reduction in the frequency of the vomiting while taking the medication but frequency has increased with its discontinuation and it has been inappetent the past two days. The owner agrees to additional tests.

PE: Same as initial examination.

Notable Laboratory Findings:
   Hematology: neutrophil count = 15,500/μL.
   Chemistries: ALT = 142 U/L; ALP = 95 U/L; glucose = 340 mg/dL; total bile acids (presumably fasted) = 5.5; fructosamine 295 μmol/L (within reference range).
   Urinalysis: glucosuria (+1).

Assessment: The serum fructosamine concentration is consistent with a stress hyperglycemia (consistent with the neutrophilia). The serum bile acid concentration is at the upper end of the reference range and only indicates that component of hepatic function has not been markedly altered. Extrahepatic diseases can cause abnormal hepatic tests (refer to Fig. 7–16), and the patient is referred for ultrasonography of the pancreas and endoscopy.

Comment: Ultrasonography of the abdomen was unremarkable (an enlarged gall bladder was noted). Visual examination of the duodenum was unremarkable. Histopathologic findings from multiple biopsy specimens was consistent with lymphocytic-plasmacytic enteritis (moderate severity).

Case 9–1

Patient: German shepherd, female, spayed, 5 years of age.

History: Weakness, lethargy, inappetence, weight loss, and vomiting (unrelated to meals) present for approximately 2 months; more pronounced periodically the past several weeks. Vitamin supplements and herbal medications prescribed at another veterinary hospital did not seem to help.

PE: Lethargic and thinner than expected for size.

Notable Laboratory Findings:

Hematology: Hct = 34%, reticulocyte count = 39,000/μL.

Chemistries: urea nitrogen = 32 mg/dL, creatinine = 1.4, glucose = 63 mg/dL, ALT = 86 U/L, ALP = 210, cholesterol = 99 mg/dL, albumin 2.3 mg/dL (total protein = 7.0 mg/dL).

Urinalysis: specific gravity = 1.038.

Assessment: There is a normocytic, normochromic, nonregenerative anemia (mild). There is a mild azotemia (with the serum creatinine concentration within the reference range) and moderately concentrated urine consistent with prerenal azotemia. However, with the protracted history of lack of oral intake of adequate food or water one might expect the urine specific gravity to be raised more than it is. Consequently, early primary renal disease should remain as a differential diagnosis especially with the presence of a nonregenerative anemia and a reduced muscle mass which could affect the plasma creatinine concentration. The serum ALT and ALP activities are slightly raised and the serum albumin concentration is slightly reduced, suggestive of a hepatopathy (hepatic insufficiency). Hypocholesterolemia and hypoglycemia can be associated with congenital portosystemic shunts, one cause of hepatic insufficiency. Consequently, the serum bile acid concentration should be measured. A value of 6.5 μmol/L (presumably fasting) was determined the next day, eliminating hepatic insufficiency as the primary disease process.

The constellation of nonspecific, persistent clinical signs and multiorgan system involvement is suggestive of hypoadrenocorticism (glucocorticoid deficiency only). Because the mineralocorticoid secretion is not affected, the plasma sodium and potassium concentrations remain within the reference range. The basal plasma cortisol concentration was 1.2 μg/dL and the 2-hour post-ACTH stimulation concentration was 1.6 μg/dL. The absence of a notable rise supports the diagnosis. The clinical response to glucocorticoid treatment was rapid and maintained.

Comment: While we know that endogenous glucocorticoids affect all organ systems in health, we do not understand all the reasons for the changes in the clinicopathologic measurements when there is a deficiency. They have a positive effect on hematopoiesis and gluconeogenesis, and enhance the response of the renal collecting tubules to antidiuretic hormone (vasopressin). A deficiency would result in the nonregenerative anemia, hypoglycemia, and inappropriate urine specific gravity. Lack of adequate nutrition may be the cause of the hypoalbuminemia. Because the albumin value was reduced, the total protein value remained in the reference range and did not support the suspected subclinical dehydration. The hypocholesterolemia may also be a result of inadequate nutrition. The reason for the abnormal serum hepatic enzyme activities are not known.

Case 10–1

Patient: Lhasa apso, female, 18 months of age.

History: Marked increase in water intake during the past 6 months, occasionally urinated in the house as a puppy but now frequently voids large volumes during the night, not interested in eating the past 2 weeks, difficulty breathing for 2 to 3 days.

PE: Quiet, mucous membranes are slightly pale, 6 to 8% dehydrated, mild dyspnea observed in the waiting room which was amplified by the exertion of handling, possible decreased lung sounds on the right side.

Notable Laboratory Findings:

Hematology: Hct = 29%, MCV = 64 fL, reticulocyte count = 45,000/μL, plasma protein = 5.1 g/dL.

Chemistries: urea nitrogen = 126 mg/dL, creatinine = 6.5 mg/dL, total protein = 5.3, albumin = 2.2 g/dL, cholesterol = 395 mg/dL, calcium = 7.7 mEq/L (corrected 9.0 mEq/L), phosphorous = 11.5 mg/dL, total CO_2 = 11 mEq/L.

Urinalysis: specific gravity = 1.009, protein = 4+, casts (coarse granular, waxy) = 2 to 5/hpf (reference <1 hyaline or fine granular per hpf), urine protein to creatinine ratio = 4.4 (reference <0.4).

Radiology: Abdomen—both kidneys are small; thorax—possible increased interstitial pattern on the right side.

Assessment: The laboratory findings are indicative of chronic renal insufficiency. The nonregenerative anemia is due to a deficiency of erythropoietin. The markedly raised serum urea nitrogen, creatinine, and phosphorous (initially) concentrations reflect an insufficient glomerular filtration rate while the marked proteinuria develops when the glomeruli can no longer adequately retain larger molecules (MW greater than ~40,000; MW of albumin is 66,000). The reduced serum albumin concentration is a consequence of increased loss. The loss of antithrombin III of approximately the same molecular weight can predispose to hypercoagulability and thromboembolism. The pulmonary vasculature is a common site for thromboembolism and it is probably the cause of dyspnea in this dog. The lesion is difficult to observe radiographically early in its development.

The specific gravity indicates that the tubules can neither concentrate nor dilute urine in response to antidiuretic hormone (ADH). Decreased tubular function contributes to the hyperphosphatemia in concert with secondary hyperparathyroidism in the more chronic cases. The reduction of viable renal tissue results in a decreased formation of calcitriol, the active form of vitamin D. Calcitriol provides negative feedback inhibition of the synthesis parathyroid hormone (PTH). The increased serum PTH concentration is responsible for many of the pathophysiologic consequences of chronic renal insufficiency. The reduction of the serum calcitriol concentration causes skeletal resistance to the action of PTH promoting a decrease in the plasma ionized calcium concentration.

The reduced total carbon dioxide suggests metabolic acidosis, a common consequence of chronic renal failure due to the tubules' decreased ability to excrete hydrogen ion and regenerate bicarbonate. The acidemia causes more of the albumin-bound calcium to exist in the physiologically active ionized state; it helps explain the absence of clinical signs of hypocalcemia when the total calcium is reduced. Care should be taken not to acutely alkalinize these patients; it causes a "shift" of the ionized calcium back to the bound form and could precipitate hypocalcemic tetany. The granular and waxy casts form in the damaged, poorly functioning tubules (with reduced filtrate flow) from the large quantities of "escaped" proteins together with the degenerating cells.

The hypercholesterolemia is probably related to the loss of albumin (and possibly other proteins). A persistent reduction in the plasma albumin concentration signals the liver to increase its production of albumin. The stimulus for enhanced albumin synthesis appears to nonspecifically activate other synthetic pathways including those involved in the formation of lipoproteins. The cholesterol-rich particles contribute to the increased serum cholesterol concentration.

Part **III**

ALGORITHMS

*It is common error to infer that things which are consec-
utive in order of time have necessarily the relations of
cause and effect.*

Jacob Bigelow

Algorithm 1

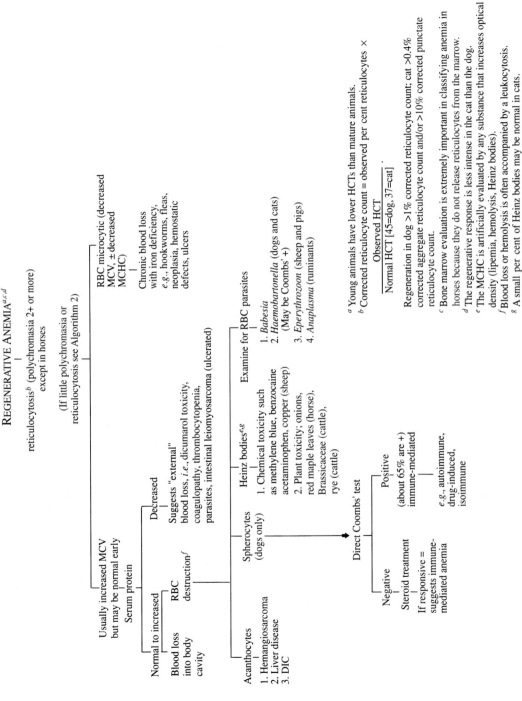

REGENERATIVE ANEMIA[a,c,d]
|
reticulocytosis[b] (polychromasia 2+ or more) except in horses

(If little polychromasia or reticulocytosis see Algorithm 2)

Usually increased MCV but may be normal early — Serum protein

- **Normal to increased**
  - RBC destruction[f]
  - Blood loss into body cavity
- **Decreased** — Suggests "external" blood loss, i.e., dicumarol toxicity, coagulopathy, thrombocytopenia, parasites, intestinal leiomyosarcoma (ulcerated)
- **RBC microcytic (decreased MCV, ± decreased MCHC)** — Chronic blood loss with iron deficiency, e.g., hookworms, fleas, neoplasia, hemostatic defects, ulcers

RBC destruction[f]

- Acanthocytes
  1. Hemangiosarcoma
  2. Liver disease
  3. DIC
- Spherocytes (dogs only) → Direct Coombs' test
  - Negative — Steroid treatment. If responsive = suggests immune-mediated anemia
  - Positive (about 65% are +) immune-mediated — e.g., autoimmune, drug-induced, isoimmune
- Heinz bodies[e,g]
  1. Chemical toxicity such as methylene blue, benzocaine acetaminophen, copper (sheep)
  2. Plant toxicity; onions, red maple leaves (horse), Brassicaceae (cattle), rye (cattle)
- Examine for RBC parasites
  1. *Babesia*
  2. *Haemobartonella* (dogs and cats) (May be Coombs' +)
  3. *Eperythrozoon* (sheep and pigs)
  4. *Anaplasma* (ruminants)

[a] Young animals have lower HCTs than mature animals.

[b] Corrected reticulocyte count = observed per cent reticulocytes ×

$$\frac{\text{Observed HCT}}{\text{Normal HCT [45=dog, 37=cat]}}.$$

Regeneration in dog >1% corrected reticulocyte count; cat >0.4% corrected aggregate reticulocyte count and/or >10% corrected punctate reticulocyte count.

[c] Bone marrow evaluation is extremely important in classifying anemia in horses because they do not release reticulocytes from the marrow.

[d] The regenerative response is less intense in the cat than the dog.

[e] The MCHC is artificially evaluated by any substance that increases optical density (lipemia, hemolysis, Heinz bodies).

[f] Blood loss or hemolysis is often accompanied by a leukocytosis.

[g] A small per cent of Heinz bodies may be normal in cats.

Algorithm 2

POORLY REGENERATIVE OR NONREGENERATIVE ANEMIA[a,c,d]

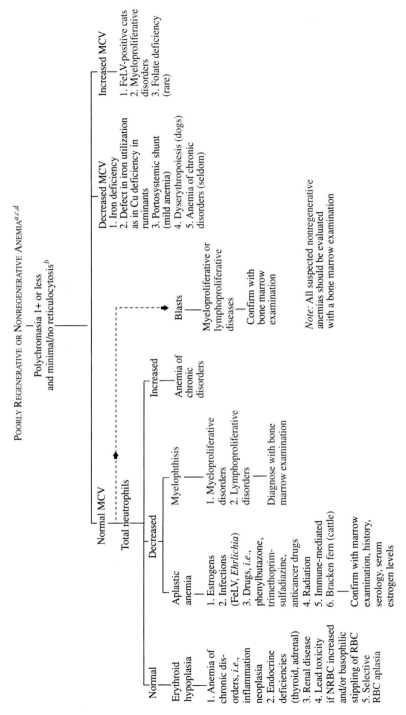

Polychromasia 1+ or less
and minimal/no reticulocytosis[b]

Normal MCV

Total neutrophils

Decreased

Aplastic anemia

1. Estrogens
2. Infections (FeLV, *Ehrlichia*)
3. Drugs, *i.e.*, phenylbutazone, trimethoprim-sulfadiazine, anticancer drugs
4. Radiation
5. Immune-mediated
6. Bracken fern (cattle)

Confirm with marrow examination, history, serology, serum estrogen levels

Myelophthisis

1. Myeloproliferative disorders
2. Lymphoproliferative disorders

Diagnose with bone marrow examination

Increased

Anemia of chronic disorders

Blasts

Myeloproliferative or lymphoproliferative diseases

Confirm with bone marrow examination

Note: All suspected nonregenerative anemias should be evaluated with a bone marrow examination

Normal

Erythroid hypoplasia

1. Anemia of chronic disorders, *i.e.*, inflammation neoplasia
2. Endocrine deficiencies (thyroid, adrenal)
3. Renal disease
4. Lead toxicity if NRBC increased and/or basophilic stippling of RBC
5. Selective RBC aplasia

Decreased MCV

1. Iron deficiency
2. Defect in iron utilization as in Cu deficiency in ruminants
3. Portosystemic shunt (mild anemia)
4. Dyserythropoiesis (dogs)
5. Anemia of chronic disorders (seldom)

Increased MCV

1. FeLV-positive cats
2. Myeloproliferative disorders
3. Folate deficiency (rare)

---

[a] Young animals have lower HCTs than mature animals.

[b] Corrected reticulocyte count = observed % reticulocyte × $\dfrac{\text{Observed HCT}}{\text{Normal HCT [45=dog, 37=cat]}}$.

Regeneration in dog >1% corrected reticulocyte count; cat >0.4% corrected aggregate reticulocyte count and/or >10% corrected punctate reticulocyte count.

[c] Bone marrow evaluation is especially important in the diagnosis of nonregenerative anemia.

[d] All cats with anemias should be tested for FeLV and FIV.

322

Algorithm 3

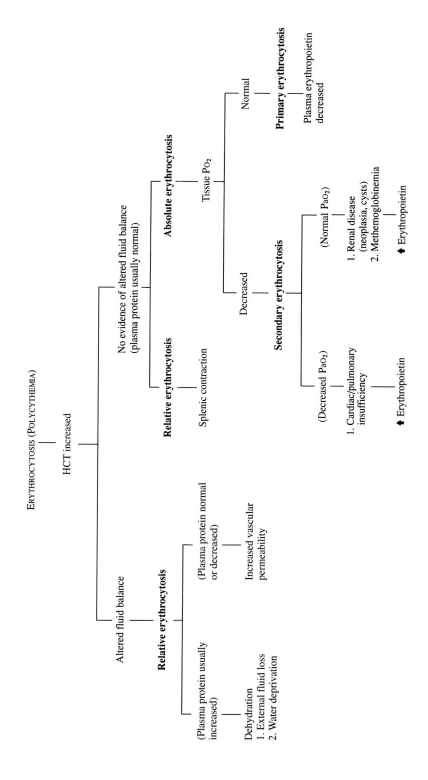

ERYTHROCYTOSIS (POLYCYTHEMIA)

HCT increased

Altered fluid balance

Relative erythrocytosis

(Plasma protein usually increased)

Dehydration
1. External fluid loss
2. Water deprivation

(Plasma protein normal or decreased)

Increased vascular permeability

No evidence of altered fluid balance
(plasma protein usually normal)

Relative erythrocytosis

Splenic contraction

Absolute erythrocytosis

Tissue Po_2

Decreased

Secondary erythrocytosis

(Decreased Pao_2)

1. Cardiac/pulmonary insufficiency

↑ Erythropoietin

(Normal Pao_2)

1. Renal disease (neoplasia, cysts)
2. Methemoglobinemia

↑ Erythropoietin

Normal

Primary erythrocytosis

Plasma erythropoietin decreased

Algorithm 4

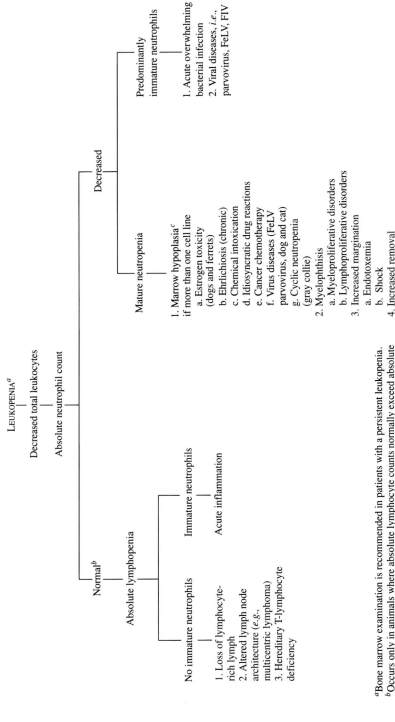

LEUKOPENIA[a]

Decreased total leukocytes

Absolute neutrophil count

Normal[b]

Absolute lymphopenia

Immature neutrophils

Acute inflammation

No immature neutrophils

1. Loss of lymphocyte-rich lymph
2. Altered lymph node architecture (e.g., multicentric lymphoma)
3. Hereditary T-lymphocyte deficiency

Decreased

Mature neutropenia

1. Marrow hypoplasia[c] if more than one cell line
   a. Estrogen toxicity (dogs and ferrets)
   b. Ehrlichiosis (chronic)
   c. Chemical intoxication
   d. Idiosyncratic drug reactions
   e. Cancer chemotherapy
   f. Virus diseases (FeLV parvovirus, dog and cat)
   g. Cyclic neutropenia (gray collie)
2. Myelophthisis
   a. Myeloproliferative disorders
   b. Lymphoproliferative disorders
3. Increased margination
   a. Endotoxemia
   b. Shock
4. Increased removal
   a. Immune-mediated
   b. Hypersplenism

Predominantly immature neutrophils

1. Acute overwhelming bacterial infection
2. Viral diseases, i.e., parvovirus, FeLV, FIV

[a]Bone marrow examination is recommended in patients with a persistent leukopenia.
[b]Occurs only in animals where absolute lymphocyte counts normally exceed absolute neutrophil counts (ruminants, occasionally horses).
[c]Marrow hypoplasia frequently involves more than one cell line. Anemia and/or thrombocytopenia are often present.

Algorithm 5

NORMAL OR INCREASED TOTAL LEUKOCYTE COUNT
WITH ABNORMAL DIFFERENTIAL COUNTS[a]

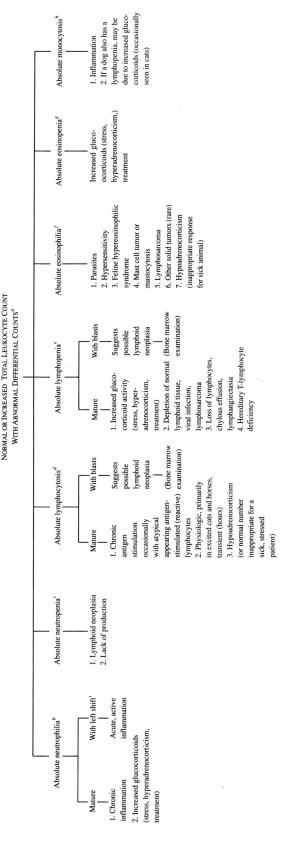

Absolute neutrophilia[b]

- Mature
  1. Chronic inflammation
  2. Increased glucocorticoids (stress, hyperadrenocorticism, treatment)
- With left shift[i]
  - Acute, active inflammation

Absolute neutropenia[c]

1. Lymphoid neoplasia
2. Lack of production

Absolute lymphocytosis[d]

- Mature
  1. Chronic antigen stimulation occasionally with atypical appearing antigen-stimulated (reactive) lymphocytes
  2. Physiologic, primarily in excited cats and horses, transient (hours)
  3. Hypoadrenocorticism (or normal number inappropriate for a sick, stressed patient)
- With blasts
  - Suggests possible lymphoid neoplasia (Bone marrow examination)

Absolute lymphopenia[e]

- Mature
  1. Increased glucocorticoid activity (stress, hyperadrenocorticism, treatment)
  2. Depletion of normal lymphoid tissue, viral infection, lymphosarcoma
  3. Loss of lymphocytes, chylous effusion, lymphangiectasia
  4. Hereditary T-lymphocyte deficiency
- With blasts
  - Suggests possible lymphoid neoplasia (Bone marrow examination)

Absolute eosinophilia[f]

1. Parasites
2. Hypersensitivity
3. Feline hypereosinophilic syndrome
4. Mast cell tumor or mastocytosis
5. Lymphosarcoma
6. Other solid tumors (rare)
7. Hypoadrenocorticism (inappropriate response for sick animal)

Absolute eosinopenia[g]

Increased glucocorticoids (stress, hyperadrenocorticism,) treatment

Absolute monocytosis[h]

1. Inflammation
2. If a dog also has a lymphopenia, may be due to increased glucocorticoids (occasionally seen in cats)

[a] Leukocytosis: Dog = 17,000; Cat = 20,000; Horse = 13,000; Cow = 12,000; Pig = 22,000; Sheep = 12,000; Goat = 13,000.
[b] Neutrophilia: Dog = 12,000; Cat = 12,500; Horse = 7000; Cow = 5000; Pig = 10,000; Sheep = 6000; Goat = 7500.
[c] Neutropenia: Dog = <3000; Cat = <2500; Horse = <2700; Cow = <1500; Pig = <3200; Sheep = <700; Goat = <1200.
[d] Lymphocytosis: Dog = 5000; Cat = 7000; Horse = 6000; Cow = 7500; Pig = 13,000; Sheep = 9000; Goat = 9000.
[e] Lymphopenia: Dog = 1000; Cat = 1500; Horse = 1500; Cow = 3000; Pig = 4500; Sheep = 2000; Goat = 2000.
[f] Eosinophilia: Dog = 1500; Cat = 800; Horse = 1000; Cow = 1500; Pig = 2000; Sheep = 1000; Goat = 700.
[g] Eosinopenia: Dog = 100; Cat = 100; Horse = 1100; Cow = 100; Pig = 100; Sheep = 100; Goat = 100.
[h] Monocytosis: Dog = 1450; Cat = 800; Horse = 1000; Cow = 1500; Pig = 2000; Sheep = 1000; Goat = 700.
[i] Left shift (band cells or younger): Dog = 300; Cat = 300; Horse = 100; Cow = 200; Pig = 800; Sheep = 100; Goat = 100.

Algorithm 6

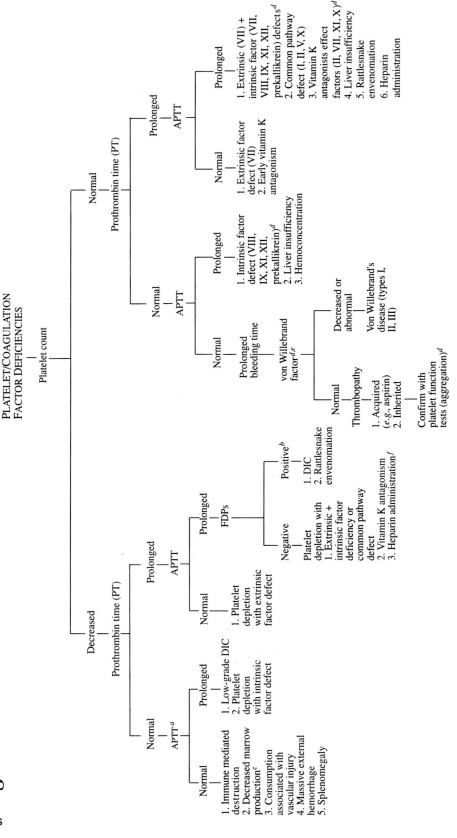

PLATELET/COAGULATION
FACTOR DEFICIENCIES

Platelet count

Decreased

Prothrombin time (PT)

Normal — APTT[a]

Normal
1. Immune mediated destruction
2. Decreased marrow production[c]
3. Consumption associated with vascular injury
4. Massive external hemorrhage
5. Splenomegaly

Prolonged
1. Low-grade DIC
2. Platelet depletion with intrinsic factor defect

Prolonged — APTT

Normal
1. Platelet depletion with extrinsic factor defect

Prolonged — FDPs

Negative
Platelet depletion with intrinsic factor deficiency or common pathway defect
1. Extrinsic + intrinsic factor deficiency or common pathway defect
2. Vitamin K antagonism
3. Heparin administration[f]

Positive[b]
1. DIC
2. Rattlesnake envenomation

Normal

Prothrombin time (PT)

Normal — APTT

Normal
Prolonged bleeding time

von Willebrand factor[d,e]

Normal
Thrombopathy
1. Acquired (e.g., aspirin)
2. Inherited

Confirm with platelet function tests (aggregation)[d]

Decreased or abnormal
Von Willebrand's disease (types I, II, III)

Prolonged
1. Intrinsic factor defect (VIII, IX, XI, XII, prekallikrein)[d]
2. Liver insufficiency
3. Hemoconcentration

Prolonged — APTT

Normal
1. Extrinsic factor defect (VII)
2. Early vitamin K antagonism

Prolonged
1. Extrinsic (VII) + intrinsic factor (VII, VIII, IX, XI, XII, prekallikrein) defects[d]
2. Common pathway defect (I, II, V, X)
3. Vitamin K antagonists effect factors (II, VII, XI, X)[d]
4. Liver insufficiency
5. Rattlesnake envenomation
6. Heparin administration

[a] APTT = Activated partial thromboplastin time.
[b] Some animals with DIC will have low or undetectable levels of fibrin degradation products (FDP).
[c] Specific tests may be necessary, e.g., Ehrlichia and RMSF serologic tests.
[d] Tests for these defects should be conducted at a special hemostasis laboratory.
[e] Formerly called factor VIII–related antigen.
[f] Especially if heparin is used to keep intravenous line open and blood is taken from it.

Algorithm 7

HEPATIC TEST ABNORMALITIES WITH
MODERATE TO MARKEDLY INCREASED ALT, AST, OR SD[a,b]

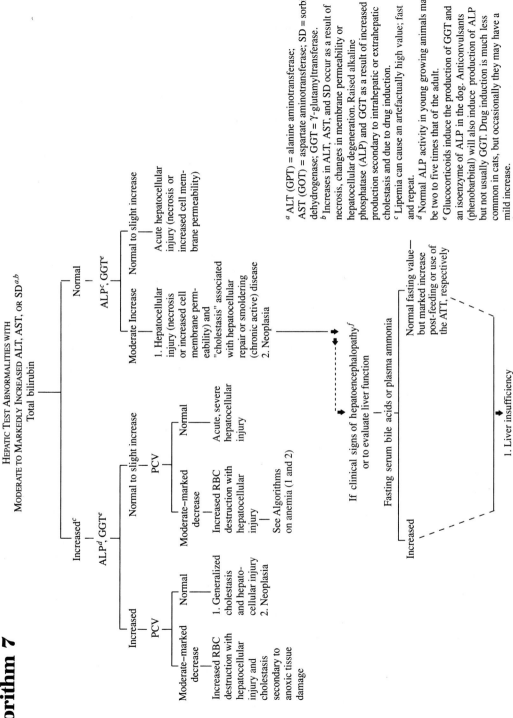

[a] ALT (GPT) = alanine aminotransferase; AST (GOT) = aspartate aminotransferase; SD = sorbitol dehydrogenase; GGT = γ-glutamyltransferase.

[b] Increases in ALT, AST, and SD occur as a result of necrosis, changes in membrane permeability or hepatocellular degeneration. Raised alkaline phosphatase (ALP) and GGT as a result of increased production secondary to intrahepatic or extrahepatic cholestasis and due to drug induction.

[c] Lipemia can cause an artefactually high value; fast and repeat.

[d] Normal ALP activity in young growing animals may be two to five times that of the adult.

[e] Glucocorticoids induce the production of GGT and an isoenzyme of ALP in the dog. Anticonvulsants (phenobarbital) will also induce production of ALP but not usually GGT. Drug induction is much less common in cats, but occasionally they may have a mild increase.

[f] Function test not needed if bilirubin is increased except in the horse; bile acid concentration is diagnostically helpful in the differential diagnosis of fasting hyper-bilirubinemia and hepatic disease in the horse.

Algorithm 8

HEPATIC TEST ABNORMALITIES WITH NORMAL OR MILDLY INCREASED ALT, AST, OR SD[a,b]

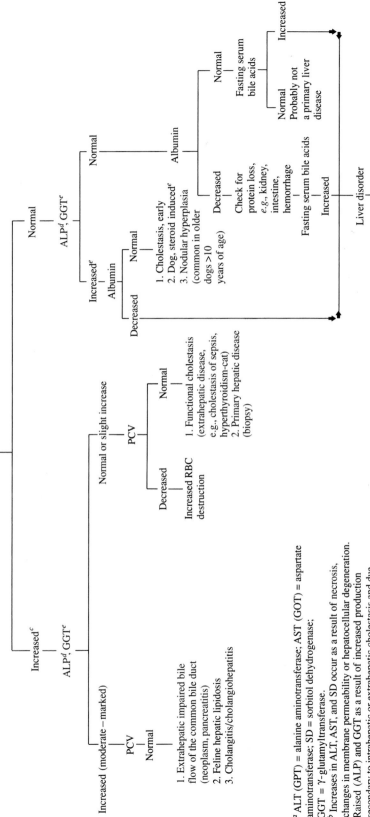

Total bilirubin

Increased[c]
— ALP[d], GGT[e]
  — PCV
    — Normal
      1. Extrahepatic impaired bile flow of the common bile duct (neoplasm, pancreatitis)
      2. Feline hepatic lipidosis
      3. Cholangitis/cholangiohepatitis

Normal or slight increase
— PCV
  — Decreased — Increased RBC destruction
  — Normal
    1. Functional cholestasis (extrahepatic disease, e.g., cholestasis of sepsis, hyperthyroidism–cat)
    2. Primary hepatic disease (biopsy)

Normal
— ALP[d], GGT[e]
  — Increased[e]
    — Albumin
      — Decreased
        1. Cholestasis, early
        2. Dog, steroid induced[e]
        3. Nodular hyperplasia (common in older dogs >10 years of age)
      — Normal
  — Normal
    — Albumin
      — Decreased — Check for protein loss, e.g., kidney, intestine, hemorrhage — Fasting serum bile acids — Increased — Liver disorder
      — Normal — Fasting serum bile acids — Normal — Probably not a primary liver disease / Increased

If clinical signs of hepatoencephalopathy[f] or to further evaluate liver function
— Fasting serum bile acids or plasma ammonia
  — Increased
    — Normal fasting value— marked increase post-feeding or use of the ATT, respectively
      1. Liver insufficiency
      2. Portosystemic venous anomaly—congenital or acquired

[a] ALT (GPT) = alanine aminotransferase; AST (GOT) = aspartate aminotransferase; SD = sorbitol dehydrogenase; GGT = γ-glutamyltransferase.

[b] Increases in ALT, AST, and SD occur as a result of necrosis, changes in membrane permeability or hepatocellular degeneration. Raised (ALP) and GGT as a result of increased production secondary to intrahepatic or extrahepatic cholestasis and due to drug induction.

[c] Lipemia can cause an artefactually high value; fast and repeat.

[d] Normal ALP activity in young growing animals may be two to five times that of the adult.

[e] Glucocorticoids induce the production of GGT and an isoenzyme of ALP in the dog. Anticonvulsants (phenobarbital) will also induce production of ALP but not GGT. Drug induction is much less common in cats, but occasionally they may have a mild increase.

[f] Function test not needed if bilirubin is increased except in the horse; bile acid concentration is diagnostically helpful in the differential diagnosis of fasting hyperbilirubinemia and hepatic disease in the horse.

Algorithm 9*

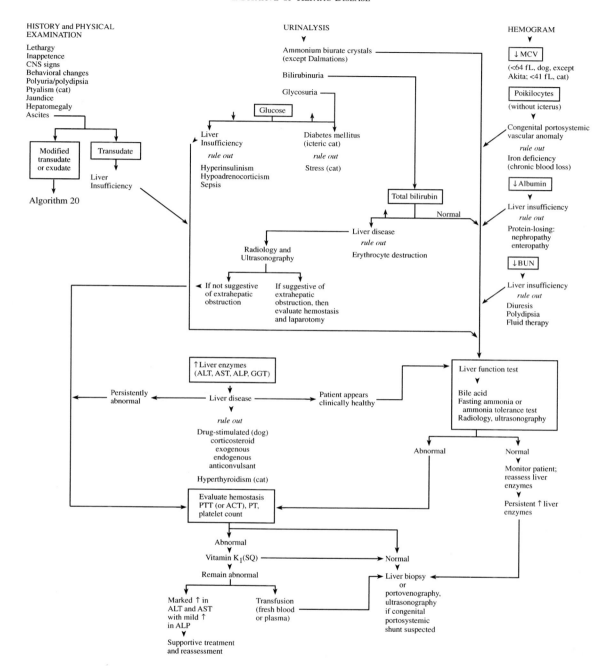

Dr. Watson: "How absurdly simple!" Sherlock Holmes: "Quite so! Every problem becomes childish once it is explained to you."
— A. Conan Doyle, *The Adventures of the Dancing Men*. Modified from Meyer DJ, Center SA: Approach to the diagnosis of
liver disorders in dogs and cats. *Comp Cont in Educ Pract Vet*, 1986;8:880–888, with permission.
*Link the components of this Algorithm to the more detailed Algorithms 7 and 8.

Algorithm 10

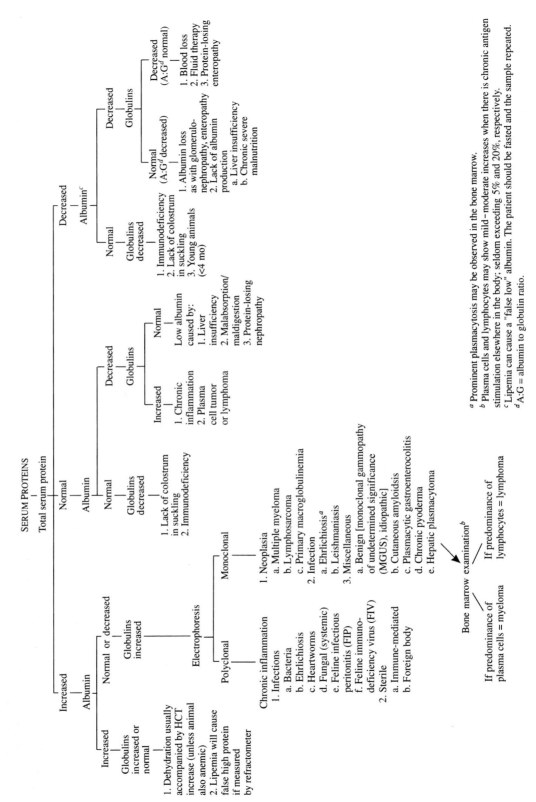

SERUM PROTEINS
Total serum protein

Increased

- Albumin
  - Increased
    - Globulins increased or normal
      1. Dehydration usually accompanied by HCT increase (unless animal also anemic)
      2. Lipemia will cause false high protein if measured by refractometer
  - Normal or decreased
    - Globulins increased
      - Electrophoresis
        - Polyclonal — Chronic inflammation
          1. Infections
             a. Bacteria
             b. Ehrlichiosis
             c. Heartworms
             d. Fungal (systemic)
             e. Feline infectious peritonitis (FIP)
             f. Feline immuno-deficiency virus (FIV)
          2. Sterile
             a. Immune-mediated
             b. Foreign body
        - Monoclonal
          1. Neoplasia
             a. Multiple myeloma
             b. Lymphosarcoma
             c. Primary macroglobulinemia
          2. Infection
             a. Ehrlichiosis[a]
             b. Leishmaniasis
          3. Miscellaneous
             a. Benign [monoclonal gammopathy of undetermined significance (MGUS), idiopathic]
             b. Cutaneous amyloidsis
             c. Plasmacytic gastroenterocolitis
             d. Chronic pyoderma
             e. Hepatic plasmacytoma

          Bone marrow examination[b]
          - If predominance of plasma cells = myeloma
          - If predominance of lymphocytes = lymphoma

Normal

- Albumin
  - Normal
    - Globulins decreased
      1. Lack of colostrum in suckling
      2. Immunodeficiency
  - Decreased
    - Globulins
      - Increased
        1. Chronic inflammation
        2. Plasma cell tumor or lymphoma
      - Normal
        - Low albumin caused by:
          1. Liver insufficiency
          2. Malabsorption/maldigestion
          3. Protein-losing nephropathy

Decreased

- Albumin[c]
  - Normal
    - Globulins decreased
      1. Immunodeficiency
      2. Lack of colostrum in suckling
      3. Young animals (<4 mo)
  - Decreased
    - Globulins
      - Normal (A:G[d] decreased)
        1. Albumin loss as with glomerulo-nephropathy, enteropathy
        2. Lack of albumin production
           a. Liver insufficiency
           b. Chronic severe malnutrition
      - Decreased (A:G[d] normal)
        1. Blood loss
        2. Fluid therapy
        3. Protein-losing enteropathy

[a] Prominent plasmacytosis may be observed in the bone marrow.

[b] Plasma cells and lymphocytes may show mild-moderate increases when there is chronic antigen stimulation elsewhere in the body; seldom exceeding 5% and 20%, respectively.

[c] Lipemia can cause a "false low" albumin. The patient should be fasted and the sample repeated.

[d] A:G = albumin to globulin ratio.

Algorithm 11

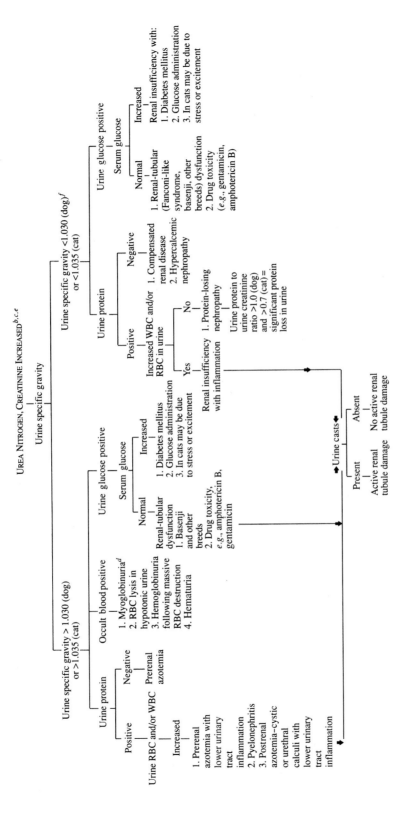

UREA NITROGEN, CREATININE INCREASED[b,c,e]

Urine specific gravity

Urine specific gravity > 1.030 (dog) or >1.035 (cat)

Urine protein
- Positive
  - Urine RBC and/or WBC Increased
    1. Prerenal azotemia with lower urinary tract inflammation
    2. Pyelonephritis
    3. Postrenal azotemia–cystic or urethral calculi with lower urinary tract inflammation
- Negative
  - Prerenal azotemia

Occult blood positive
1. Myoglobinuria[d]
2. RBC lysis in hypotonic urine
3. Hemoglobinuria following massive RBC destruction
4. Hematuria

Urine glucose positive

Serum glucose
- Normal
  - Renal-tubular dysfunction
    1. Basenji and other breeds
    2. Drug toxicity, e.g., amphotericin B, gentamicin
- Increased
  1. Diabetes mellitus
  2. Glucose administration
  3. In cats may be due to stress or excitement

Urine specific gravity <1.030 (dog)[f] or <1.035 (cat)

Urine protein
- Positive
  - Increased WBC and/or RBC in urine
    - Yes
      - Renal insufficiency with inflammation
    - No
      1. Protein-losing nephropathy

      Urine protein to urine creatinine ratio >1.0 (dog) and >0.7 (cat) = significant protein loss in urine
- Negative
  1. Compensated renal disease
  2. Hypercalcemic nephropathy

Urine glucose positive

Serum glucose
- Normal
  1. Renal-tubular (Fanconi-like syndrome, basenji, other breeds) dysfunction
  2. Drug toxicity (e.g., gentamicin, amphotericin B)
- Increased
  Renal insufficiency with:
  1. Diabetes mellitus
  2. Glucose administration
  3. In cats may be due to stress or excitement

→ Urine casts
- Present
  - Active renal tubule damage
- Absent
  - No active renal tubule damage

---

[a] The type of kidney disease can be confirmed only with a renal biopsy.

[b] In the dog and cat phosphate levels are also increased when there is a reduction in glomerular filtration. In the horse (occasionally in dogs) serum calcium may be increased while phosphate is normal.

[c] Azotemia may be accompanied by hyperamylasemia in dogs.

[d] Differentiate from hemoglobin by precipitation test with ammonium sulfate.

[e] Advanced renal disease may lead to secondary hyperparathyroidism (see Fig. 9–3).

[f] Fluid administration will decrease the urine specific gravity.

331

Algorithm 12

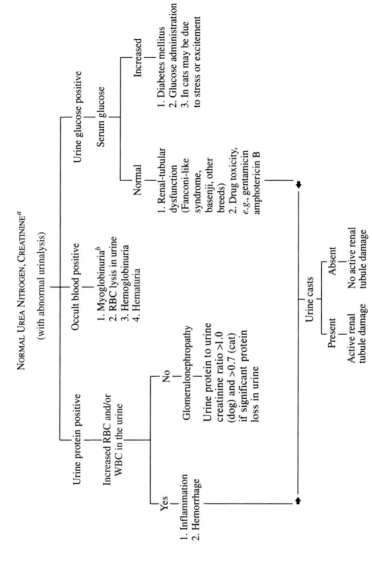

NORMAL UREA NITROGEN, CREATININE[a]

(with abnormal urinalysis)

Urine protein positive

Increased RBC and/or WBC in the urine

Yes
1. Inflammation
2. Hemorrhage

No

Glomerulonephropathy

Urine protein to urine creatinine ratio >1.0 (dog) and >0.7 (cat) if significant protein loss in urine

Occult blood positive

1. Myoglobinuria[b]
2. RBC lysis in urine
3. Hemoglobinuria
4. Hematuria

Urine glucose positive

Serum glucose

Normal
1. Renal-tubular dysfunction (Fanconi-like syndrome, basenji, other breeds)
2. Drug toxicity, e.g., gentamicin amphotericin B

Increased
1. Diabetes mellitus
2. Glucose administration
3. In cats may be due to stress or excitement

Urine casts

Present
Active renal tubule damage

Absent
No active renal tubule damage

[a] The type of kidney disease can be confirmed only with a renal biopsy.
[b] Differentiate from hemoglobin by precipitation test with ammonium sulfate.

Algorithm 13

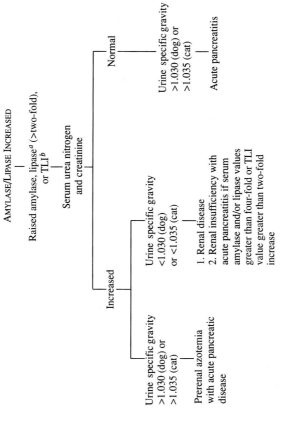

AMYLASE/LIPASE INCREASED

Raised amylase, lipase[a] (>two-fold), or TLI[b]

Serum urea nitrogen and creatinine

Increased

Urine specific gravity >1.030 (dog) or >1.035 (cat)

Prerenal azotemia with acute pancreatic disease

Urine specific gravity <1.030 (dog) or <1.035 (cat)

1. Renal disease
2. Renal insufficiency with acute pancreatitis if serum amylase and/or lipase values greater than four-fold or TLI value greater than two-fold increase

Normal

Urine specific gravity >1.030 (dog) or >1.035 (cat)

Acute pancreatitis

[a] Serum amylase and lipase are not raised usually in feline pancreatitis; lipase activity may be raised in peritoneal fluid.
[b] TLI = trypsin-like immunoreactivity.

333

Algorithm 14

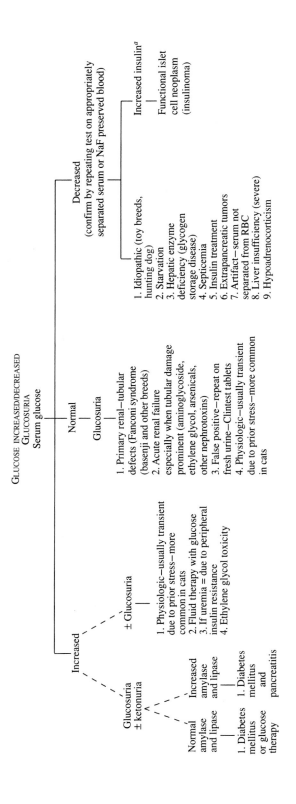

GLUCOSE INCREASED/DECREASED
GLUCOSURIA
Serum glucose

Increased

— ± Glucosuria

1. Physiologic—usually transient due to prior stress—more common in cats
2. Fluid therapy with glucose
3. If uremia = due to peripheral insulin resistance
4. Ethylene glycol toxicity

— Glucosuria ± ketonuria

Normal amylase and lipase
1. Diabetes mellitus or glucose therapy

Increased amylase and lipase
1. Diabetes mellitus and pancreatitis

Normal

— Glucosuria

1. Primary renal–tubular defects (Fanconi syndrome (basenji and other breeds)
2. Acute renal failure especially when tubular damage prominent (aminoglycoside, ethylene glycol, arsenicals, other nephrotoxins)
3. False positive—repeat on fresh urine—Clinest tablets
4. Physiologic—usually transient due to prior stress—more common in cats

Decreased
(confirm by repeating test on appropriately separated serum or NaF preserved blood)

1. Idiopathic (toy breeds, hunting dog)
2. Starvation
3. Hepatic enzyme deficiency (glycogen storage disease)
4. Septicemia
5. Insulin treatment
6. Extrapancreatic tumors
7. Artifact—serum not separated from RBC
8. Liver insufficiency (severe)
9. Hypoadrenocorticism

Increased insulin[a]

Functional islet cell neoplasm (insulinoma)

[a] or if the insulin value is within the reference range in association with hypoglycemia; an inappropriate relationship

334

Algorithm 15

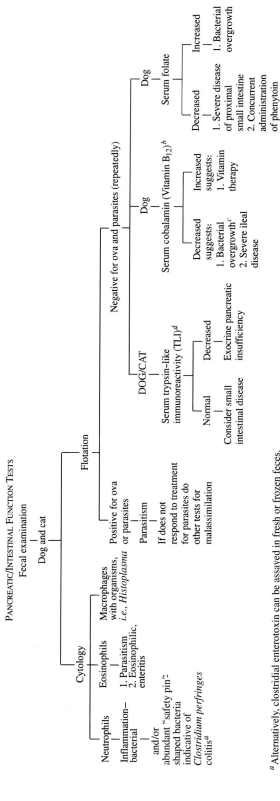

PANCREATIC/INTESTINAL FUNCTION TESTS

Fecal examination

- Dog and cat
  - **Cytology**
    - Neutrophils
      - Inflammation—bacterial
      - and/or abundant "safety pin"-shaped bacteria indicative of *Clostridium perfringes* colitis[a]
    - Eosinophils
      - 1. Parasitism
      - 2. Eosinophilic enteritis
    - Macrophages with organisms, i.e., *Histoplasma*
  - **Flotation**
    - Positive for ova or parasites
      - Parasitism
      - If does not respond to treatment for parasites do other tests for malassimilation
    - Negative for ova and parasites (repeatedly)
      - DOG/CAT
        - Serum trypsin-like immunoreactivity (TLI)[d]
          - Normal
            - Consider small intestinal disease
          - Decreased
            - Exocrine pancreatic insufficiency
      - Dog
        - Serum cobalamin (Vitamin B₁₂)[b]
          - Decreased suggests:
            - 1. Bacterial overgrowth[c]
            - 2. Severe ileal disease
          - Increased suggests:
            - 1. Vitamin therapy
      - Dog
        - Serum folate
          - Decreased
            - 1. Severe disease of proximal small intestine
            - 2. Concurrent administration of phenytoin sulfasalazine
          - Increased
            - 1. Bacterial overgrowth

[a] Alternatively, clostridial enterotoxin can be assayed in fresh or frozen feces.
[b] Parenteral administration of B₁₂ (in B complexes) will increase the value.
[c] Bacterial overgrowth may be associated with multiple causes of malabsorption.
[d] TLI = trypsin-like immunoreactivity.

Algorithm 16

CALCIUM NORMAL/INCREASED; PHOSPHORUS
Total calcium or corrected calcium[a] (dog)

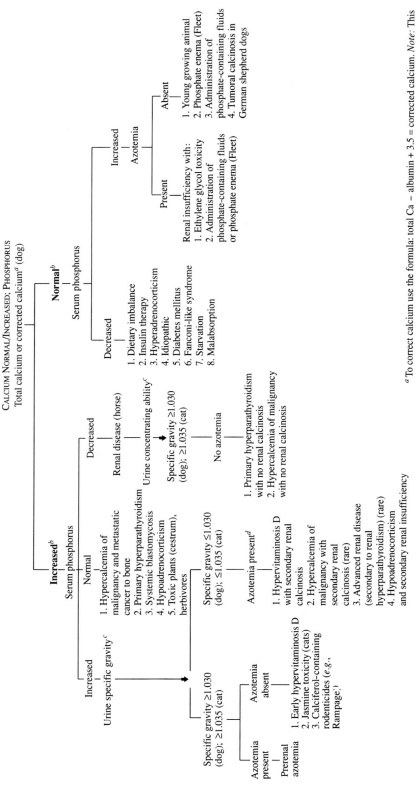

[a] To correct calcium use the formula: total Ca − albumin + 3.5 = corrected calcium. *Note:* This formula has been established for the dog and may not be applicable to other species.
[b] Age is important in evaluating minerals. Very young growing animals tend to have slightly higher values than adults.
[c] Ability to concentrate urine must be related to the patient's hydration state.
[d] Any hypercalcemia may be accompanied be renal problems (azotemia) notably when calcium × phosphorus = >70.

Algorithm 17

CALCIUM DECREASED; PHOSPHORUS

Total calcium or corrected calcium[a] decreased[b,c]

Serum phosphorus

Increased

Azotemia

- **Present**

  Renal insufficiency with
  1. Ethylene glycol toxicity
  2. Hypoparathyroidism
  3. Administration of phosphate-containing fluids or phosphate enema (Fleet)

- **Absent**

  1. Young growing animal
  2. Hypoparathyroidism
  3. Phosphate enema (Fleet)
  4. Administration of phosphate-containing fluids

Normal

1. EDTA treatment
2. Hypovitaminosis D
3. Malabsorption
4. Blister beetle toxicosis (horse)
5. Thyroid C-cell tumors (bull)

Decreased

1. Eclampsia
2. Hypovitaminosis D
3. Dietary lack of minerals
4. Hypomagnesemia
5. Parturient paresis (cow)

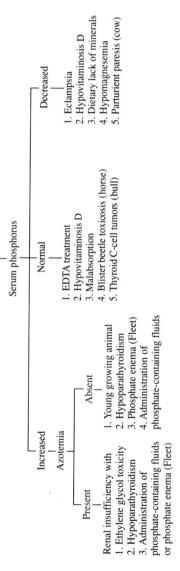

[a] To correct calcium, use the formula: total calcium − albumin + 3.5 = corrected calcium. *Note:* This formula has been established for the dog and may not be applicable to other species.

[b] Age is important in evaluating minerals. Very young growing animals tend to have slightly higher values than adults.

[c] Artifacts that may influence serum calcium include a reduced value sample is contaminated with EDTA or if sample is diluted, and a raised value if lipemia is present.

Algorithm 18

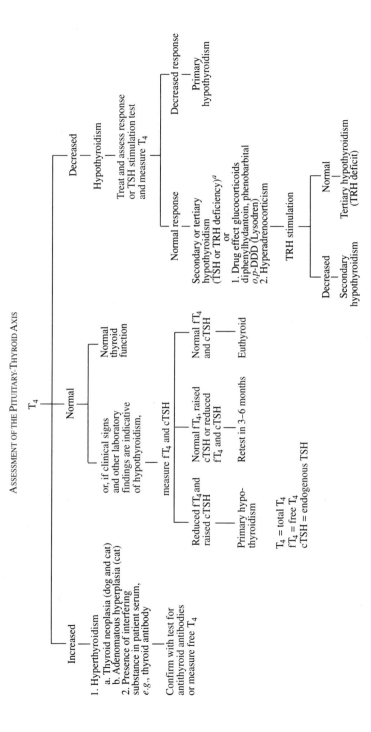

ASSESSMENT OF THE PITUITARY-THYROID AXIS

T4

Increased

1. Hyperthyroidism
   a. Thyroid neoplasia (dog and cat)
   b. Adenomatous hyperplasia (cat)
2. Presence of interfering substance in patient serum, *e.g.*, thyroid antibody

Confirm with test for antithyroid antibodies or measure free T4

Normal

or, if clinical signs and other laboratory findings are indicative of hypothyroidism,

measure fT4 and cTSH

Reduced fT4 and raised cTSH

Primary hypothyroidism

Normal fT4, raised cTSH or reduced fT4 and cTSH

Retest in 3–6 months

Normal thyroid function

Normal fT4 and cTSH

Euthyroid

T4 = total T4
fT4 = free T4
cTSH = endogenous TSH

Decreased

Hypothyroidism

Treat and assess response or TSH stimulation test and measure T4

Normal response

Secondary or tertiary hypothyroidism (TSH or TRH deficiency)[a]
or
1. Drug effect glucocorticoids diphenylhydantoin, phenobarbital *o,p*-DDD (Lysodren).
2. Hyperadrenocorticism

TRH stimulation

Decreased

Secondary hypothyroidism

Normal

Tertiary hypothyroidism (TRH deficit)

Decreased response

Primary hypothyroidism

[a] Secondary and tertiary hypothyroidism are rare.

Algorithm 19

ASSESSMENT OF THE PITUITARY-ADRENOCORTICAL AXIS

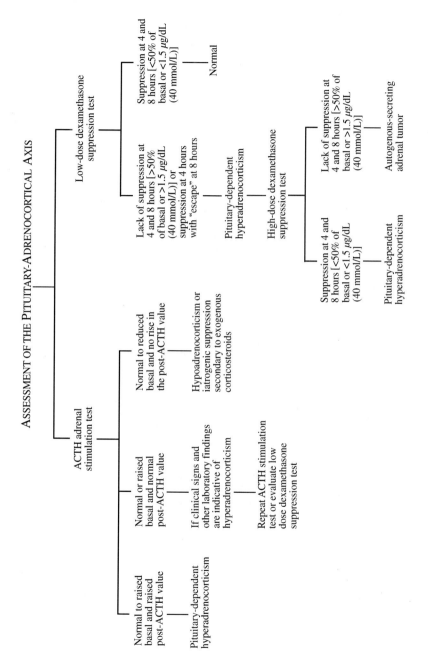

ACTH adrenal stimulation test

Normal to raised basal and raised post-ACTH value

Pituitary-dependent hyperadrenocorticism

Normal or raised basal and normal post-ACTH value

If clinical signs and other laboratory findings are indicative of hyperadrenocorticism

Repeat ACTH stimulation test or evaluate low dose dexamethasone suppression test

Normal to reduced basal and no rise in the post-ACTH value

Hypoadrenocorticism or iatrogenic suppression secondary to exogenous corticosteroids

Low-dose dexamethasone suppression test

Lack of suppression at 4 and 8 hours [>50% of basal or >1.5 μg/dL (40 mmol/L)] or suppression at 4 hours with "escape" at 8 hours

Pituitary-dependent hyperadrenocorticism

High-dose dexamethasone suppression test

Suppression at 4 and 8 hours [<50% of basal or <1.5 μg/dL (40 mmol/L)]

Pituitary-dependent hyperadrenocorticism

Lack of suppression at 4 and 8 hours [>50% of basal or >1.5 μg/dL (40 mmol/L)]

Autogenous-secreting adrenal tumor

Suppression at 4 and 8 hours [<50% of basal or <1.5 μg/dL (40 mmol/L)]

Normal

In problematic cases, the endogenous ACTH is measured along with a basal cortisol.
Raised ACTH value and normal or raised basal cortisol value indicates pituitary-dependent hyperadrenocorticism.
Reduced ACTH value and normal or raised basal cortisol value indicates autogenous secreting adrenal tumor.
Reduced ACTH value and normal or reduced basal cortisol value indicates hypoadrenocorticism (primary or iatrogenic); note that if prednisone is being given, it is measured as cortisol resulting in a reduced ACTH value and a raised basal cortisol value.

Algorithm 20

EVALUATION OF EFFUSIONS

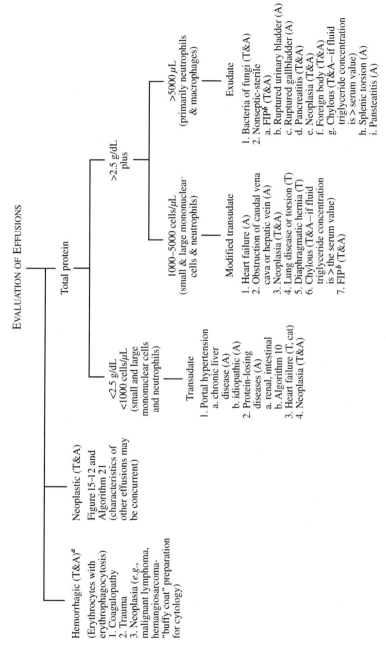

Hemorrhagic (T&A)[a]
(Erythrocytes with erythrophagocytosis)
1. Coagulopathy
2. Trauma
3. Neoplasia (*e.g.*, malignant lymphoma, hemangiosarcoma—"buffy coat" preparation for cytology)

Neoplastic (T&A)
Figure 15–12 and Algorithm 21
(characteristics of other effusions may be concurrent)

Total protein

<2.5 g/dL
<1000 cells/µL
(small and large mononuclear cells and neutrophils)

Transudate
1. Portal hypertension
   a. chronic liver disease (A)
   b. idiopathic (A)
2. Protein-losing diseases (A)
   a. renal, intestinal
   b. Algorithm 10
3. Heart failure (T, cat)
4. Neoplasia (T&A)

>2.5 g/dL
plus

1000–5000 cells/µL
(small & large mononuclear cells & neutrophils)

Modified transudate
1. Heart failure (A)
2. Obstruction of caudal vena cava or hepatic vein (A)
3. Neoplasia (T&A)
4. Lung disease or torsion (T)
5. Diaphragmatic hernia (T)
6. Chylous (T&A—if fluid triglyceride concentration is > the serum value)
7. FIP[b] (T&A)

>5000/µL
(primarily neutrophils & macrophages)

Exudate
1. Bacteria of fungi (T&A)
2. Nonseptic-sterile
   a. FIP[b] (T&A)
   b. Ruptured urinary bladder (A)
   c. Ruptured gallbladder (A)
   d. Pancreatitis (T&A)
   e. Neoplasia (T&A)
   f. Foreign body (T&A)
   g. Chylous (T&A—if fluid triglyceride concentration is > serum value)
   h. Splenic torsion (A)
   i. Pansteatitis (A)

[a] Location of effusion: T = thorax; A = abdomen.
[b] FIP = feline infectious peritonitis; an effusion albumin to globulin ratio (A:G) of < 0.81 provides additional diagnostic criteria for FIP.

Algorithm 21

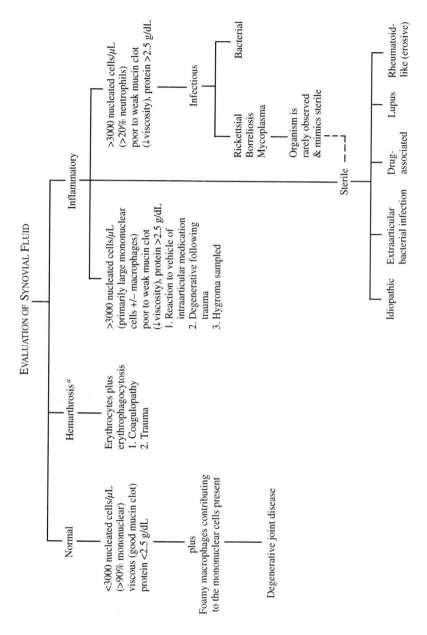

EVALUATION OF SYNOVIAL FLUID

Normal
<3000 nucleated cells/μL (>90% mononuclear) viscous (good mucin clot) protein <2.5 g/dL

plus
Foamy macrophages contributing to the mononuclear cells present

Degenerative joint disease

Hemarthrosis[a]
Erythrocytes plus erythrophagocytosis
1. Coagulopathy
2. Trauma

Inflammatory

>3000 nucleated cells/μL (primarily large mononuclear cells +/– macrophages) poor to weak mucin clot (↓viscosity), protein >2.5 g/dL
1. Reaction to vehicle of intraarticular medication
2. Degenerative following trauma
3. Hygroma sampled

>3000 nucleated cells/μL (>20% neutrophils) poor to weak mucin clot (↓viscosity), protein >2.5 g/dL

Infectious

Rickettsial Borreliosis Mycoplasma

Organism is rarely observed & mimics sterile

Bacterial

Sterile

Idiopathic

Extraarticular bacterial infection

Drug-associated

Lupus

Rheumatoid-like (erosive)

[a]Contamination of synovial fluid during the collection process makes this classification problematic since erythrophagocytosis is not always associated with hemarthrosis. The operator is in the best position to determine whether or not the blood is iatrogenic.

341

Algorithm 22

342

MICROSCOPIC EXAMINATION OF THE CYTOLOGY SPECIMEN

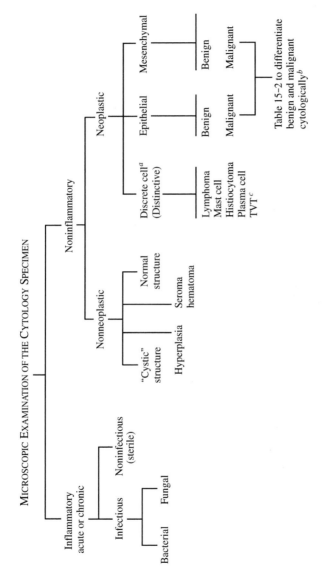

Modified from Meyer DJ: Diagnostic cytology in clinical oncology. In Withrow SJ, MacEwen GE (eds); *Veterinary Clinical Oncology*, 2nd ed. Philadelphia, WB Saunders Co, 1996, pp 43–51.

[a]Commonly referred to as "round cell" tumors; the term can be misleading cytologically because both epithelial and mesenchymal neoplasms can have a "round cell" appearance occasionally. Cell discreteness (not attached to each other to form clusters or sheets) or distinctive cellular features is emphasized by this nomenclature.

[b]Knowledge of the biological behavior of the specific type of neoplasm contributes to the classification as benign or malignant. For example, the apocrine gland adenocarcinoma appears relatively benign by cytologic criteria yet has a malignant behavior. In contrast, the typically self-limiting histiocytoma can demonstrate criteria of malignancy cytologically.

[c]TVT = transmissable venereal cell tumor.

Part **IV**

APPENDIX: REFERENCE INTERVALS AND CONVERSION TABLES

TABLE 1. Reference Intervals for Hematology Values of Adult Animals[a,b]

Test	Units	Canine	Feline	Equine	Bovine	Porcine	Ovine
RBC	$\times 10^6/\mu L$	5.4–7.8	5.8–10.7	6.4–10.0	5.0–10.0	5.0–8.0	8.0–15.0
Hemoglobin	g/dL	13–19	9–15	11–17	8–15	10–18	8–16
Hct	%	37–54	30–47	32–47	24–46	33–50	24–49
MCV	fL	62–74	41–51	43–54	37–51	50–67	23–48
MCHC	g/dL	32–36	31–35	34–37	33–37	30–34	31–34
MCH	pg	22–27	13–18	15–19	13–18	17–21	8–12
RDW	%	12–15	14–19	18–22	16–24		
Platelets	$\times 10^5/\mu L$	1.6–4.3	3–8	1–2.7	2–7.3	2–8	3–8
MPV	fL	6.7–11.1	ND	4.6–7.3	4.5–6.7		
Fibrinogen	mg/dL	100–400	100–300	100–500	200–700	100–500	100–500
Icterus index	units	<5	<5	5–25	0–20	<5	<5
Plasma protein	g/dL	6.0–7.8	6.2–8.0	6.1–8.0	7.0–8.5	6.0–8.0	6.0–7.5
Reticulocytes	$\times 10^3/\mu L$	<80	<30 agg <500 punc	0	0	<70	0
WBC	$\times 10^3/\mu L$	6.0–17.0	5.5–19.5	5.2–13.9	4.0–12.0	10–22	4.0–12.0
Bands	$\times 10^3/\mu L$	0–0.3	0–0.3	0–0.1	0–0.12		
Segmented	$\times 10^3/\mu L$	3.0–11.5	2.5–12.5	2.2–7.4	0.6–4.0	3.2–10.0	1.0–5.0
Lymphocytes	$\times 10^3/\mu L$	1.0–4.8	1.5–7.0	1.1–5.3	2.5–7.5	4.4–13.5	2.0–9.0
Monocytes	$\times 10^3/\mu L$	0.15–0.135	0–0.85	0–0.9	0.03–0.8	0.2–2.2	0–0.75
Eosinophils	$\times 10^3/\mu L$	0.1–1.25	0–1.5	0–0.6	0–2.4	0.2–2.0	0.1–0.75
Basophils	$\times 10^3/\mu L$	<0.1	<0.1	<0.3	<0.2	Rare	Rare

Erythrocyte morphology[c]

	1+	2+	3+	4+
Anisocytosis				
Canine	7–15[d]	16–20	21–29	>30
Feline	5–8	9–15	16–20	>20
Bovine	10–20	21–30	31–40	>40
Equine	1–3	4–6	7–10	>10
Polychromasia				
Canine	2–7	8–14	15–29	>30
Feline	1–2	3–8	9–15	>15
Bovine	2–5	6–10	11–20	>20
Equine	Rare	Rare	Rare	Rare
Hypochromasia (all species)	1–10	11–50	51–200	>200
Poikilocytosis (all species)	3–10	11–50	51–200	>200
Codocytes (canine only)	3–5	6–15	16–30	>30
Spherocytes (all species)	5–10	11–50	51–150	>150
Echinocytes (all species)	5–10	11–100	101–250	>250
Acanthocytes, schistocytes (all species)	1–2	3–8	9–20	>20

[a]From the Veterinary Teaching Hospital-University of Florida.

[b]Platelet counts determined electronically for all species except the cat. Reference range for canine platelet counts determined by manual method is $2–5 \times 10^5/\mu L$.

[c]Weiss DJ: Uniform evaluation and semiquantitative reporting of hematologic data in veterinary laboratories. Vet Clin Pathol 1984;13:27.

[d]Number of affected cells/1000× microscopic field.

TABLE 2. Reference Intervals for Serum Chemistry for Adult Animals[a]

Test	Units	Canine	Feline	Equine	Bovine	Porcine	Ovine
Ammonia	μmol/L	0–40	0–40	0–40			
ALP	U/L	10–73	15–92	102–257	29–99	26–362	68–387
ALT	U/L	15–58	30–100	4–12	17–37	32–84	60–84
AST	U/L	16–43	12–56	152–294	48–100	9–113	98–278
Amylase	U/L	510–1864	365–948	9–34	12–107		
Anion gap	mEq/L	11–26	13–24	7–16	12–22		
Bile acid–fast	μmol/L	<5	<2	<15	See text		
Postprandial	μmol/L	<15	<15				
Bilirubin (total)	mg/dL	0.1–0.3	0.1–0.2	0.5–2.1	0.1–0.3	0.1–0.2	0.1–0.4
Calcium	mg/dL	9.0–10.8	7.4–10.5	10.6–13.0	7.9–10.0	8–12	10.4–13
CO_2	mEq/L	20–27	15–25	26–35	24–34	18–26	21–28
Chloride	mEq/L	110–118	116–125	97–104	94–104	100–105	98–115
Cholesterol	mg/dL	108–266	38–186	50–143	87–254	36–54	50–140
Cholinesterase	U/L	1347–2269	1000–2000				
Cortisol (basal)	μg/dL	1.0–6.8	0.3–2.6				
CK (CPK)	U/L	40–254	59–527	113–333	44–228		
Creatinine	mg/dL	0.5–1.4	0.7–1.8	1.0–1.9	0.7–1.1	1.0–2.7	1.2–1.9
Folate	μg/L	7.5–17.5	13.4–38				
GGT	U/L	1–5	0–2	9–25	20–48		
Glucose	mg/dL	77–120	58–120	76–127	37–71	65–95	50–80
Iron	μg/dL	84–233	65–233	74–209	57–162	91–199	166–222
Lipase	U/L	13–200	0–83				
Magnesium	mEq/L	1.2–2.0	1.5–3.5	1.3–2.0	1.4–2.3		
Osmolality	mOsm/kg	291–315	292–356	282–302			
Phosphorus, inorganic	mg/dL	2.4–6.1	2.6–7.9	2.0–4.3	4.6–9.0	5.3–9.6	5.0–7.3
Potassium	mEq/L	4.2–5.6	4.0–5.3	2.4–5.2	4.0–5.3	4.9–7.1	4.0–6.0
Protein (total)	g/dL	5.4–7.1	5.7–7.9	5.5–7.3	5.9–7.7	7.0–8.9	6.0–7.9
Albumin	g/dL	2.5–3.6	2.3–3.4	2.7–4.2	2.7–4.3	1.9–3.3	2.4–3.9
Globulin	g/dL	2.4–4.0	2.6–4.5	2.1–3.8	2.5–4.1	5.3–6.4	3.5–5.7
Sodium	mEq/L	145–153	151–158	136–142	136–144	139–152	136–154
SD (SDH)	U/L	2.9–8.2	3.9–7.7	1.9–5.8	4.3–15.3	1–6	6–28
T_3	ng/dL	85–250	85–250				
T_4	μg/dL	1.2–3.0	1.2–3.0				
T_4 (free)	ng/dL	0.7–3.3					
TLI	μg/L	5–35					
Triglycerides	mg/dL	20–112	10–114	4–44	0–14		
Urea nitrogen	mg/dL	7–25	18–33	12–26	10–26	8–24	18–31

[a]From the Veterinary Teaching Hospital-University of Florida, with permission.

**TABLE 3. Conversion of Conventional Units to SI Units
in Serum Chemistry**

Component	Conventional Unit	Factor	SI Units
ACTH	pg/mL	0.22	pmol/L
Albumin	g/dL	10	g/L
Aminotransferases (ALT, AST)	IU/L	1	U/L
Ammonia	μg/dL	0.5872	μmol/L
Amylase	Somogyi units	1.85	U/L
Bicarbonate	mEq/L	1	mmol/L
Bilirubin	mg/dL	17.1	μmol/L
Calcium	mg/dL	0.25	mmol/L
CO_2	mEq/L	1	mmol/L
Chloride	mEq/L	1	mmol/L
Cholinesterase	IU/L	1	U/L
Cholesterol	mg/dL	0.026	mmol/L
Cortisol	μg/dL	27.6	nmol/L
Creatine kinase (CK)	IU/L	1	U/L
Creatinine	mg/dL	88.4	μmol/L
Creatinine clearance	mL/min	0.0167	mL/sec
Fibrinogen	mg/dL	0.01	g/L
γ-Glutamyltransferase (GGT γ-glutamyl-transpeptidase GGTP)	IU/L	1	U/L
Globulin	g/dL	10	g/L
Glucose	mg/dL	0.055	mmol/L
Insulin	μIU/L	7.175	pmol/L
Iron-binding capacity	μg/dL	0.179	μmol/L
Iron (total)	μg/dL	0.179	μmol/L
Lipase	IU/L	1	U/L
Magnesium	mEq/L	0.5	mmol/L
Magnesium	mg/dL	0.41	mmol/L
Osmolality	Osm/kg	1	mmol/L
Phosphatase, alkaline (ALP)	IU/L	1	U/L
Phosphorus, inorganic	mg/dL	0.323	mmol/L
Potassium	mEq/L	1	mmol/L
Protein (total)	g/dL	10	g/L
Sodium	mEq/L	1	mmol/L
T_4	μg/dL	12.87	nmol/L
fT_4	ng/dL	12.87	pmol/L
T_3	mg/dL	0.0154	nmol/L
Triglycerides	mg/dL	0.011	μmol/L
Urea nitrogen (BUN)	mg/dL	0.357	mmol/L
Uric acid	mg/dL	0.059	mmol/L
Xylose	mg/dL	0.0666	mmol/L
Zinc	μg/dL	0.1530	μmol/L

TABLE 4. **Reference Intervals for Hematology Values for Adult Animals Expressed in SI Units**

Test	Units	Canine	Feline	Equine	Bovine	Porcine	Ovine
RBC	$\times 10^{12}$/L	5.4–7.8	5.8–10.7	6.4–10.0	5.0–10.0	5.0–8.0	8.0–15.0
Hemoglobin	g/L	130–190	90–150	110–170	80–150	100–180	80–160
Hct	Volume fraction	37–54	30–47	32–47	24–46	33–50	24–49
MCV	fL	64–74	41–51	43–54	37–51	50–67	23–48
MCHC	g/L	340–360	310–350	340–370	330–370	300–340	310–340
MCH	pg	22–27	13–18	15–19	13–18	17–21	8–12
RDW	%	12–15	14–19	18–22	16–24		
Platelets	$\times 10^9$/L	160–430	300–800	100–270	200–730	200–800	300–800
MPV	fL	6.7–11.1	ND	4.6–7.3	4.5–6.7		
Fibrinogen	g/L	1–4	1–3	1–5	2–7	1–5	1–5
Icterus index	units	<5	<5	5–25	0–20	<5	<5
Plasma protein	g/L	60–78	62–80	61–80	70–85	60–80	60–75
Reticulocytes	$\times 10^9$/L	<80	<30 agg <500 punc	0	0	<70	0
WBC	$\times 10^9$/L	6.0–17.0	5.5–19.5	5.2–13.9	4.0–12.0	10–22	4.0–12.0
Bands	$\times 10^9$/L	0–0.3	0–0.3	0–0.1	0–0.12		
Segmented	$\times 10^9$/L	3.0–11.5	2.5–12.5	2.2–7.4	0.6–4.0	3.2–10.0	1.0–5.0
Lymphocytes	$\times 10^9$/L	1.0–4.8	1.5–7.0	1.1–5.3	2.5–7.5	4.4–13.5	2.0–9.0
Monocytes	$\times 10^9$/L	0.15–1.35	0–0.85	0–0.9	0.03–0.8	0.2–2.2	0–0.75
Eosinophils	$\times 10^9$/L	0.1–1.25	0–1.5	0–0.6	0–2.4	0.2–2.0	0.1–0.75
Basophils	$\times 10^9$/L	<0.1	<0.1	<0.3	<0.2	Rare	Rare

TABLE 5. Reference Intervals for Serum Chemistry Values for Adult Animals Expressed in SI Units

Test	Units	Canine	Feline	Equine	Bovine	Porcine	Ovine
Ammonia	μmol/L	0–40	0–40	0–40			
ALP	U/L	10–73	15–92	102–257	29–99	26–362	68–387
ALT	U/L	15–58	30–100	4–12	17–37	32–84	60–84
AST	U/L	16–43	12–56	152–294	48–100	9–113	98–278
Amylase	U/L	510–1864	365–948	9–34	12–107		
Anion gap	mmol/L	11–26	13–24	7–16	12–22		
Bile acids	μmol/L	<5	<2	<15	See text		
Postprandial	μmol/L	<15	<10				
Bilirubin (total)	μmol/L	1.7–5.1	1.7–3.4	9–36	1.7–5.1	1.7–3.4	1.7–7
Calcium	mmol/L	2.25–2.7	1.85–2.6	2.65–3.25	1.98–2.5	2–3	2.6–3.25
CO_2	mmol/L	20–27	15–25	26–35	24–34	18–26	21–28
Chloride	mmol/L	110–118	116–125	97–104	94–104	100–105	98–115
Cholesterol	mmol/dL	2.8–6.9	1.0–4.8	1.3–3.7	2.3–6.6	1.0–1.4	1.3–3.6
Cholinesterase	U/L	1347–2269	1000–2000				
Cortisol (basal)	nmol/L	28–188	5–72				
CK (CPK)	U/L	40–254	59–527	113–333	44–228		
Creatinine	μmol/L	44–124	62–159	88–168	62–97	88–239	106–168
GGT	U/L	1–5	0–2	9–25	20–48		
Glucose	mmol/L	4.3–6.7	3.2–6.7	4.2–7.0	2.1–3.9	3.6–5.2	2.8–4.4
Iron	μmol/L	15–42	12–42	13–37	10–29	16–36	30–40
Lipase	U/L	13–200	0–83				
Magnesium	mmol/L	0.6–1.0	0.7–1.7	0.6–1.0	0.7–1.1		
Osmolality	mmol/kg	291–315	292–356	282–302			
Phosphorus, inorganic	mmol/L	0.8–2	0.8–2.6	0.7–1.4	1.5–2.9	1.7–3	1.6–2.4
Potassium	mmol/L	4.2–5.6	4.0–5.3	2.4–5.2	4.0–5.3	4.9–7.1	4.0–6.0
Protein (total)	g/L	54–71	57–79	55–73	59–77	70–89	60–79
Albumin	g/L	25–36	23–34	27–42	27–43	19–33	24–39
Globulin	g/L	24–40	26–45	21–38	25–41	53–41	35–57
Sodium	mmol/L	145–153	151–158	136–142	136–144	139–152	136–154
SD (SDH)	U/L	3–8	4–8	2–6	4–15	1–6	6–28
T_3	nmol/L	0.9–1.3	0.7–1.2	0.9–1.2			
T_4	μmol/L	1.6–2.4	1.2–3.0	1.4–1.7			
fT_4	pmol/L	1.2–2.4	1.8–2.7	0.7–0.9			
Triglycerides	mmol/L	0.2–1.3	0.1–1.3	0.1–0.5	0–0.2		
Urea nitrogen	mmol/L	2.5–8.9	6.4–11.8	4.3–9.3	3.6–9.3	2.86–8.6	6.4–11

TABLE 6. Age Related Changes in Serum Chemistry Analytes in Beagle Dogs During First Year of Life[a]

Age:	2 weeks		4 weeks		6 weeks		8 weeks		3 months		6 months		9 months		12 months	
Sex:	M	F	M	F	M	F	M	F	M	F	M	F	M	F	M	F
Analytes that change rapidly during first 12 weeks																
Urea N	24.7	24.1	20.1	15.9	14.6	15.5	14.0	15.1	11.5	10.3						
mg/dL	(9.8)	(6.3)	(3.6)	(3.5)	(2.9)	(2.2)	(5.0)	(4.0)	(2.6)	(2.4)						
Cholesterol	247.0	233.3	268.5	271.9	196.4	159.5	145.6	125.2	146.5	146.5						
mg/dL	(37.9)	(37.9)	(8.5)	(53.1)	(49.6)	(47.5)	(37.2)	(28.3)	(20.6)	(19.9)						
Triglyceride	98.0	97.8	100.2	73.3	65.2	54.3	63.0	68.7	31.4	33.4						
mg/dL	(42.0)	(59.4)	(31.4)	(30.7)	(31.1)	(19.8)	(17.1)	(19.2)	(5.3)	(8.2)						
LDH	86.1	86.9	106.5	51.9	71.1	45.3	49.4	54.5	35.2	33.6						
IU/L	(41.7)	(83.0)	(70.4)	(31.4)	(28.1)	(21.5)	(15.6)	(23.6)	(9.5)	(9.8)						
T$_4$	9.9	9.7	7.4	8.4	5.5	5.6	4.4	4.1	2.8	2.8						
μg/dL	(2.2)	(1.5)	(1.7)	(2.7)	(1.1)	(3.3)	(1.3)	(1.4)	(0.5)	(0.6)						
Glucose	132.8	132.2	134.5	139.5	130.5	125.3	121.8	115.3	108.5	104.5						
mg/dL	(13.1)	(12.5)	(12.5)	(17.6)	(11.9)	(14.3)	(6.3)	(10.7)	(7.9)	(11.0)						
GGT	10.8	6.8	0.0	0.2	0.0	0.0	0.0	0.0	0.0	0.0						
IU/L	(9.6)	(8.6)	(0.0)	(0.6)	(0.0)	(0.0)	(0.0)	(0.0)	(0.0)	(0.0)						
Bilirubin	0.5	0.8	0.5	0.3	0.4	0.4	0.3	0.4	0.3	0.3						
mg/dL	(0.3)	(0.6)	(0.2)	(0.2)	(0.2)	(0.2)	(0.1)	(0.1)	(0.1)	(0.1)						
ALT	9.0	7.3	12.1	9.9	18.2	16.8	22.5	21.3	21.9	23.9						
IU/L	(3.8)	(1.8)	(6.0)	(3.3)	(7.8)	(7.9)	(10.3)	(10.7)	(7.6)	(6.9)						

Analytes that change gradually during the first year of life

Age:	2 weeks		4 weeks		6 weeks		8 weeks		3 months		6 months		9 months		12 months	
Sex:	M	F	M	F	M	F	M	F	M	F	M	F	M	F	M	F
ALP IU/L	149 (33)	127 (23)	88 (24)	99 (23)	103 (24)	112 (28)	122 (22)	125 (39)	145 (20)	143 (29)	93 (16)	90 (17)	66 (17)	64 (12)	43 (13)	59 (35)
Phosphorus$_i$ mg/dL	8.8 (0.9)	8.8 (1.0)	8.1 (1.2)	8.1 (0.6)	8.4 (0.8)	8.5 (0.3)	8.9 (0.4)	9.0 (0.8)	8.0 (0.9)	7.8 (0.5)	7.2 (0.6)	7.0 (0.9)	5.5 (0.7)	5.3 (0.4)	3.9 (0.9)	4.3 (0.7)
Calcium mg/dL	12.8 (2.0)	13.3 (1.3)	13.1 (1.1)	12.4 (0.9)	12.7 (0.7)	12.4 (0.9)	13.5 (0.8)	12.9 (1.0)	11.8 (0.5)	12.0 (0.9)	12.8 (0.8)	12.2 (1.1)	11.7 (1.0)	11.3 (0.8)	10.9 (0.6)	11.0 (0.4)
Creatinine mg/dL	0.5 (0.1)	0.4 (0.1)	0.4 (0.1)	0.4 (0.1)	0.4 (0.1)	0.4 (0.1)	0.5 (0.1)	0.5 (0.1)	0.6 (0.1)	0.6 (0.1)	0.9 (0.1)	0.8 (0.1)	0.9 (0.1)	0.9 (0.1)	1.0 (0.1)	0.9 (0.1)
AST IU/L	16 (4)	16 (5)	14 (3)	13 (2)	18 (4)	15 (4)	20 (5)	18 (5)	21 (3)	20 (4)	29 (5)	27 (5)	28 (6)	26 (4)	24 (3)	22 (4)
Protein g/dL	3.8 (0.2)	4.0 (0.2)	3.8 (0.3)	4.0 (0.3)	4.3 (0.4)	4.2 (0.2)	4.4 (0.4)	4.2 (0.4)	4.9 (0.2)	4.6 (0.2)	5.3 (0.3)	5.4 (0.3)	5.8 (0.4)	5.7 (0.2)	5.9 (0.2)	5.8 (0.3)

[a]Wolford ST, Schroer RA, Gohs FX, et al: Effect of age on serum chemistry profile, electrophoresis and thyroid hormones in beagle dogs two weeks to one year of age. Vet Clin Pathol 1988;17:35–42. Mean values (1 S.D.). M = male, F = female.

TABLE 7. Variations in Reference Intervals for Serum Chemistry Values by Age: Beagle Dogs, 3 to 14 Years Old[a]

Laboratory Test[b]	3 Years	6 Years	9 Years	12 Years	14 Years
ALP (U/L)	40–75	39–115	51–140	58–112	44–143
ALT (U/L)	35–61	30–55	27–51	58–141	41–68
AST (U/L)	24–32	21–29	24–40	30–50	25–34
Bilirubin, total (mg/dL)	0–0.1	0.1–0.1	0.05–0.1	0.05–0.1	0.05–0.1
Calcium (mg/dL)	10–11	10–10	9–10	10–11	10–11
Chloride (mEq/L)	109–114	103–110	107–112	105–108	107–111
Cholesterol (mg/dL)	139–171	154–224	126–300	156–248	159–231
Triglycerides (mg/dL)	23–36	24–54	19–87	34–102	26–38
Creatinine (mg/dL)	0.8–1.0	0.6–1.0	0.5–0.7	0.7–0.9	0.5–0.8
GGT (U/L)	0–17	0–2	2–4	0–7	0–5
Glucose (mg/dL)	91–102	89–104	92–104	80–95	83–100
Iron (µg/dL)	137–285	187–276	41–233	119–189	91–192
LDH (U/L)	74–112	58–145	134–261	179–360	91–216
Phosphorus, inorganic (mg/dL)	3.9–5.1	3.2–4.4	3.9–5.0	3.7–5.2	3.9–4.5
Potassium (mEq/L)	4.6–5.0	4.5–5.1	4.6–5.2	5.0–5.5	4.7–5.3
Protein (g/dL)	5.4–5.9	6.0–6.3	5.8–6.6	6.0–6.6	5.8–6.7
Albumin (g/dL)	3.3–3.6	3.1–3.5	3.0–3.5	3.0–3.3	2.7–3.4
Globulin (g/dL)	2.2–2.6	2.5–2.9	2.6–3.3	3.1–3.5	2.9–3.5
Sodium (mEq/L)	150–154	143–149	149–151	145–149	145–149
Urea nitrogen (mg/dL)	19–22	9–16	10–13	10–18	10–19

[a]From Loweth LA, et al: The effects of aging on hematology and serum chemistry values in the beagle dog. Vet Clin Pathol 1990;19:13.
[b]Limits represent the 10th and 90th percentile values.

TABLE 8. Variations in Reference Intervals for Hematology Values by Age: Beagle Dogs, 3 to 14 Years Old[a]

Laboratory Test[b]	3 Years	6 Years	9 Years	12 Years	14 Years
RBC × 10^6/µL	6.6–7.8	6.5–7.6	5.9–7.4	6.1–7.3	5.7–7.1
Hemoglobin (g/dL)	15–18	16–18	14–18	14–17	14–17
PCV (%)	43–50	44–49	38–50	40–49	40–47
Band neutrophils/µL	0	0	0–63	0–68	0–54
Segmented neutrophils/µL	3944–9287	3605–7724	4207–7217	4724–9587	4464–10,255
Lymphocytes/µL	2185–3318	1334–2467	1667–2702	1676–2658	1628–2453
Monocytes/µL	101–769	173–626	149–620	181–521	189–688
Eosinophils/µL	208–1010	217–500	275–711	99–721	201–408
Basophils/µL	0	0–70	0–102	0	0

[a]From Loweth LA, et al: The effects of aging on hematology and serum chemistry values in the beagle dog. Vet Clin Pathol 1990;19:13.
[b]Limits represent the 10th and 90th percentile values.

TABLE 9. Erythrocyte Changes During Pregnancy in Beagles, Brittany Spaniels, and Labrador Retrievers[a]

	Gestation Week 1			Gestation Week 8			Lactation Week 8		
	Beagles	*Brittany Spaniels*	*Labrador Retrievers*	*Beagles*	*Brittany Spaniels*	*Labrador Retrievers*	*Beagles*	*Brittany Spaniels*	*Labrador Retrievers*
RBC × 10^6/μL									
Mean	7.2	6.2	7.3	5.1	5.0	5.6	7.0	5.6	6.7
Range	6.2–9.2	5.2–7.2	5.5–9.1	4.1–6.1	4.1–6.0	4.4–6.8	5.8–8.2	4.4–6.8	5.7–7.7
PCV (%)									
Mean	47	43.3	50	34.3	33.0	38.2	46.6	40.8	44.1
Range[b]	38.4–54.6	38.5–48.1	42.4–57.6	39.2–50.8	25.2–40.8	30.4–46.0	39.2–54.0	32.8–48.8	36.1–52.1
Hemoglobin (g/dL)									
Mean	17.2	15.9	18.1	12.3	11.8	13.9	16.5	14.7	15.9
Range[b]	15.2–19.2	14.1–17.7	15.3–20.9	10.3–14.3	9.2–14.4	11.7–16.1	13.9–19.1	11.7–17.7	13.1–18.7
MCV (fL)									
Mean	66.6	70.3	69.2	67.3	72.6	67.9	67.3	73.3	65.9
Range[b]	59.2–76	59.7–80.9	50.6–87.8	60.7–73.6	58.6–86.6	52.9–82.9	60.7–73.6	63.1–83.4	55.8–76.0
MCHC (g/dL)									
Mean	36.8	36.6	36.2	36	36.4	36.8	35.5	36	36.1
Range[b]	30.6–43	34.4–38.8	34.2–38.2	31.2–40.8	34.6–38.2	31.8–41.4	31.7–39.4	33.0–39.0	32.7–39.5

[a]From Allard RL, Carlos AD, and Faltin EC: Canine hematological changes during gestation and lactation. Comp Anim Pract 1989;19:3–6.
[b]Range is ± 2 standard deviations.

TABLE 10. Hematologic Values of Growing Healthy Beagle Dogs from Birth to 8 Weeks of Age: Range and (Median)[a]

Hematology Parameter	Birth	1 Week	2 Weeks	3 Weeks	4 Weeks	6 Weeks	8 Weeks
RBC $\times 10^6/\mu L$	4.7–5.6 (5.1)	3.6–5.9 (4.6)	3.4–4.4 (3.9)	3.5–4.3 (3.8)	3.6–4.9 (4.1)	4.3–5.1 (4.7)	4.5–5.9 (4.9)
Hemoglobin (g/dL)	14–17 (15.2)	10.4–17.5 (12.9)	9–11 (10.0)	8.6–11.6 (9.7)	8.5–10.3 (9.5)	8.5–11.3 (10.2)	10.3–12.5 (11.2)
PCV (%)	45–52.5 (47.5)	33–52 (40.5)	29–34 (31.8)	27–37 (31.7)	27–33.5 (29.9)	26.5–35.5 (32.5)	31–39 (34.8)
MCV (fL)	93.0	89.0	81.5	83.0	73.0	69.0	72.0
MCH (pg)	30.0	28.0	25.5	25.0	23.0	22.0	22.5
MCHC (g/dL)	32.0	32.0	31.5	31.0	32.0	31.5	32.0
NRBC/100 WBC	0–13 (2.3)	0–11 (4.0)	0–6 (2.0)	0–9 (1.6)	0–4 (1.2)	0–0	0–1 (0.2)
WBC $\times 10^3/\mu L$	6.8–18.4 (12.0)	9–23 (14.1)	8.1–15.1 (11.7)	6.7–15.1 (11.2)	8.5–16.4 (12.9)	12.6–26.7 (16.3)	12.7–17.3 (15)
Band neutrophils $\times 10^3/\mu L$	0–1.5 (0.23)	0–4.8 (0.50)	0–1.2 (0.21)	0–0.5 (0.09)	0–0.3 (0.06)	0–0.3 (0.05)	0–0.3 (0.08)
Segmented neutrophils $\times 10^3/\mu L$	4.4–15.8 (8.6)	3.8–15.2 (7.4)	3.2–10.4 (5.2)	1.4–9.4 (5.1)	3.7–12.8 (7.2)	4.2–17.6 (9.0)	6.2–11.8 (8.5)
Lymphocytes $\times 10^3/\mu L$	0.5–4.2 (1.9)	1.3–9.4 (4.3)	1.5–7.4 (3.8)	2.1–10.1 (5.0)	1.0–8.4 (4.5)	2.8–16.6 (5.7)	3.1–6.9 (5.0)
Monocytes $\times 10^3/\mu L$	0.2–2.2 (0.9)	0.3–2.5 (1.1)	0.2–1.4 (0.7)	0.1–1.4 (0.7)	0.3–1.5 (0.8)	0.5–2.7 (1.1)	0.5–2.7 (1.1)
Eosinophils $\times 10^3/\mu L$	0–1.3 (0.4)	0.2–2.8 (0.8)	0.08–1.8 (0.6)	0.07–0.9 (0.3)	0–0.7 (0.25)	0.1–1.9 (0.5)	0–1.2 (0.4)
Basophils $\times 10^3/\mu L$	0.0	0–0.2 (0.01)	0.0	0.0	0.015 (0.01)	0.0	0.0

[a]From Earl FL, Melvegar BA, Wilson RL: The hemogram and bone marrow profile of normal neonatal and weaning beagle dogs. Lab Anim Sci 1973;23:690.

TABLE 11. Hematologic Values of Growing Healthy Kittens from Birth to 17 Weeks of Age: Mean (Range)[a]

Hematology Parameter	0–2 Weeks	2–4 Weeks	4–6 Weeks	6–8 Weeks	8–9 Weeks	12–13 Weeks	16–17 Weeks
RBC × 10^6/µL	5.29 (4.81–5.77)	4.67 (4.47–4.87)	5.89 (5.43–6.35)	6.57 (6.05–7.09)	6.95 (6.77–7.13)	7.43 (6.97–7.89)	8.14 (7.60–8.68)
Hemoglobin (g/dL)	12.1 (10.9–13.3)	8.7 (8.3–9.1)	8.6 (8.0–9.2)	9.1 (8.5–9.7)	9.8 (9.4–10.2)	10.1 (9.5–10.7)	11.0 (10.2–11.9)
PCV (%)	35.3 (31.9–38.7)	26.5 (24.9–28.1)	27.1 (25.5–28.7)	29.8 (27.2–32.4)	33.3 (31.9–34.7)	33.1 (29.9–36.3)	34.9 (32.7–37.1)
MCV (fL)	67.4 (63.6–71.2)	53.9 (51.5–56.3)	45.6 (43.0–48.2)	45.6 (43.6–47.6)	47.8 (46.0–49.6)	44.5 (40.9–48.1)	43.1 (40.1–46.1)
MCH (pg)	23.0 (21.8–24.2)	18.8 (17.2–20.4)	14.8 (13.7–16.0)	13.9 (13.3–14.5)	14.1 (13.7–14.5)	13.7 (12.9–14.5)	13.5 (12.7–14.3)
MCHC (g/dL)	34.5 (32.9–36.1)	33.0 (31.0–34.0)	31.9 (30.7–33.1)	30.9 (29.9–31.9)	29.5 (28.7–30.3)	31.3 (29.5–32.1)	31.6 (30.0–33.2)
WBC × 10^3/µL	9.67 (8.53–10.81)	15.31 (12.89–17.73)	17.45 (14.71–20.19)	18.07 (14.19–21.95)	23.68 (19.9–27.46)	23.10 (16.48–29.92)	19.7 (17.46–21.94)
Band neutrophils × 10^3/µL	0.06 (0.02–0.10)	0.11 (0.03–0.19)	0.20 (0.08–0.32)	0.22 (0.06–0.38)	0.12 (0.0–0.30)	0.15 (0.01–0.27)	0.16 (0.020–0.30)
Neutrophils × 10^3/µL	5.96 (4.60–7.32)	6.92 (5.38–8.46)	9.57 (6.27–12.87)	6.75 (4.69–8.81)	11.0 (8.18–13.82)	11.0 (7.46–14.54)	9.74 (7.90–11.58)
Lymphocytes × 10^3/µL	3.73 (2.69–4.77)	6.56 (5.38–7.74)	6.41 (4.87–7.95)	9.59 (6.45–12.73)	10.17 (6.75–13.59)	10.46 (5.24–15.68)	8.7 (6.58–10.82)
Monocytes × 10^3/µL	0.01 (0.0–0.03)	0.02 (0.0–0.06)	0.0	0.01 (0.0–0.03)	0.11 (0.0–0.23)	0.0	0.02 (0.0–0.06)
Eosinophils × 10^3/µL	0.96 (0.10–1.82)	1.40 (1.08–1.72)	1.47 (0.97–1.97)	1.08 (0.68–1.48)	2.28 (1.66–2.90)	1.55 (0.85–2.25)	1.00 (0.62–1.38)
Basophils × 10^3/µL	0.02 (0.0–0.04)	0	0	0.02 (0.0–0.06)	0	0.03 (0.0–0.09)	0

[a]From Meyers-Wallen VN, Haskins ME, Patterson DF: Hematologic values in healthy neonatal, weanling and juvenile kittens. Am J Vet Res 1984;45:1322. Range calculated from mean ±2 standard deviations.

TABLE 12. Normal Values for Biochemical Indicators of Hepatobiliary Disorders in Young Dogs and Cats: Median and (Range)[a]

Test	Puppies					Kittens		
	1–3 Days	2 Weeks	4 Weeks	8 Weeks	Adult	2 Weeks	4 Weeks	Adult
BSP (%, 30 min)	<5	<5	<5	<5	05	ND[b]	ND	0–3
Bile acids (μmol/L)	<15	<15	<15	<15	0–15	ND	<10	0–10
Bilirubin (mg/dL)	0.5 (0.2–1.0)	0.3 (0.1–0.5)	0 (0–0.1)	0.1 (0.1–0.2)	(0–0.04)	0.3 (0.1–1.0)	0.2 (0.1–0.2)	(0–0.2)
ALT (IU/L)	69 (17–337)	15 (10–21)	21 (20–22)	21 (9–24)	(12–94)	18 (11–24)	17 (14–26)	(25–91)
AST (IU/L)	108 (44–194)	20 (10–40)	18 (14–23)	22 (10–32)	(13–56)	18 (8–48)	17 (12–24)	(9–42)
ALP (IU/L)	3845 (618–8760)	236 (176–541)	144 (135–210)	158 (144–177)	(4–107)	123 (68–269)	111 (90–135)	(10–77)
GGT (IU/L)	1111 (163–3558)	24 (4–77)	3 (2–7)	1 (0–7)	(0–7)	1 (0–3)	2 (0–3)	(0–4)
Protein (g/dL)	4.1 (3.4–5.2)	3.9 (3.6–4.4)	4.1 (3.9–4.2)	4.6 (3.9–4.8)	(5.4–7.4)	4.4 (4.0–5.2)	4.8 (4.6–5.2)	(5.8–8.0)
Albumin (g/dL)	2.1 (1.5–2.8)	1.8 (1.7–2.0)	1.8 (1.0–2.0)	2.5 (2.1–2.7)	(2.1–2.7)	2.1 (2.0–2.4)	2.3 (2.2–2.4)	(2.5–3.0)
Cholesterol (mg/dL)	136 (221–204)	282 (223–344)	328 (266–352)	155 (111–258)	(103–299)	229 (164–443)	361 (222–434)	(150–270)
Glucose (mg/dL)	88 (52–127)	129 (111–146)	109 (86–115)	145 (124–272)	(65–110)	117 (76–129)	110 (99–112)	(63–144)

[a]From Center SA, Hornbuckle WE, Hoskins JD: The liver and pancreas. In Hoskins JD (ed): Veterinary Pediatrics: Dogs and Cats from Birth to Six Months. Philadelphia, WB Saunders Co, 1990, Chapter 8.

[b]BSP, sulfobromophthalein; ALT, alanine aminotransferase; AST, aspartate aminotransferase; ALP, alkaline phosphatase; GGT, γ-glutanyltransferase; ND, not determined.

TABLE 13. Age-Related Changes in Plasma and Urine Values in Young Cats: Mean and (Range)[a]

Laboratory Test	4–6 Weeks	7–12 Weeks	13–19 Weeks	20–24 Weeks
Plasma sodium (mEq/L)	152 (147–158)	151 (144–160)	154 (148–161)	155 (149–162)
Plasma potassium (mEq/L)	4.7 (3.7–5.6)	4.9 (3.6–7.1)	4.7 (3.3–6.5)	4.4 (3.5–6.0)
Plasma chloride (mEq/L)	122 (118–127)	122 (113–128)	123 (118–130)	124 (117–129)
Plasma protein (g/dL)	4.6 (4.2–5.1)	5.2 (4.2–6.7)	5.9 (4.8–6.8)	6.2 (5.4–7.1)
Plasma calcium (mg/dL)	9.7 (8.4–11.0)	9.9 (8.8–11.2)	10.1 (8.8–11.1)	9.9 (8.9–10.9)
Plasma phosphorus (mg/dL)	7.4 (5.0–9.9)	8.2 (6.0–10.5)	7.8 (6.4–9.7)	7.1 (4.9–9.8)
Endogenous creatinine clearance (mL/min/kg)	2.19 (0.1–4.2)	4.1 (2.4–5.7)	3.96 (2.6–5.9)	3.38 (2.1–4.7)
FE sodium (%)	0.25 (0.02–0.46)	0.50 (0.01–1.08)	0.57 (0.34–0.79)	0.55 (0.32–0.75)
FE potassium (%)	12.84 (2.37–25.15)	22.56 (12.61–41.51)	22.64 (11.91–37.64)	23.21 (13.51–31.26)
FE chloride (%)	0.62 (0.25–1.13)	1.10 (0.54–1.79)	1.14 (0.6–1.73)	1.16 (0.76–1.62)
FE calcium (%)	0.39 (0.02–2.11)	0.32 (0.04–2.01)	0.12 (0.02–0.50)	0.06 (0.01–0.13)
FE phosphorus (%)	17.10 (1.51–43.76)	27.43 (9.30–48.88)	30.14 (13.95–53.84)	36.20 (12.35–96.19)
24-Hour urinary protein excretion (mg/dL)	4.62 (0.23–16.43)	9.09 (2.54–27.57)	7.34 (3.15–27.93)	6.80 (2.55–17.28)
Plasma osmolality (mOsm/kg)	307 (275–334)	316 (277–343)	313 (187–333)	309 (264–333)
Urine osmolality (mOsm/kg)	1424 (618–2680)	2432 (1214–3474)	2792 (1408–3814)	2383 (918–3384)
Urine production (ml/kg/24 hours)	25.3 (10.4–66.2)	32.1 (4.3–62.3)	26.2 (12.6–53.4)	20.9 (10.2–30.9)

[a]From Crawford MA: The urinary system. In Hoskins JD (ed): Veterinary Pediatrics: Dogs and Cats from Birth to Six Months. Philadelphia, WB Saunders Co, 1990, Chapter 10.

FE, urinary fractional excretion.

TABLE 14. Erythrogram of Foals Up to 1 Year of Age[a,b]

Age	PCV (%)	Hemoglobin (g/dL)	RBC × 10⁶/μL	MCV (fL)	MCHC (g/dL)
<12 hours	43 ± 3	15.4 ± 1.2	10.7 ± 0.8	40 ± 2	36 ± 2
1 day	40 ± 3	14.2 ± 1.1	9.9 ± 0.6	41 ± 3	35 ± 2
3 days	38 ± 3	14.1 ± 1.3	9.6 ± 0.7	39 ± 2	37 ± 1
1 week	35 ± 3	13.3 ± 1.2	8.8 ± 0.6	39 ± 2	38 ± 1
2 weeks	34 ± 3	12.6 ± 1.4	8.9 ± 0.9	38 ± 2	38 ± 1
3 weeks	34 ± 3	12.6 ± 1.1	9.2 ± 0.6	37 ± 2	37 ± 1
1 month	34 ± 4	12.5 ± 1.2	9.3 ± 0.8	36 ± 1	37 ± 1
2 months	37 ± 4	13.6 ± 1.5	10.8 ± 1.7	35 ± 2	37 ± 1
3 months	36 ± 2	13.4 ± 0.9	10.5 ± 0.9	35 ± 1	37 ± 2
4 months	36 ± 3	13.4 ± 1.1	10.4 ± 0.9	34 ± 1	38 ± 2
5 months	35 ± 3	12.7 ± 1.2	10.2 ± 0.6	35 ± 2	37 ± 2
6 months	34 ± 2	12.2 ± 0.8	9.5 ± 0.7	36 ± 2	36 ± 1
9 months	36 ± 3	12.6 ± 1.0	9.4 ± 0.8	39 ± 2	35 ± 1
12 months	36 ± 3	13.3 ± 1.0	9.5 ± 0.7	38 ± 2	37 ± 2

[a]From Harvey JW, et al: Haematology of foals up to one year old. Equine Vet J 1984;16:347.
[b]Values are mean ± 1 standard deviation.

TABLE 15. Hemostasis Values for Healthy Horses[a]

Laboratory Test	Mean ± SD	Range
Prothrombin time (seconds)	9.8 ± 0.34	9.2–10.5
APPT (seconds)	46.5 ± 9.2	31–93
Antithrombin III (%)	193 ± 28	115–239
Plasminogen (%)	110 ± 23	63–146
Fibrinogen (mg/dL)	192 ± 80	120–490
Fibrin(ogen) degradation products (μg/dL)	24 ± 19	0–64
Platelet count × 10⁵/μL	1.33 ± 0.34	0.89–2.32

[a]From Prasse KW, et al: Evaluation of coagulation and fibrinolysis during the prodromal stages of carbohydrate-induced acute laminitis in horses. Am J Vet Res 1990;51:1950.

TABLE 16. Leukograms of Foals Up to 1 Year of Age[a]

Age	Total WBC × 10³/μL	Neutrophils × 10³/μL	Lymphocytes × 10³/μL	Monocytes × 10³/μL	Eosinophils × 10³/μL	Basophils × 10³/μL
<12 hours	9.5 ± 2.44	7.94 ± 2.22	1.34 ± 0.60	0.19 ± 0.12	0	0.002 ± 0.007
1 day	8.44 ± 1.77	6.80 ± 1.72	1.43 ± 0.42	0.19 ± 0.10	0.11 ± 0.027	0.003 ± 0.010
3 days	7.55 ± 1.50	5.70 ± 1.44	1.45 ± 0.36	0.32 ± 0.13	0.045 ± 0.062	0.032 ± 0.046
1 week	9.86 ± 1.79	7.45 ± 1.55	2.10 ± 0.63	0.27 ± 0.11	0.028 ± 0.042	0.058 ± 0.069
2 weeks	8.53 ± 1.68	6.00 ± 1.54	2.22 ± 0.45	0.24 ± 0.13	0.063 ± 0.063	0.012 ± 0.021
3 weeks	8.57 ± 1.90	5.66 ± 1.64	2.59 ± 0.63	0.22 ± 0.10	0.078 ± 0.066	0.026 ± 0.032
1 month	8.14 ± 2.02	5.27 ± 2.00	2.46 ± 0.45	0.29 ± 0.17	0.121 ± 0.148	0.016 ± 0.032
2 months	9.65 ± 2.13	5.70 ± 1.88	3.46 ± 0.63	0.31 ± 0.15	0.092 ± 0.092	0.018 ± 0.039
3 months	11.69 ± 2.51	6.43 ± 1.96	4.73 ± 1.21	0.38 ± 0.19	0.184 ± 0.181	0.018 ± 0.028
4 months	10.18 ± 1.99	4.78 ± 1.36	4.70 ± 1.31	0.32 ± 0.17	0.353 ± 0.319	0.018 ± 0.027
5 months	10.07 ± 2.29	4.60 ± 1.90	4.92 ± 1.48	0.27 ± 0.12	0.272 ± 0.152	0.010 ± 0.027
6 months	9.03 ± 1.13	4.00 ± 0.84	4.53 ± 0.74	0.23 ± 0.11	0.247 ± 0.150	0.014 ± 0.024
9 months	8.68 ± 1.19	3.82 ± 0.78	4.39 ± 1.10	0.22 ± 0.10	0.234 ± 0.232	0.021 ± 0.024
12 months	9.19 ± 1.36	4.28 ± 0.81	4.27 ± 1.13	0.20 ± 0.12	0.339 ± 0.221	0.019 ± 0.037

[a]From Harvey JW, et al: Haematology of foals up to one year old. Equine Vet J 1984;16:347. Values are mean ±1 standard deviation.

TABLE 17. Per Cent Fractional Urinary Excretion of Electrolytes in Cows: Mean and (Standard Error)[a]

Electrolyte	Summer	Autumn	Winter	Spring
Sodium	1.3	0.68	0.63	0.33
	(0.13)	(0.09)	(0.13)	(0.06)
Potassium	55.16	47.41	32.44	21.65
	(4.12)	(3.80)	(3.15)	(3.41)
Chloride	2.12	2.25	1.80	0.68
	(0.11)	(0.12)	(0.17)	(0.12)
Osmolality	4.70	3.84	3.71	1.82
	(0.25)	(0.19)	(0.16)	(0.18)

[a]From Itoh N: Fractional electrolyte excretion in adult cows: Establishment of reference ranges and evaluation of seasonal variations. Vet Clin Pathol 1989;18:86–87.

TABLE 18. Normal Per Cent Fractional Urine Creatinine/Electrolyte Clearance of Domestic Animals[a]

Electrolyte	Dog	Cat	Horse	Cow	Sheep
Sodium	0–0.7	0.24–0.1	0.02–1.0	0.2–1.43	0–0.071
Potassium[b]	0–20	6.7–23.9	15–65	15–63	80–180
Chloride	0–0.8	0.41–1.3	0.04–1.6	0.4–2.3	0–4.7
Phosphorus	3–39	17–73	0–0.2		0–0.53

[a]Calculated using the formula:

$$\% \; CrCl(Fc)(E) = \frac{Cr \; serum}{Cr \; urine} \times \frac{E \; urine}{E \; serum} \times 100$$

[b]The Fc for potassium in herbivorous animals is largely dependent upon the diet.

INDEX

Page numbers in *italics* refer to illustrations; page numbers followed by t refer to tables.